ESSENTIAL OPHTHALMIC SURGERY

Commissioning editor: Melanie Tait
Desk editor: Claire Hutchins
Production Controller: Chris Jarvis
Development editor: Zoë A. Youd
Cover designer: Fred Rose

ESSENTIAL OPHTHALMIC SURGERY

Alexander J. E. Foss

DM MA FRCOphth MRCP BM BCh

Consultant Ophthalmic Surgeon, University Hospital,
Queen's Medical Centre, Nottingham, UK

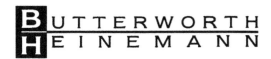

OXFORD AUCKLAND BOSTON JOHANNESBURG MELBOURNE NEW DELHI

Butterworth-Heinemann
Linacre House, Jordan Hill, Oxford OX2 8DP
225 Wildwood Avenue, Woburn, MA 01801-2041
A division of Reed Educational and Professional Publishing Ltd

A member of the Reed Elsevier plc group

First published 2001

Every effort has been made to ensure that the drug doses within the text are
accurate and conform to the standards accepted at time of publication.
However, drug doses must always be checked in a formulary before
administration. The author and publisher do not accept responsibility for
any inaccuracies, errors or omissions.

British Library Cataloguing in Publication Data
Foss, A.J.E.
    Essential Ophthalmic Surgery
    1. Eye – Surgery
    I. Title
    617.7′1

Library of Congress Cataloguing in Publication Data
A catalogue record for this book is available from the Library of Congress

ISBN 0 7506 4197 5

For information on all Butterworth–Heinemann publications visit our
website at www.bh.com

Designed and typeset by Keyword Typesetting Services Ltd,
Wallington, Surrey

Transferred to digital printing 2006

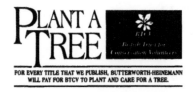

FOR EVERY TITLE THAT WE PUBLISH, BUTTERWORTH-HEINEMANN
WILL PAY FOR BTCV TO PLANT AND CARE FOR A TREE.

CONTENTS

PREFACE

Surgery is about learning monkey tricks, but finding a good monkey can be difficult

Luke Herbert,
Western Eye Hospital, London (1999)

A good friend provided the above quotation, and he is absolutely right. The initial purpose of this book was to cover 'all that we would like to know, but are afraid to ask'. Since then, it has become more ambitious. Surgery is about learning tricks, and I have attempted to collect as many of these tricks as possible, in addition to the basic principles, for the most commonly performed ophthalmic operations. The scientific basis has been emphasized where possible.

This book is divided into three parts: the first explains the basic principles of surgery; the second describes ocular anaesthesia (with particular emphasis on local anaesthetic techniques) and the third describes specific surgical techniques. The range of operations described is limited to those with which a candidate for the Royal College of Ophthalmologist's fellowship examination is expected to be familiar. Vitreo-retinal surgery is becoming the exclusive domain of the subspecialist, and is therefore not covered.

I have tried to describe the rationale behind the most commonly performed procedures, the relevant clinical anatomy, the procedures themselves, the complications that may be encountered, and suggestions regarding their management. In surgery as in most activities, 'the devil is in the detail'; I hope that the devilish detail is covered in sufficient depth so that the objectives are made clear.

Surgery is an evolving subject, and I have done my best to ensure that this book is accurate; however, I am sure that I can rely on my colleagues to point out where I have gone astray and to suggest improvements.

A. J. E. Foss

ACKNOWLEDGEMENTS

Many details of surgical practice are passed on orally, and I am clearly indebted to all those who have trained me, especially the consultants at the Oxford Eye Hospital (1988–1990) and Moorfields Eye Hospital (1991–1997), and my colleagues at Nottingham. I would particularly like to thank Peter Shah for reviewing the text and co-authoring Chapter 23, Stephen Tuft for writing Chapter 22, Ken Hoffer for trying to teach me about biometry, Richard Gregson for reviewing Chapter 21 and Emmanuel Rosen and Paul Chell for reviewing Chapter 27.

I have also absorbed information from a large number of sources, and cannot always recall from whom or where; I hope that this will not cause offence to those concerned, and I fully acknowledge their help.

PART 1

BASIC PRINCIPLES OF SURGERY

1

GENERAL CONSIDERATIONS

THE OPERATING THEATRE

The early history of surgery is dominated by one obstacle, that of postoperative wound infection, and theatre design reflects this. The second problem has been organizational, reflecting the need to be able to carry out complex tasks with multiple pieces of equipment. It is axiomatic that **most postoperative infections occur as a result of inoculation with micro-organisms at the time of surgery**, and ophthalmology is no exception. Even delayed onset endophthalmitis following cataract surgery is usually due to low-grade and slowly growing pathogens, which are thought to be introduced by direct inoculation at the time of surgery.

MAINTAINING ASEPSIS

Theatres are organized into the following 'zones' with varying degrees of access:

1. General access zone. This includes the theatre reception, holding areas and changing rooms.
2. Limited access zone. This includes staff rest rooms, recovery area and theatre administration offices.
3. Restricted access zone. This consists of the operating suite, comprising the operating room, the anaesthetic room, scrub area, preparation room (or clean utility) and the utility room (for cleaning and/or disposal of used instruments).

The zone concept is similar to the counter-current principle for urine concentration in the kidney (see Figure 1.1). The cleaning effort is the same in each zone, and the effect is multiplied by having several zones. Within the restricted access zone similar principles apply, so that those scrubbed and the instruments at the actual operation site are much cleaner than the rest of the operating room. This idea of zones has superseded the idea of one-way traffic with clean and dirty streams, which is similar to the way in which the bladder maintains sterility (which is by the flow of urine being greater than the speed of migration

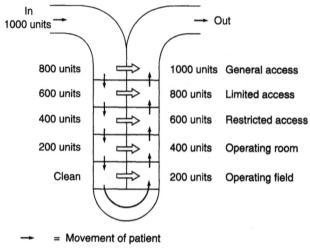

Figure 1.1   The zone concept acts in a manner similar to the counter-current mechanism for concentrating urine in the kidney.

of organisms from the urethra, which is far from clean – see Figure 1.2), but requires strict organization and staff discipline to ensure that there is no crossing of personnel from the dirty stream into the clean stream.

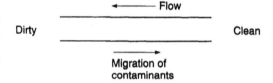

Figure 1.2   The bladder principle for maintaining cleanliness. If the flow rate exceeds the migration ability of organisms, then sterility can be maintained.

Ultimately, there are several limiting factors that determine the level of asepsis that can be achieved. These are:

1. The patient's own flora (eyelid and conjunctival flora in ophthalmic surgery)
2. The surgeon's flora – these are minimized by the use of protective clothing, but the facial skin is not completely covered (in orthopaedic surgery, where postoperative infection of joint implants is so devastating, the facial skin is also covered)
3. Handling technique – direct transfer of organisms can be avoided by a meticulous handling technique
4. The air – airborne spores are potentially infectious but of uncertain importance.

VENTILATION

The purposes of theatre ventilation are to provide clean air, dispose of airborne pollutants (mainly exhaust anaesthetic gases) and control temperature and humidity.

There are three main types of theatre ventilation systems, but the plenum turbulent airflow system is used almost universally. This system draws air in at roof level by fans, and this is filtered, humidified, warmed or cooled as appropriate, and finally ducted into the theatre at wall or ceiling level. The air pressure in theatre is kept slightly higher than the rest of the department, thus creating a unidirectional airflow from clean to dirty areas. The pressure is therefore highest in the preparation room and lowest in the utility and disposal areas, and the aim is to achieve 20–30 air changes per hour with a low air velocity of 0.1–0.3 m/s[1]. A meaningful pressure differential can of course only be achieved with the theatre doors closed.

The other two systems, the ultraclean ventilation system and the high-input/high-exhaust enclosures, are used mainly for orthopaedic surgery. The importance of air as a source of wound contamination for hip replacements was stressed by Professor Sir John Charnley, who advocated the use of the ultraclean air system[2]. An MRC committee confirmed his views; ultraclean air systems halved the sepsis rate and quartered the infection rate when used in combination with occlusive clothing[3,4].

The risk of infection is increased by the presence of an implant. While it takes an inoculum of 1 million *S. aureus* to cause skin sepsis, this drops to 100 in the presence of a suture[5] and to just a single organism for a hip implant. Although cataract surgery is a clean operation and generally uses an implant, the infection rate is much lower than for total hip replacements with conventional theatre ventilation. This is due to a combination of factors, including a much smaller wound area, the shorter duration of the operation, and the circulation of aqueous in the anterior chamber washing itself out repeatedly. While poor draping technique has been shown to be associated with an increased rate of endophthalmitis, there is no evidence that ultraclean systems improve the current sepsis rate of 0.1–0.4 per cent[6,7]. The current trend for endophthalmitis prophylaxis is toward prophylactic antibiotics in the infusion solutions, with two large series[8,9] reporting an endophthalmitis rate of around 0.01 per cent; with such low rates it would be virtually impossible to demonstrate any further improvement and it is therefore likely that most ophthalmic theatres will continue to use the plenum turbulent airflow system.

The risk of patient hypothermia is quite considerable under general anaesthetic, due to reduced heat production from loss of muscle activity, increased heat loss from vasodilatation, and fluid loss from ventilation. Thus, most theatres are run at 20–22°C with a humidity of 4–60 per cent.

NOISE

It would appear that the natural state of (wo)man is to talk. The advantage of allowing people to talk in theatre is that they tend to be more relaxed, which is good for 'team bonding', while complete silence is intimidating. The disadvantages include the following:

- The act of speaking sheds bacteria
- Noise can be distracting to the surgeon
- Noise can impede surgeon–patient communication
- Sudden noise may elicit a startle reflex.

A good compromise is appropriate background music. Music is an excellent way of conveying mood, and must be chosen with care to help generate an atmosphere of calm. For this, the patient's own wishes should be taken into consideration when operating under local or topical anaesthesia.

LIGHTING

It is clearly important to be able to see the field of surgery. Daylight is the best illumination for appreciating subtle colour differences and, accordingly, the light source must be of the correct colour temperature (4000 K). General background illumination is usually in the region of 500 lux, and additional lighting is provided by luminaires (multi-reflector or multi-lamp types) to ensure that the lighting comes from a broad source in order to minimize the problems of shadows.

Most intraocular procedures require special lighting arrangements for two reasons: first, the lighting intensity declines with the square of the magnification; and secondly, co-axial illumination is required for cataract surgery. Co-axial illumination results in retro-illumination, which provides optimal visualization of small or translucent objects. Under retro-illumination, any edge will appear black, not due to absorption, but from light scattering (and therefore less coming back in a straight line) or, if slightly off-axis, bright from the scatter against a dark background! Small particles are also more visible for the same reason (Figure 1.3).

Contrast is everything and, when using retro-illumination, can be enhanced by reducing direct illumination. Accordingly, it must be possible to dim or turn off the background lights in theatre (and to black out any windows).

MAGNIFICATION

The limiting factor in performing tasks in everyday life is visual discrimination, and the use of either loupes or a microscope for surgery (microsurgery) helps to overcome this limitation.

Increasing magnification gives increased discrimination up to a limit defined as the minimum separation of two points, which is determined by the wave nature of light. In light microscopy this occurs at a magnification of around ×1000, but is never reached in surgical practice due to two other limiting factors:

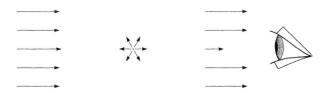

Figure 1.3 The effect of scattering of light from a particle viewed by retro-illumination. Although no light has been absorbed, very little light is scattered in a forward direction and the particle accordingly appears as a dark image against a bright background. Equally, if the illumination is slightly off-axis, the background will appear dark and the scattering particle will 'light up'.

1. The illumination diminishes proportionately to the square of the magnification
2. The depth of the focus falls proportionately to the square of the magnification.

The problem of illumination can be overcome by increasing the strength of the light source; however, this is limited by light toxicity. The loss of depth of focus is truly limiting. For these reasons, it is therefore a good principle to use the lowest magnification power necessary.

Loupes are spectacle-mounted Gallilean telescopes, which give limited magnification of ×2 − ×4. They are suitable for minor procedures, but are limited in lacking a light source. A second limitation is the need to keep one's head still as a tremor in any direction will be likewise magnified. An operating microscope solves both of these problems. It has its own illumination system and is independently mounted to provide good stability and a zoom system is now standard to provide variable magnification. An important design feature of a zoom system is that a change in magnification should not alter the point of focus.

RETINAL PHOTOTOXITY

A limiting factor on the level of illumination is light toxicity, particularly retinal phototoxicity from co-axial illuminated operating microscopes, which is most commonly reported following cataract surgery.

Tso[10] has divided photic injury into three phases:

1. The immediate phase, when the retina looks normal.
2. Within 48 hours a mild disturbance at the level of the retinal pigment epithelium may be seen (sometimes with frank retinal oedema), and fluorescein angiography shows early hyperfluorescence and late staining. The lesion itself reflects the shape of the light source; a tungsten bulb tends to give an oval burn while a fibre-optic cable gives a round burn. The lesion is usually located just above or below the fovea due to the fact that most systems are not exactly co-axial (e.g. 6° for the Zeiss microscope and 1.5° for the Wild microscope).
3. The reparative stage, which is characterized by a combination of pigment hyperplasia/clumping and pigment loss at the level of the retinal pigment epithelium.

Although the power and light wavelength used and host factors must all have a role to play, the factor that is best correlated with clinical phototoxicity is exposure time[11]. In one study[12] the incidence of phototoxicity following cataract surgery was 0.9 per cent for cases taking less than 100 minutes and 39 per cent for cases taking longer, but other case reports suggest that the critical cut-off time may be nearer 60 minutes[11]. Almost certainly a significant number of cases of phototoxicity are undiagnosed, and a further proportion are likely to be misdiagnosed as Irvine–Gass syndrome, given the similar fluorescein angiogram appearances.

PREPARING THE INSTRUMENTS

The single most important requirement in preparing instruments is to ensure their sterility. Sterilization used to be defined as the inactivation or removal of all living organisms, but this definition will have to be slightly modified with the discovery of prions, which can only be destroyed by incineration. Sterilization must be distinguished from disinfection, which applies to inanimate objects and is the removal of vegetative micro-organisms but not necessarily spores, and antisepsis, which implies the use of bacteriostatic agents primarily designed to remove potentially pathogenic bacteria from skin and wounds.

Nowadays there is increased use of single-use disposable instruments, whose cleanliness is guaranteed. For non-disposable instruments, the inability to remove prions means that there will be increasing emphasis on tracking systems in order to allow identification and destruction of any instrument that has been in contact with a patient who subsequently contracted a prion-related disorder.

STERILIZATION

It is important that all instruments and inanimate objects are clean prior to being sterilized for several reasons:

1. Cleaning reduces the bacterial load – killing occurs on a log scale, and a large microbial load increases the chance of failing to achieve complete sterility
2. Organic material can interfere with sterilization – this especially applies to chemical methods where blood in particular is an effective 'quencher' and will protect the bacteria
3. Dead bacteria can still cause inflammation due to the endotoxins they contain.

Sterilization can be achieved by heat, exposure to chemicals or gases, filtration, and irradiation.

Heat
The hot air oven is the method often used for instruments that cannot be sterilized by moist heat, such as powders, oils, cotton wool swabs and paraffin gauze dressings. The oven consists of a closed chamber

heated to 160°C for 1 hour, although the time can be reduced to 22 minutes by increasing the temperature to 180°C.

The autoclave is the most commonly used method of heat sterilization, and uses moist heat in the form of pressurized steam; when the steam condenses it gives up a large amount of heat and therefore provides a very rapid and efficient way of heating instruments to the required temperature. Twelve minutes at the holding temperature of 121°C is sufficient, but most have a holding period of 18 minutes to allow for a 50 per cent margin of error.

Autoclaves need to be inspected at regular intervals to ensure that they achieve the correct temperature and pressure; however, an important routine check is the use of the Bowie–Dick test, which involves a tape patterned with grey stripes that darken on exposure to a given amount of heat and allow a quick visual inspection.

Gases

Only two gases are used with any frequency for sterilization. Formaldehyde vapour is used largely in the disinfection of rooms and bulky objects such as blankets and mattresses. Ethylene oxide is used for delicate instruments that cannot withstand autoclaving, and will sterilize equipment in a humid atmosphere at 55°C although sterilization times are relatively lengthy (1 hour in a high pre-vacuum chamber or 12 hours using a plastic bag method). Evidence of sterility is provided by the spore test, which takes a further 2 days; a further disadvantage is that some materials such as rubber and plastic can absorb the gas and should not be used for 5 days afterwards. Ethylene oxide takes a gaseous form at room temperature, when it is potentially explosive and is toxic to both skin and mucous membranes.

Chemicals

Chemicals can be used for sterilization, but they tend to be very toxic and corrosive. Weaker agents are suitable for human use, but are only suitable for disinfection or antisepsis.

Glutaraldehyde (Cidex®, Gigasept®) will kill bacteria, fungi and viruses rapidly, tubercle bacilli in about 60 minutes and spores in 3–10 hours; it can therefore be considered a high-level disinfectant when used for 10–60 minutes and a form of sterilization when used for a minimum of three hours. Glutaraldehyde is not as effective as autoclaving, but it is non-corrosive and does not damage lensed instruments; its major use is for delicate instruments such as endoscopes for which other techniques are unsuitable. Aqueous solutions of glutaraldehyde are acidic and this form will not kill spores; to make it sporicidal it must be made alkaline (pH 7.5–8.5). It is an irritant to nasal and ocular mucosa, and there is an occupational exposure limit of 0.2 ppm.

Other methods

Micro-organisms can be removed from air and fluid by filters. This technique has a long history and is employed to sterilize air and gases used for intraocular injections. The pore size used for filtration is

0.22 μm or less; cocci are about 1 μm in diameter and bacilli are larger. The Chlamydiae, Rickettsiae and Coxiellae are in the region of 0.3–0.5 μm and so should be safely removed, but this technique will not remove viruses, bacterial spores or all the mycoplasms (0.05–0.3 μm). Accordingly, the Medicines Control Agency does not consider filtration to be sufficient when an alternative method of sterilization is possible.

Organisms can also be inactivated by exposure to irradiation. This is the preferred method for many commercial applications and is how most disposable instruments are sterilized.

PREPARING THE PATIENT

CONSENT

There are two categories of consent: 'expressed' and 'implied'. Implied consent pertains to situations when the patient's action appears to indicate consent (like stretching out his arm to a phlebotomist); in such situations consent has been inferred rather than sought. This type of consent should be avoided, as the patient may have been acting on a misunderstanding (e.g. he may have been preparing to shake hands in the above example!). Express consent should always be obtained. There are three main issues in consent[13]:

1. Has the patient the intellectual capacity to give consent?
2. Was appropriate information given beforehand?
3. Was consent given voluntarily?

The large majority of ophthalmic operations are elective, and difficult issues such as consent in unconscious patients hardly ever arise. A perennial issue is how informed consent must be. The defence for not offering detailed descriptions of all the risks is that giving such detail provokes needless anxiety, but the existing evidence, on British patients, directly opposes this stance: a full explanation with full details of the risks as well as benefits reduces rather than increases anxiety[14]. Clearly it is impractical (and may be impossible) to obtain fully informed consent, but patients should be told the risks at least in outline. For example, for cataract surgery the patient should be told:

- The success rate of surgery and how success is defined (e.g. 95 per cent chance of achieving driving vision or better).
- The risks of surgery (e.g. 1/100 of being worse off, 1/100 of requiring a second operation and 1/1000 of going blind in the eye in question).
- The major alternatives to a particular course of action, including inaction (vision may remain at its current level for years).

There is a theoretical risk of bilateral visual loss from an operation on just one eye from sympathetic ophthalmitis and is an example of when a complete discussion might provoke undue anxiety considering the magnitude of risk that it represents during, for example, routine cataract surgery. (A suggestion is that a risk need not be specifically mentioned if it is equal to or less than 'background' rates – e.g. 1/2000 people are registered blind or partially sighted each year for whatever reason, whilst the risk of sympathetic ophthalmitis following cataract surgery has been estimated at 1/10 000[15] but is now probably considerably less). Of course, if there is a situation where sympathetic ophthalmitis is a significant risk, then clearly the patient must be informed.

The final issue is that consent should be given voluntarily, and this aspect arises mainly in connection with clinical trials. A patient may be persuaded to enter a trial, but not coerced. Any trial should be approved by the local ethics committee, and the members will often decide how much information should be provided to the patient.

CLOTHING

Both patients and surgeons change into clean clothes before surgery. This is for reasons of basic hygiene, and because clothing worn should be easily washable.

In the operating theatre the patient will be cleaned and/or covered with drapes, so low-level contamination of patients' clothes with micro-organisms is not a major issue for extraocular procedures. It is certainly acceptable to allow patients to enter the theatre for minor surgical procedures in everyday clothing. For operations during which significant mess is generated, cheap clothing that is easily cleaned and potentially expendable is desirable. For intraocular surgery (and particularly implant procedures) even low-level contamination is not acceptable, and patients should change into clean clothing before coming to theatre.

PREPARING THE SURGEON

SCRUBBING

It is not possible to sterilize skin, and the pores in particular act as a sanctuary for microbial organisms. Of greater concern are the pathogens that can be carried by surgeons from the wards to the theatre (as Dr Semmelwiess showed in Vienna in the 1860s when the mortality rate was 12 per cent in the maternity wards from puerperal fever due to doctors seeing patients after working in the pathology laboratories without washing their hands). However, the rate of infection is dependent on microbial load, and scrubbing will therefore reduce infectivity.

The two most commonly used agents for scrubbing are povidone-iodine (Betadine®) and chlorhexidine (Hibiscrub®). These agents have been shown to reduce bacterial counts by 98 per cent following two 2-minute scrubs[16]. There is some evidence to suggest that chlorhexidine may be the more effective[17,18].

MASKS, GOWNS AND CAPS

The purpose of gowns, masks and caps is to provide a barrier to micro-organisms. They are used to protect the patient from being contaminated by micro-organisms originating from the surgeon and *vice versa*.

Masks prevent wound infection by bacteria shed from the nose and throat. Facemasks were introduced around the turn of the twentieth century, when it was found that nasal carriers were important in the spread of contagious diseases[19,20] and that haemolytic streptococci isolated from wounds and puerperal fever were the same as those isolated from the throats of surgical and obstetric teams[21,22]. While it has been straightforward to demonstrate that masks reduce shedding of bacteria[23-27] it has not been possible to correlate mask use with a reduction in wound infections in general surgery[28].

The barrier function of masks is assessed in one of two ways[29]. The first is by measuring the bacterial filtration efficiency, which can be done either *in vitro* (the mask is challenged with a nebulized aerosol of *S. aureus* in peptone water) or *in vivo* (the bacteria shed by someone coughing is compared with and without a mask). Like all biological-based tests there is considerable inter-test variation and it is slow – it takes 2 days for the bacteria to grow to form colonies. The second test is the filtration efficiency test, where a suspension of polystyrene latex spheres similar in size to *S. aureus* is filtered through a mask; the spheres are easily counted and results can be obtained within 5 minutes. Most masks show filtration efficiencies of greater than 99 per cent, and accordingly they give excellent protection against direct expulsion. However, all masks have a face fit leakage of around 5 per cent, which reduces the overall filtration efficiency to 95 per cent. Face fit and correct positioning is therefore a vital factor in assessing the overall efficiency of masks (Figure 1.4). Most facemasks have a mouldable strip at the top to conform to the shape of the surgeon's face, and the purpose of this is to improve the seal of the mask and prevent humid air steaming up the lenses of the surgeon and/ or operating microscope. There are also anti-fog masks available, which have a flap of plastic film at the top to further reduce the problem.

The barrier function of masks decreases when they are damp, so their function fails with time. However, the barrier function lasts at least 20 minutes, which is generally long enough for an experienced cataract surgeon to perform an operation, suggesting that facemasks may be more useful than in other forms of surgery. **The corollary of this is that the mask should be changed between cases.** There is evidence that facial movements behind a mask may increase bacterial contamination[30], and there has been the suggestion that operating in silence may be more effective than using a facemask[28].

The theatre gown should cover the surgeon from the neck to the knee, and is fastened at the back. The rear fastening has a flap that can be wrapped round the back to ensure a sterile covering. The cuffs of the sleeve should be elasticated so that the theatre glove can be fitted

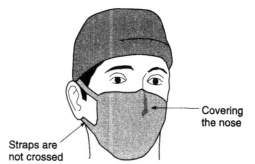

Figure 1.4 The correct way to wear a facemask, with the nose covered and the straps uncrossed.

Covering the nose

Straps are not crossed

over it, ensuring a tight junction. When fully scrubbed, it is axiomatic that everything below the waist is potentially dirty, and that the hands should be kept above waist level.

GLOVES

The introduction of surgical gloves is usually attributed to William Halsted, although the first recorded use is by Johann Walbaum in 1758. The first material used was a sheep's caecum, but nowadays most gloves are made of latex.

Gloves protect the operator from exposure to toxins and infection, and the patient from infection. However, it should be noted that gloves are a toxic risk in their own right.

The ideal glove should be non-toxic, present a barrier to cross-infection, and be strong enough to resist accidental perforation by sharp instruments whilst having a good grip and preserving the sense of touch. For ophthalmic surgery grip and touch sensitivity are particularly important, and there are gloves designed with these particular properties in mind (e.g. Biogel M®).

Glove powder
The problems of glove powder are well known[31]. There are five recognized hazards, of which the first three are particularly relevant to ophthalmic surgery:

1. Powder-related allergy
2. Increased risk of infection
3. Sterile postoperative inflammation
(4. Delayed wound healing)
(5. Misdiagnosis).

Originally gloves were sterilized by boiling and then put on wet and powders were introduced with the transition to dry sterilization techniques to prevent the surfaces sticking together. The first powders to be used, talc and lycopodium, were recognized to cause granulomatous inflammation, leading to the introduction of starch (being biodegradeable) in 1947. However, starch has since been found to cause similar complications and, more significantly, it is a risk factor for the development of latex allergy.

Postoperative inflammation

There are three ways by which gloves can cause postoperative inflammation, and the first two are a consequence of glove powder:

1. Powders can cause a sterile granulomatous inflammation. Sterile endophthalmitis as a consequence of glove powder is rare, but has been described[32].
2. Powders are a risk factor for infection and can reduce the inoculum of bacteria required to produce an infection. Starch and related powders have not been implicated as a risk factor for bacterial endophthalmitis, but work on abdominal surgery has shown that powders reduce the required inoculum of bacteria to generate an abscess by a factor of 10.
3. Absorbed endogenous pyrogens can cause sterile inflammation. Endogenous pyrogens are endotoxins that come from gram-negative bacteria, and are essentially bacterial breakdown products that are generated during sterilization. Patients with pre-existing sepsis may be sensitized to the presence of endotoxins (i.e. the Schwartzman reaction).

These problems are relatively minor. Of far greater importance is that of latex allergy.

Latex allergy

Latex allergy is becoming increasingly common, and can be both career and lifestyle limiting. It is important to distinguish between an irritant or toxic reaction and an allergic reaction. Irritant reactions have a shallow dose–response relationship, are non-specific, require relatively high exposure, are relatively predictable and are reversible on reduction of exposure. They are characterized by irritation or itching, dry skin, peeling and flaking. Allergic reactions show a very steep dose–response curve, are highly specific, idiosyncratic, and require not just reduction but complete avoidance of the stimulus. Once sensitization occurs, the tendency to allergy is not easily reversed.

Two types of allergic reactions have been described with gloves; type 1 (or IgE) mediated allergy, and type 4 (or delayed contact) hypersensitivity. Type 4 reactions are delayed by 6–8 hours following exposure and are characterized by localized rash and symptoms. The allergens responsible are thought be the residual accelerators, which are chemicals introduced to help the polymerization process, and reducing these has led to a reduction in Type 4 reactions[33]. Type 1 reactions, however, are on the increase. The allergen(s) for type 1 reactions are the protein impurities present in rubber. Type 1 allergic reactions range from mild (localized contact urticaria) to severe (affecting the mucous membranes and causing anaphylaxis), and recognized risk factors are an atopic predisposition, hand dermatitis, and the use of glove powders. Standard skin prick tests show a prevalence of positive reactions of 7–17 per cent among health care workers. The incidence is particularly high among theatre nurses using powdered gloves, at 22 per cent, dropping to 3 per cent in a hospital that did not use powdered gloves[34].

Non-latex, non-powdered gloves are available for those who develop severe contact reactions and for use on sensitive patients.

Glove perforation

Glove perforation compromises the safety of both the patient and the surgeon. As the standard glove used in ophthalmic surgery is thinner than that used for general surgery so as to improve tactility and fine handling, it is clearly less resistant to accidental puncture. The rate of punctures varies from 5–50 per cent, and the majority occur on the left hand, suggesting that perforation may be related to suturing technique[35]. Using forceps for suturing and dissection reduces the risk[36].

POSITIONING THE PATIENT

THE OPERATING TABLE

The operating table must be stable, comfortable and adjustable. It must also have an antistatic covering (to prevent sparks) and protect pressure points.

Headrests

The correct head position for most intraocular procedures is with the head absolutely horizontal (i.e. the tip of the chin and the forehead on the same level and the eyes looking straight up). If the head tilts away from the eye being operated on there is a tendency for a pool of fluid to collect over the medial canthus, and this can make life difficult. For other procedures, access can be improved by head tilt – for example, both temporal artery biopsy and DCR surgery are facilitated by a degree of head tilt away from the surgical site.

The headrest can be considered to be an extension of the operating table, and its functions are very similar. The most commonly used are the Reubens and the Halliday pillows; the Halliday pillow is much deeper and the edges are at the same level as the eye, so this makes a good hand rest if required.

There are situations where a head clamp may be preferable, particularly for patients under general anaesthesia; this is the securest way of immobilizing the head and accordingly tends to be favoured by vitreo-retinal surgeons.

POSITIONING THE SURGEON

There are two conflicting principles when positioning the surgeon; the first is the requirement for surgeon mobility, and the second is the need for support to suppress tremor.

Classically the surgeon stands, which allows easy movement around the patient. A chair is a convenience but can make the surgeon too static, and for such procedures as lid surgery it is better to be standing. For a DCR, by contrast, there is only one good position to be operating from, and it really does not matter if the surgeon sits or stands. However, sitting is preferable when using a microscope. The presence of the microscope limits the surgeon's mobility anyway, and sitting helps to eliminate one source of tremor.

A requirement for fine surgery is support for the surgeon's forearms. If operating from above the patient's head, the patient's forehead can be used as a forearm/hand rest. When operating from the side (as for temporal incision cataract surgery) this option is not available, and it is important for the operating chair to have arms.

PREPARING THE SURGICAL FIELD

The aim of preparing the surgical field is to minimize wound infections while optimizing access.

ANTISEPSIS

A large number of agents have been used as antiseptics, but this section is limited to those that may be encountered in surgical practice.

Phenols

Lister initiated the use of antiseptic agents with a phenol (carbolic acid) spray. Phenol works by coagulating proteins and is highly effective against both bacteria and viruses, but it is toxic, unpleasant to work with and expensive, so it is no longer used. The cresols are alkyl phenols, and these are still used. For example, Lysol is a solution of cresols in soap and the domestic disinfectant Dettol is a chlorinated xylenol (a methyl cresol).

Alcohols

Alcohols act as protein coagulants and are also used as antiseptics at 70 per cent concentration. They act rapidly, and are clear fluids that readily evaporate and leave no stain. However, they do not penetrate organic matter well. Isopropyl alcohol tends to be used in clinical practice; ethanol is just as effective, but its use is expensive due to excise duty!

Isopropyl alcohol is the antiseptic of choice for such outpatient procedures as venepuncture (it is the active agent in Medi-swabs®).

Dyes

There are two types of dyes used as antiseptics; anilines and acridines. However, only the acridines proflavine and acriflavine are routinely used. They are non-toxic and have bactericidal activity against both gram-positive and gram-negative bacteria which resists quenching

('quenching' refers to the loss of antimicrobial activity in the presence of proteins). Their commonest use is incorporation into dressings such as flavine wool.

Halogens

Agents that release chlorine and iodine show good antiviral and antibacterial activity. The iodophor Betadine® is most commonly used in clinical practice. An iodophor is a solution of iodine in a surface-active detergent (most commonly povidone), and betadine is a mixture of povidone and iodine. Iodophors work by oxidizing SH groups. One disadvantage is that allergy to iodine is relatively common which is a contra-indication to their use.

Detergents

Detergents with antiseptic properties are cationic detergents (neutral and anionic detergents have little antibacterial activity). They show good activity against gram-positive organisms (i.e. the major skin commensals), but are of no value against mycobacteria, viruses, spores, and many gram-negative organisms. The best known cationic detergent is benzalkonium chloride, which is used as a preservative in many eye-drop preparations. The limitations of these agents should be recognized; not only do they have activity against a limited range of organisms, they are also easily quenched and are incompatible with soap.

Cationic agents can be combined with other agents such as chlorhexidine (Savlon®) and iodophors (Betadine surgical scrub®) to increase the antimicrobial activity.

Chlorhexidine

Chlorhexidine is a chlorinated biphenyl, which is active against gram-positive and gram-negative bacteria and mycobacteria. It is non-toxic and allergic reactions are not a problem. It is used in a number of disinfectant preparations.

Hibitane® contains 1% chlorhexidine, and Hibiscrub® contains 4% chlorhexidine in a detergent base.

DRAPES

Drapes and surgeons' gowns are made of broadly similar materials, and they serve identical functions – to provide a sterile covering to those areas of surgeon and patient that may come into direct contact with each other but are not formally cleaned. The material must provide a barrier to fluids (particularly blood) and micro-organisms, and be lint- and particulate-free, sterilizable and fire safe.

The earliest material used for gowns and drapes was linen, but this has now largely been replaced by cotton. The major advantages of these materials are that they fold and are air-permeable, and accordingly are extremely comfortable to wear. Unfortunately, the features that make them comfortable also make them poor barriers to micro-organisms. There is only a 30 per cent reduction in bacterial dispersion rate with a surgical gown[36], but it will be more effective against larger particles, which may be of greater importance in causing wound infections. Worse still, these materials are easily wetted and, once wet, lose much of their barrier function and may even enhance bacterial transfer due to 'wick' formation[38].

Barrier function is partly a function of weave density, and tight weaves are functionally superior but less comfortable as they are warmer to wear and less permeable. The properties can be improved by suitable surface chemical treatment (the equivalent of Scotchgarding®), but this tends to decline with repeated washings.

A review by AORN suggested that many cotton gowns and drapes have often lost their barrier properties after only 30 washings[39], and a further disadvantage of natural fabrics is that they tear easily, which severely compromises barrier function. They also tend to shed lint.

Disposable drapes

It is perhaps not surprising that there has been a trend towards single-use disposable drapes, which are made of cellulose and reinforced with synthetic polymers. While these can be relatively stiff and uncomfortable to wear, there is no doubt that their barrier functions are superior and they are 10 times more effective than ordinary cotton in preventing bacterial dispersion[40]. Two studies have shown an almost three-fold reduction in wound infection rates when using disposable drapes and gowns, compared to cotton[41,42].

Plastic incision drapes

These are adhesive plastic drapes that are placed over the incision site, and the drape is then cut in order to make the incision. They are transparent, adhesive, elastic, non-irritating and easily cut. They were initially used for abdominal surgery, and the idea was to immobilize bacteria adjacent to the skin. This antibacterial action can be enhanced by including an antibacterial agent such as an iodophor in the adhesive. Plastic incision drapes are particularly useful for intraocular surgery as, when correctly applied, they allow the eyelashes to be covered. Failure to drape the eyelashes is a risk factor for postoperative endophthalmitis.

Dust and micro-organisms

Dust is particularly important when discussing dissemination of micro-organisms from skin. Bacteria are not shed from skin as unicellular organisms, but on desquamated skin cells. The outermost layer of skin cells is shed every 24 hours, amounting to 10^9 cells/day per day[43,44], and each cell is around 40 μm across but will fragment on being shed to give even more particles; the average size of bacteria-carrying particles in a hospital is 12–14 μm[45]. The major site of S. aureus carriage is the nose, where it is found in about 40 per cent of the population, but the next most common site is the perineum, where it is found in 12 per cent[46]. For the unclothed subject, occlusive underpants will reduce airborne dispersion by 80 per cent[47].

THE SPECULUM

The major function of the lid speculum is to provide access. The specula available can be subdivided into two major classes; the rigid specula (e.g. Clarke's) and the wire specula. The rigid specula give the best access as they can be opened wide and then locked in that position, but they are more bulky than the wire specula and, if the lids are forced too far apart, can cause the lateral canthus to press on the eye and increase the intraocular pressure. The problem of a speculum causing a rise in the intraocular pressure is particularly important for cases of a penetrating eye injury. The best solution to this problem is the use of lid clips, which can be individually adjusted.

The wire specula are most commonly used for intraocular surgery, and give good access without over-opening the lids. There is the standard speculum and a version designed for phakoemulsification with the crossbar removed to prevent catching on the phako probe. The Pierce speculum is a compromise between wire and rigid speculum. It is designed for use in children or in any situation where the interpalpebral fissure is not of standard size, as it allows for adjustment.

A secondary function provided by guarded specula (such as the Lang's) is to keep the eyelashes out of the operative field. These specula differ from standard specula in having lash guards. However, they dislodge relatively easily, particularly in situations where the lids become 'floppy' (e.g. enucleation procedures). Guarded specula have been largely superseded by the use of plastic incision drapes which, when correctly applied, are more effective at keeping eyelashes out of the operating field.

For the majority of intraocular surgery, the most commonly used system is a plastic incision drape with a wire speculum.

In some situations, particularly lid surgery, the surgeon wants to be able to close or evert the lids; in these situations lid margin traction sutures (e.g. 4/0 silk) are used either on their own (for traction) or in combination with a Desmarres retractor (for eversion) rather than a speculum.

PREPARING FOR INTRAOCULAR SURGERY

Draping for intraocular surgery poses a particular problem, as the cornea must remain transparent for most procedures. It is not possible to scrub the ocular surface and, while it is traditional to clean the eyelid skin, this is not the incision site.

Most postoperative intraocular infections result from inoculation of bacteria at the time of surgery. The pilosebaceous units are particularly rich in bacteria, and cleaning systems will not penetrate to the depths of these units. In ophthalmology, eyelashes are an obvious cause for concern, and an adequate draping system must remove them from the operative field. There was a time when eyelashes used to be routinely shaved off before intraocular surgery, but this is rarely done nowadays.

To prepare an eye for intraocular surgery:

1. Use routine preoperative anti-microbial drops (e.g. a drop of chloramphenicol in the anaesthetic room).
2. When the patient is on the table, clean the cheek, forehead and eyelid skin (including the roots of the eyelashes) with aqueous povidone-iodine (or chlorhexidine if the patient is allergic to iodine).
3. Drape the hair.
4. Apply a plastic incision drape to the eye, with the lids open and the lashes everted. It is easier to start with the upper lid; once the lid margin is stuck the drape may be used to retract it in order to open the eye. The process can then be repeated on the lower lashes and lid.
5. Incise the drape. This creates two flaps. The upper lashes are usually much more troublesome than the lower lashes, and accordingly the flaps created are designed with the upper flap being larger than the lower. A central relieving incision in the centre of each flap can help them fold properly.
6. Insert the speculum so that the plastic drape flaps wrap around and completely cover the lid margin. This is important both to prevent infection and to reduce sensation. Exposed eyelashes are very sensitive to touch and, when they are not anaesthetized (as occurs with topical anaesthesia), irrigation of the ocular surface is sufficient to provoke a blink reflex and a Bell's phenomenon.
7. Finally, consider a drop of either aqueous povidone-iodine, diluted chlorhexidine or chloramphenicol directly into the fornices.

The installation of povidone-iodine into the conjunctival fornices has been reported significantly to reduce postoperative endophthalmitis from 0.24 to 0.06 per cent, but the two groups in the trial were neither randomized nor controlled for other such factors as use of antibiotics[48]. More importantly, perhaps, no toxicity has been reported with the use of a drop of either chloramphenicol or povidone-iodine in the conjunctival fornices, and it is difficult to justify not using them.

REFERENCES

1. Humphreys, H. (1993). Infection control and the design of the operating suite. *J. Hosp. Infect.*, 23, 61–70.
2. Charnley, J. (1979). *Low Friction Arthroplasty of the Hip*. Springer-Verlag.
3. Lidwell, O. M., Lowbury, E. J. L., Whyte, W. *et al.* (1983). Airborne contamination of wounds in joint replacement operations: the relation to sepsis rates. *J. Hosp. Infect.*, 4, 111–31.
4. Lidwell, O. M., Lowbury, E. J. L., Whyte, W. *et al.* (1984). Infection and sepsis after operations for total hip or knee-joint replacement: influence of ultra-clean air, prophylactic antibiotics and other factors. *J. Hygiene*, 93, 505–29.
5. (6)Elek, S. D. and Cohen, P. E. (1957). The virulence of Staphylococcus pyogenes for man. A study of the problem of wound infection. *Br. J. Exp. Path.*, 38, 573–86.
6. Kattan, H. M., Flynn, H. W., Pflugfelder, S. C. *et al.* (1991). Nosocomial endophthalmitis survey: current incidence of infection after intraocular surgery. *Ophthalmology*, 98, 227–38.

7. Menikoff, J. A., Speaker, M. G., Marmor, M. and Raskin, E. M. (1991). A case–control study of risk factors for postoperative endophthalmitis. *Ophthalmology*, **98**, 1761–68.
8. Gills, J. P. (1991). Filters and antibiotics in irrigating solutions for cataract surgery. *J. Cataract Refract. Surg.*, **17**, 385.
9. Gimbel, H. V., De Brof, R. S. and De Brof, B. M. (1994). Prophylactic intracameral antibiotics during cataract surgery: the incidence of endophthalmitis and corneal oedema. *Eur. J. Implant Refract. Surg.*, **6**, 280–85.
10. Tso, M. O. M. (1973). Photic maculopathy in rhesus monkeys: a light and electron microscope study. *Invest. Ophthalmol.* **12**, 17–34.
11. Michels, M. and Sternberg, P., Jr. (1990). Operating microscope-induced retinal phototoxicity: pathophysiology, clinical manifestations and prevention. *Surv. Ophthalmol.*, **34**, 237–52.
12. Khwarg, S. G., Linstone, F. A., Daniels, S. A. *et al.* (1984). Incidence, risk factors and morphology in operating microscope light retinopathy. *Am. J. Ophthalmol.*, **103**, 255–63.
13. Kennedy, I. and Grubb, A. (1994). *Medical Law: Text with Materials*, 2nd edn. Butterworths.
14. Kerrigan, D. D., Thevasagayam, R. S., Woods, T. O. *et al.* (1993). Who's afraid of informed consent? *Br. Med. J.*, **306**, 298–300.
15. Marak, G. E. J. (1979). Recent advances in sympathetic ophthalmia. *Surv. Ophthalmol.*, **24**, 141–56.
16. Connell, J. F. J. and Rousselot, L. M. (1964). Povidone-iodine. *Am. J. Surg.*, **108**, 849–55.
17. Kobayashi, H. (1991). Evaluation of surgical scrubbing. *J. Hosp. Infect.*, **18** (Suppl. B), 29–34.
18. Lowbury, E. J. L. and Lilly, H. A. (1973). Use of 4% chlorhexidine detergent solution (Hibiscrub) and other methods of skin disinfection. *Br. Med. J.*, **1**, 510–15.
19. Hamilton, A. (1905). Dissemination of streptococci through invisible sputum in relation to scarlet fever and sepsis. *J. Am. Med. Assoc.*, **1905**, 1108–11.
20. Teague, O. (1913). Some experiments bearing upon droplet infection in diphtheria. *J. Infect. Dis.*, **12**, 398–414.
21. Paine, C. G. (1935). The aetiology of puerperal infection with special reference to droplet infection. *Br. Med. J.*, i, 24–6.
22. Meleney, F. L. and Stevens, F. A. (1926). Postoperative haemolytic streptococcus wound infections and their relation to haemolytic streptococcus carriers among operating personnel. *Surg. Gynecol. Obstet.*, **43**, 338–42.
23. Berger, S. A., Kramer, M., Nagar, H. *et al.* (1993). Effect of surgical mask position on bacterial contamination of the operative field. *J. Hosp. Infect.*, **23**, 51–4.
24. Ford, C. R. and Peterson, D. E. (1963). The efficiency of surgical face masks. *Am. J. Surg. Pathol.*, **106**, 954–7.
25. Greene, V. W. and Vesley, D. (1962). Method for evaluating the effectiveness of surgical masks. *J. Bacteriol.*, **83**, 663–7.
26. Hirschfield, J. W. and Laube, P. J. (1941). Surgical masks, an experimental study. *Surgery*, **9**, 720–30.
27. Quesnel, L. B. (1975). The efficiency of surgical masks of varying design and composition. *Br. J. Surgery.*, **62**(12) 936–40.
28. Orr, N. W. M. (1981). Is a mask necessary in the operating theatre? *Ann. R. Coll. Surg. Engl.*, **63**, 390–92.
29. Davis, W. T. (1991). Filtration efficiency of surgical masks: the need for more meaningful standards. *Am. J. Infect. Control*, **19**, 16–18.
30. Schweizer, R. T. (1976). Mask wriggling as a potential cause of wound contamination. *Lancet*, **2**, 1129–30.
31. Haglund, U. and Junghanns, K. (1997). Glove powder – the hazards which demand a ban. *Eur. J. Surg.*, **167**(S579), 1–55.
32. Aronson, S. (1972). Starch endophthalmitis. *Am. J. Ophthalmol.*, **73**, 570–79.
33. Heese, A., Peters, K.-P. and Koch, H. U. (1997). Type 1 allergies to latex and the aeroallergenic problem. *Eur. J. Surg.*, **579** (Suppl.), 19–22.
34. Brehler, R., Kolling, R., Webb, M. and Wastell, C. (1997). Glove powder – a risk factor for the development of latex allergy? *Eur. J. Surg.*, **579** (Suppl.), 23–25.
35. Fell, M. (1987). Failure rates in surgical gloves. In: *The Patient and Surgeon in Theatre*. The Medicine Group (UK) Ltd.
36. Brookes, A. (1994). Surgical glove perforation. *Nursing Times*, **90**, 60–62.
37. Whyte, W., Vesley, D. and Hodgson, R. (1976). Bacterial dispersion in relation to operating room clothing. *J. Hygiene*, **76**, 367–78.

38. Beck, W. C. and Collette, T. S. (1952). False faith in the surgeon's gown and drape. *Am. J. Surg.*, **83**, 125–62.
39. Lehr, P. S. and Palmer, P. N. (1999). Operating room practices: myth or science? *AORN*, **49**, 645–9.
40. Whyte, W., Bailey, P. V., Hamblen, D. L. *et al.* (1983). A bacteriologically occlusive clothing system for use in the operating room. *J. Bone Joint Surg.*, **65**, 502–6.
41. Moylan, J. A., Fitzpatrick, K. T. and Davenport, K. E. (1987). Reducing wound infections. Improved gown and drape barrier performances. *Arch. Surg.*, **122**, 152–7.
42. Moylan, J. A. and Kennedy, B. V. (1980). The importance of gown and drape barriers in the prevention of wound infection. *Surg. Gynecol. Obstet.*, **151**, 465–70.
43. Jansen, L. H., Hojyo-Tomoko, M. T. and Kligman, A. M. (1975). Improved fluorescence staining technique for estimating turnover of the human stratum corneum. *Br. J. Dermatol.*, **90**, 9–12.
44. Mackintosh, C. A., Lidwell, O. M., Towers, A. G. and Marples, R. R. (1978). The dimensions of skin fragments dispersed into the air during activity. *J. Hygiene*, **81**, 471–9.
45. Noble, W. C., Lidwell, O. M. and Kingston, D. (1963). The size distribution of airborne particles carrying micro-organisms. *J. Hygiene*, **66**, 385–91.
46. Polakoff, S., Richards, I. D. G., Parker, M. T. and Lidwell, O. M. (1967). Nasal and skin carriage of *S. aureus* by patients undergoing surgical operations. *J. Hygiene*, **65**, 559–66.
47. Hill, J., Howell, A. and Blowers, R. (1974). Effect of clothing on dispersal of *Staphylococcus aureus* by males and females. *Lancet*, **2**(7889), 1131–3.
48. Speaker, M. G. and Menikoff, J. A. (1991). Prophylaxis of endophthalmitis with topical povidone-iodine. *Ophthalmology*, **98**, 1669–75.

2

WOUND CREATION

Wound creation has two major purposes, the most important of which is to give adequate access to allow the proposed operation to be completed safely – big mistakes are caused by little holes! The second aim is to minimize subsequent scar formation. Good wound closure minimizes scar formation, and this is facilitated by thoughtful planning of the incision. Most of the following points should be self-evident:

- Although too small an incision is hazardous, a gratuitously large incision should be avoided.
- The incision should be hidden in an existing anatomical landmark (e.g. the skin crease to approach the upper lid; the hairline for temporal artery biopsies; and the eyebrow for brow-lifts).
- Wounds heal better on concave surfaces when healing by secondary intention, but can cause bowstringing due to contracture when healing by primary intention.

In contrast to many other types of surgery, Langer's lines (the lines of cleavage) are relatively unimportant. For example, the DCR excision and incisions used to make wedge resections of the eyelids run at right angles to these lines; when they are followed, it is because some anatomical structure (such as the upper lid skin crease) is in line with them.

INSTRUMENTS

KNIVES AND BLADES

Scalpel blades
The major blades used are as follows (Figure 2.1):

1. The no. 10 and 15 blades have a rounded contour and are designed for making long rather than deep incisions. As such, they are ideal for cutting skin. The no. 15 blade is smaller than the no. 10, and is therefore the one used in ophthalmic surgery. The correct grip for general surgery is with handle in the palm of the hand and the index finger held along the top of the handle, which gives a compromise between power and precision. Since great force is rarely required for ophthalmic surgery, the precision

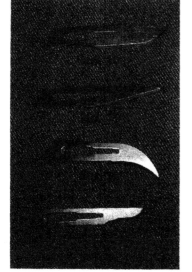

Figure 2.1 Types of scalpel blade.

grip (as in holding a pen) is usually adopted by ophthalmic surgeons.

2. The no. 11 blade is used for stabbing incisions in the skin and mucosa. It can make deep wounds with sharp corners (as in incision and curettage of Meibomian cysts, or opening the lacrimal sac and cutting the nasal flaps when performing a DCR). There are few indications for deep stabbing wounds, as these can be dangerous. These blades blunt easily.

3. The no. 12 (or sickle) blade has a sharp point and a cutting edge on the inside of the curve, and is designed for suture removal. It is also suitable for cutting lacrimal and nasal mucosa flaps when performing a DCR; the sharp point cuts the mucosa and, with the cutting edge on the inside, is effectively guarded, thereby minimizing the risk of accidental injury to the skin. This is an advantage when operating at the base of a small incision.

Disposable blades

Most corneal surgery requires deep incisions with sharp borders, and many intraocular procedures need a paracentesis (a stab incision). These incisions are particularly demanding on the knives, and a blade does not last long. Two solutions to this problem have been adopted: the first is to use a cheap blade, which can be disposed of after use and therefore a new one be used for each case; the second is to use a particularly durable material such as diamond.

Modern disposable hypodermic needles make excellent fine stabbing instruments – for example, as needed when using iris hooks.

Diamond knives

These are durable enough to be sterilized by autoclaving. They do blunt with time, and it is important that they are handled with care. In particular, the blade should not come into contact with any other metal instrument, as this will rapidly blunt them. The blades can be retracted to protect them, and it is good practice for the scrub nurse to hand the instrument over with the blade retracted and for the surgeon to return it in the same position. Diamond blades can be resharpened.

There are a number of designs for diamond blades, and the choice depends upon the requirements. Many of the designs have been generated by refractive surgeons, whose dominant concerns have been linearity of the incision and control of the depth. Many blades are designed with one edge vertical and the other at a diagonal of 15–45°, and cutting with the diagonal end tends to cause a rounded entry and a depth less than the depth dialled (if using a guarded knife). The more diagonal the blade is, the easier it is to control the cut.

Using a vertical edge makes a cut with square edges at the full depth, if using a guarded blade, but it is harder to control the direction of the cut. Once again there are variations on the theme. For example, the Thornton trifacet knife has a rectangular blade so that it cuts vertically in both directions; this is exclusively a blade for refractive surgery.

SCISSORS

Scissors may be sharp-pointed or blunt-tipped, straight or curved, right- or left-handed, and of various sizes. Spring scissors are also available. Sharp-pointed, straight scissors are useful for suture removal and when a combination of stab incision and cutting is required. Blunt-tipped scissors are more appropriate for most other situations, including blunt dissection, undermining and cutting tissue.

The correct way to hold scissors is by three-point fixation (Figure 2.2). Most scissors are designed to be held by the right hand and will cut poorly when used in the left hand. The reason for this is that two separate torques are applied in operation (Figure 2.3); the first torque is to shut the blades (the 'up and down' torque), while the second torque is a rotary torque along the long axis of the scissors and determines whether the two blades are in apposition or pulled apart when closed. The natural tendency is for the thumb to push on the handle when closing the blades, and most instruments are designed with this in mind and for use in the right hand. These instruments can be used with the left hand, but the grip and action need to be changed so that the ring finger is curled up on the inside of its handle and pushing out while the thumb is pulling in; this is an unnatural action.

Figure 2.2 Three-point fixation for holding scissors. The handles are held by the thumb and ring finger while the index finger supports the fulcrum.

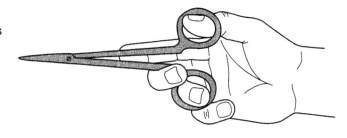

Figure 2.3 Right-handed scissors do not work well in the left hand. This is due to there being, in addition to the 'up and down' torque, a second torque that is in opposite directions for right and left hands. This second torque acts to separate or oppose the blades for right-handed scissors.

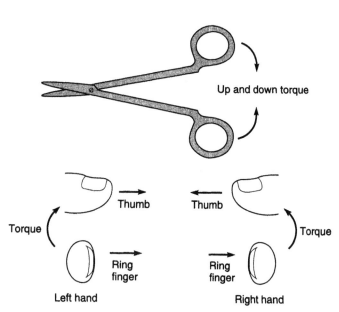

Three-point fixation is clearly not possible with the small scissors often required in ophthalmic surgery, and the solution is spring scissors, which can be held in a manner similar to forceps. There is only one torque in action ('up and down'), so they can be used in either hand; however, because they lack the second torque they are less robust.

FORCEPS AND SKIN HOOKS

Forceps and skin hooks are used for holding tissue, and their design reflects the conflicting requirements of securely holding tissue whilst not damaging or traumatizing it. For skin, hooks are superior to forceps; while microperforations are irrelevant in skin, rough handling of the skin edges may promote dieback of the tissue and lead to scar formation.

Forceps vary with regard to their tips, their size, and the presence or otherwise of blocking. Plain tips are required for holding very fragile tissue, and their grip can be improved by having horizontal grooves (e.g. Moorfields forceps). Toothed forceps are ideal for firmly gripping tissue, but will traumatize it. A compromise is the microgroove, and such forceps are ideal for most anterior segment ocular surgery.

Many forceps are blocked behind the tips, and can therefore be used for holding and tying sutures. Again, size is important, particularly in the case of plain-tipped forceps. These will only work if there is accurate apposition of the tips when closed, and are useless if the tips do not meet. Many of the fine-tipped forceps used in microsurgery are particularly delicate and readily damaged, and great care must be taken to ensure that the forceps are appropriate to the task in hand (Table 2.1).

Many surgical forceps have very fine tips, and it can be difficult to view them without magnification. Accordingly, some manufacturers,

Table 2.1 Specific examples of forceps for different tasks	
Tissue	*Forceps*
Conjunctiva	Moorfields or plain-tipped forceps
Cornea and sclera	Jail's forceps (or 'ones into twos' after the number of teeth involved in the grip), Colibri's forceps or microgroove forceps
Skin	Skin hooks and Adson's forceps
Tendon	Lister's forceps (or 'twos into threes')
Lens capsule	Utrata forceps, which are exceptionally fine-tipped and long forceps. The ends are enlarged, angled to make grabbing the capsule easier, and blunt-ended. They are extremely delicate and easily damaged
Cartilage	Non-toothed forceps (toothed tips will shred cartilage)

such as Duckworth and Kent, have developed symbols to help the scrub nurse identify the tips:

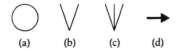

(a) Notched or microgrooved forceps (e.g. Hoskin's)
(b) Plain tips
(c) Blocked forceps for tying
(d) Toothed forceps

ELECTROSURGERY

Although electricity is most commonly used for stopping bleeding (diathermy), it can also be used for tissue destruction and wound creation.

The term 'cautery' comes from the Greek *kauterion* (literally, 'branding iron'). Heat has long been known to prevent infection and cause coagulation, and it is mainly used for the latter. Any source of heat will do, and procedures were originally performed using the 'hot iron'; 'electrocautery' simply means that electricity is the source of heat. Instruments are usually based around a wire that is heated with the aid of direct current. No electricity passes through the patient, and the effect is merely thermal.

Another use derives from the fact that burnt tissue contracts, and this effect has been used to correct lid malpositions such as medial ectropion (by retropunctal cautery) and entropion (by anterio-lamellar cautery[1,2]).

The term cautery is often used inappropriately to describe electro-surgical coagulation.

Electrosurgery differs from cautery in that current passes through the patient. The use of direct current exposes the patient to the risk of electrocution, as does the use of low frequency alternating current (the UK mains electricity runs at 50 Hz, which is too low to be used safely). However, Arsene D'Arsonval noted that electrical alternating currents of greater than 10 000 Hz failed to cause neuromuscular stimulation, and therefore at these high frequencies there is no risk of electrocution. Most surgical generators use frequencies in the range of 300 kHz, which is within the radio-wave range, and hence this is sometimes referred to as radiosurgery; this is potentially confusing because the very accurately targeted forms of radiotherapy such as the gamma knife are also referred to as radiosurgery.

MONOPOLAR VERSUS BIPOLAR DIATHERMY

These terms refer to where the return electrode is situated. In bipolar surgery, both the active electrode and the return electrode are at the surgical site (Figure 2.4a); this is the set-up that is most commonly used in ophthalmic surgery. Its use is restricted to coagulation, and the current path is confined to the tissue grasped between the two tines of the forceps.

In most forms of surgery, however, the monopolar set-up is more commonly used because it is more versatile and can be used for tissue destruction as well as for coagulation. In monopolar surgery the instrument held by the surgeon is only the active terminal, with the return electrode placed elsewhere on the body (usually in the form of a pad; Figure 2.4b). This arrangement allows for cutting as well as coagulation.

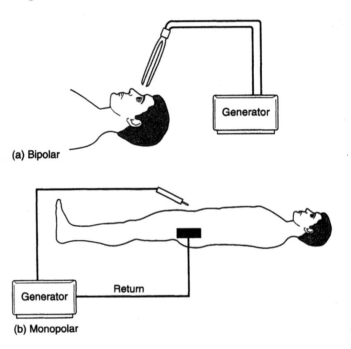

Figure 2.4 (a) Bipolar electrosurgery; (b) monopolar electrosurgery.

CURRENT WAVEFORMS

There are two distinct effects of electrosurgery; tissue vaporization (as occurs in the 'cutting' mode), and coagulation. Which of these two effects occurs depends upon the temperature reached, and this in turn depends upon the current waveform (Figure 2.5).

In the cutting mode the output is continuous, resulting in high-energy delivery but relatively low voltage, so sparking occurs only over a very short distance. In the coagulation mode the output occurs for only 6 per cent of the 'duty cycle', resulting in low heat output. The result is tissue dessication, leading to coagulation rather than vaporization. The actual energy delivered will clearly depend upon the voltage used, so at very low voltages it is possible to achieve a coagulation effect on the 'cutting' mode.

The term 'blend' refers to a modification of the duty cycle, and is not simply a mixture of coagulation and cutting currents; however, it does result in a balance between cutting and coagulation.

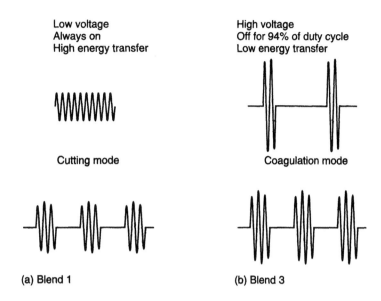

Low voltage
Always on
High energy transfer

High voltage
Off for 94% of duty cycle
Low energy transfer

Cutting mode

Coagulation mode

(a) Blend 1

(b) Blend 3

Figure 2.5 Current patterns in electrosurgery.

Blend has properties intermediate between cutting and coagulation. As blend increases, the duty cycle on time drops (from 50% for blend 1, to 40% for blend 2 to 25% for blend 3), the voltage increases and the effect changes from predominantly cutting to predominantly coagualtion.

TYPES OF ELECTROSURGERY

There are three distinct modes of tissue destruction:

1. Electrosurgical cutting, where the surgeon holds the cutting instrument a little away from the tissue (i.e. no pressure is used, in contrast to using a blade) and allows it to spark; this results in maximum current concentration and causes the cells to explode, leaving a cavity behind them, resulting in a cutting effect. The effect can be enhanced by the use of argon, which is readily ionized and will accordingly further concentrate the current. The cutting mode does not cause haemostasis and the effect is like a scalpel.
2. Fulguration, which is sparking with the coagulation waveform to produce coagulation and charring over a relatively large area. As with electrosurgical cutting, the sparking is achieved by holding the electrode a little away from the tissue, resulting in a coagulum.
3. Desiccation, which occurs when the electrode is in direct contact with the tissue. By touching the tissue, the high current concentration is lost and the cells dry out rather than vaporize, again resulting in a coagulum.

The build up of coagulum on the electrode can be reduced by using a non-stick coating.

HAZARDS

Inadvertant burns

Inadvertant burns are a particular problem with the monopolar set-up and can occur by more than one mechanism. With the monopolar set-up, current that enters a patient must exit. With the old grounded generators (like household appliances), the current eventually returns to earth and accordingly the patient, apart from the return electrode, had to be insulated from any other contact to earth (e.g. a metallic drip stand) as this would result in a return to ground and a potential burn at the point of contact. This problem has been largely solved by 'isolated generator technology' (see Figure 2.6).

The second problem is of burns at the site of the return electrode itself. The return pathway should therefore be over a large surface area so that there is sufficiently low current density to leave the tissue unaffected. Thus, the return electrode is usually a large, electrically conducting pad. If the contact between the return electrode and the patient is poor, it allows points of high current density to form.

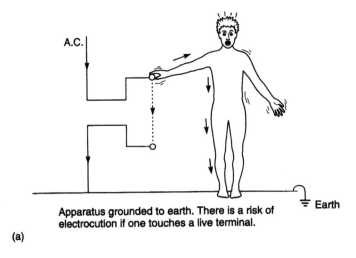

Apparatus grounded to earth. There is a risk of electrocution if one touches a live terminal.

(a)

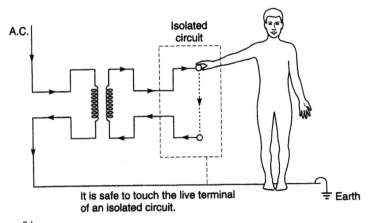

It is safe to touch the live terminal of an isolated circuit.

(b)

Figure 2.6 Circuit diagrams for (a) grounded (b) isolated circuit generators.

Modern electrolysis units have 'return electrode monitoring', which checks that there is a low resistance connection between the electrode and the patient (Figure 2.7); if it detects high resistance, it will inactivate the generator.

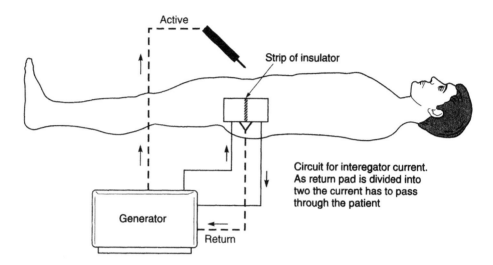

Figure 2.7 Return electrode monitoring by means of an interegator current.

Smoke and fire

Smoke from electrosurgery can carry viral DNA, bacteria and carcinogens. It is good practice to reduce exposure to it by using suction to extract it.

Fire is a particular hazard for monopolar systems, and clearly monopolar cautery should not be used in an oxygen-rich environment, in the presence of flammable agents such as alcohol, or with paper drapes. When not in use, the active electrode should be stored in an insulated safety holster.

REFERENCES

1. el-Kasaby, H. T. (1992). Cautery for lower lid entropion. *Br. J. Ophthalmol.*, **76**, 532–3.
2. Ziegler, S. L. (1909). Galvanocautery puncture in ectropion and entropion. *J. Am. Med. Assoc.*, **63**, 183.

3

BLOOD

Blood poses special problems to the surgeon:

- Excessive blood loss threatens the haemodynamic stability of the patient, although this is hardly ever a problem with ophthalmic operations.
- Blood is densely packed with pigment, and accordingly a small amount of blood can completely obscure the view and stain all tissues red.
- Postoperative haematoma formation is a risk factor for postoperative infection. In procedures in which the orbital septum has been breached there is a risk of intraorbital haematoma formation, which can lead to blindness; this is the presumed cause of reported blindness following blepharoplasty. The risk of blindness following this procedure is estimated at $1 : 10\,000$[1] and presumably applies to any procedure that results in opening of the orbital septum (e.g. ptosis repair).

Blood can also promote healing and, while this may be beneficial in most types of surgery, it is a potential hindrance in filtration surgery.

GENERAL MEASURES

If a problem with bleeding can be anticipated, then taking simple preventative measures is good practice:

1. Ask the patient to avoid aspirin and aspirin-like compounds for 1 week prior to any elective procedure
2. For those on oral anticoagulants (usually warfarin), check the prothrombin time and consider discontinuing treatment for 3 weeks prior to surgery
3. Consider using a preoperative local anaesthetic containing adrenaline, even when performing a procedure under general anaesthesia
4. Place the patient in a head-up posture on the table
5. Use hypotensive anaesthesia.

REMOVING BLOOD

SWABS

Swabs are used to absorb blood in order to allow visualization of the anatomy, and the two most commonly used materials are gauze and cellulose sponge. For microsurgery cellulose sponge swabs are preferable, because they are solid, do not fragment and tend not to leave bits behind. They can also be cut into any shape, although triangular is the most common. However, when they are dry they are very absorbent and will desiccate any tissue that they touch; they must therefore be lightly moistened before use.

Gauze is a coarse, plain-woven cotton (or cotton and viscose) cloth, and comes in a number of sizes. It is absorbent and, being pliable, can be used to hold tissue edges. Gauze soaked in saline can also be used to keep exposed tissues moist.

SUCTION

Large volumes of blood are most readily removed by suction. Suction units in theatre work on the Venturi principle and run off compressed air. A problem with suction is that tissue can be sucked up in addition to blood; therefore all suction units have a hole on the side of the sucker which, when opened, breaks the suction and allows any impacted tissue to be removed. Suction units are also easily blocked, and there is a sterile rod available with each suction unit which can be passed up or down the sucker to clear it.

CONTROLLING BLEEDING

PRESSURE

All bleeding stops with pressure. Bleeding will generally stop within 6 minutes of continuous pressure, by which time clotting mechanisms have been activated.

Intraocular surgery (particularly intra- and extracapsular cataract surgery) presents a particular problem, because making the surgical section reduces the intraocular pressure to zero. In this situation even the lowest pressure bleeding can continue unchecked, which may result in expulsive haemorrhages. The current trend in surgical practice is increasingly towards small incisions and utilizing infusion lines, which maintain the intraocular pressure throughout the procedure.

One of the purposes of a postoperative dressing is to reduce haematoma formation by pressure.

LIGATURES

Ligatures are threads used for tying off medium to large vessels. Most of the vessels encountered in ophthalmic surgery are small and best dealt with by other techniques. The one exception is a temporal artery biopsy, when the vessel should be tied off both proximal and distal to the section to be excised, using any absorbable suture material.

The general surgical technique of using artery clips and then tying the vessels with ligatures is rarely used in ophthalmic surgery.

SUTURE LIGATION

The Z-stitch (Figure 3.1) is a technique used in general surgery for control of bleeding points that are difficult to identify. A variant of this, suture ligation of vessels, is a general surgical technique used for large vessels and rarely used in ophthalmic practice[2]. However, the same technique can be used for closing congenital lacrimal fistulas. The suture is first passed through the fistula to prevent the ligature slipping, then round each side of it (Figure 3.2).

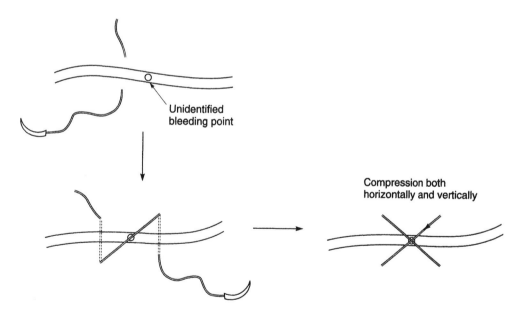

Figure 3.1 A Z-suture ligation of an unidentified bleeding point. Suture tract resembles a Z, but when tied it looks like an X.

CAUTERY

The commonest technique used for control of bleeding is diathermy (see Electrosurgery, Chapter 2).

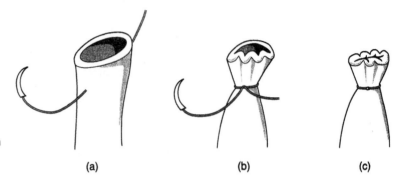

Figure 3.2 Suture ligation of a fistula. A stitch is passed through the fistula (a) and tied first one side (b) and then the other (c).

(a)   (b)   (c)

HAEMOSTATIC MATERIALS

Bone wax

Bleeding from bone is a potential problem as diathermy works poorly in this situation, and surgical bone wax has long been recognized as a good solution[3]. It is composed of white beeswax, paraffin wax and isopropyl palmitate, and is used to tamponade bleeding. It can be applied to wet surfaces, although it seems to work better if dry. The technique is to press it firmly into the bone and then smear it across the surface. The potential disadvantage is that it can act as a barrier to healing.

Oxidized cellulose, gelatin sponges and collagen felts

Oxidized sponges (e.g. Sturgiseal[TM]) are the least satisfactory way of controlling bleeding, but they can be useful when there is continuous bleeding from unidentified bleeding points. This situation is most commonly encountered from bleeding within a cavity, such as when performing a dacryocystorhinostomy (DCR). Oxidized sponges are white, porous, absorbent and haemostatic. They can be used to pack 'dead spaces', and are completely resorbed in 6 weeks.

Collagen felts and gelatin sponges have similar properties to oxidized cellulose sponges, and have similar uses. Collagen is extremely haemostatic, as it is probably the relevant stimulus for clotting *in vivo*, and accordingly the clotting times with collagen felts are significantly shorter than with oxidized cellulose. These materials are resorbed in 3–4 weeks.

Chondroitin sulphate

The viscoelastic chondroitin sulphate has been shown to be a coagulant[4], and accordingly would be an appropriate agent to tamponade intraocular bleeding (e.g. Viscoat®).

REFERENCES

1. Lowry, J. C. and Bartley, G. B. (1994). Complications of blepharoplasty (Review). *Surv. Ophthalmol.*, 38(4), 327–50.
2. Johnson, C.D. (1997). In: *Essential Surgical Technique,* 1st edn (C. D. Johnson and J. Cumming, eds), pp. 1–32. Chapman and Hall.
3. Horsley, V. (1892). Antiseptic wax. *Br. Med. J.*, 1, 1165.
4. Pandolfi, M. Hedner, U. (1984). The effect of sodium hyaluronate and sodium chondroitin sulphate on the coagulation system *in vitro*. *Ophthalmology*, 91, 864–6.

4

WOUND CLOSURE

The basic principle underlying wound closure is good approximation of tissue to allow healing by primary intention. The major advantage of healing by primary intention is that it allows healing with a minimum of scar formation. Suturing is the mainstay technique of wound closure, but other techniques all have their place.

SUTURE EQUIPMENT

TYPES OF SUTURES

Suture materials are classified according to their thickness or gauge (Table 4.1) and composition. The metric classification has been adopted by both the European and the United States Pharmacopoeia, and refers to the thickness of the suture material in tenths of a millimetre (i.e. a suture with a metric number of 0.1 has a diameter of 1/100 of a millimetre).

The suture materials can be separated into absorbable and non-(or very slowly) absorbable, and the following descriptions are of the most commonly used materials.

Table 4.1 Suture classification

Non-metric	Metric
Non-absorbable and synthetic sutures	
11/0	0.1
10/0	0.2
9/0	0.3
9/0 virgin silk	0.3
8/0 virgin silk	0.3
8/0	0.4
7/0	0.5
6/0	0.7
5/0	1
4/0	1.5
3/0	2
2/0	3
0	3.5

Absorbable sutures

Catgut

This suture is not and never has been made from cats, and comes from the submucosal layer of sheep's intestines. The name probably derives from 'kitgut', where 'kit' is an Arabian fiddle. It is one of the oldest used suture materials, with the first clear reference being made by Galen of Pergamon in about 175 AD. Its main disadvantage is that absorption, which is by phagocytosis, provokes a marked inflammatory response. It was gradually being superseded by synthetic materials such as Dexon® and Vicryl®, but the process has been hastened by the problem of variant Creutzfeld-Jakob Disease, which has resulted in catgut being withdrawn.

Polyglycolid acid (Dexon®)

First available in 1971, Dexon® is a slowly absorbable suture. It is a homopolymer of glycolic acid, and retains 55 per cent of its strength at 1 week and 20 per cent by week three. Absorption is complete by 8–14 weeks. It degrades by hydrolysis, and accordingly provokes much less inflammation than catgut. It is a multifilament suture with fair handling properties and good knot security.

Polyglycan 910 (Vicryl®)

Polyglycan 910 (Vicryl®) is a synthetic suture that was first available in 1974, and is a polymer of glycolic acid and lactic acid in the ratio of 9 : 1. It comes either undyed (tan or gold) or dyed (purple). It degrades predominantly by hydrolysis to carbon dioxide and water, aided by phagocytosis[1], and because glycolic acid and lactic acid are natural metabolites, there is minimal tissue reaction. Sutures of 8/0 or thicker come as a coated (with a mixture of calcium stearate and a copolymer made from 65 per cent lactide and 35 per cent glycolide), braided multifilament, while 9/0 and 10/0 Vicryl® are uncoated monofilaments.

Coated Vicryl® is superior to Dexon® (polyglycolic acid) in most ways, being stronger at all time points but degrading in a similar manner. It offers wound support for around 30 days, and absorption is complete by 8–14 weeks. The 9/0 and 10/0 absorb more quickly, offering wound support for only 10–15 days. It is a good choice of suture material where an absorbable suture is desired (e.g. subcutaneous or deep closure).

Vicryl Rapide® is a rapidly absorbable variant that is generated by irradiation, which partially fragments the structure[2]. Its initial strength is equivalent to that silk, but its strength is down to 50 per cent at 1 week and nothing by 2 weeks. The idea of the rapidly absorbable variant is to make it suitable for cutaneous suture in situations where suture removal may be difficult, such as in children[2].

Poliglecaprone 25 monofilament (Monocryl®)

This comes as an undyed synthetic monofilament that offers complete support for 20 days and then absorbs by hydrolysis over the next

70–90 days. It is an option for suturing muscles during strabismus procedures.

Polydioxanone (PDS® and PDS II®)

This is a more recent synthetic monofilament, which is a polymer of para-dioxanone. It also absorbs by hydrolysis. Its advantage over Vicryl® and Dexon® is that it is one-fifth stronger than these and four times more flexible.

Non-absorbable sutures

Silk

There are two types of silk used for suturing, each with remarkably different properties:

1. Twisted virgin silk is raw silk that still contains the natural gums and allows the many fine strands to stick together to form a thin and strong suture. Its advantage over braided silk is that a finer suture can be produced. Virgin silk (8/0) was once the material of choice for cataract wound closure, but the gums degrade and produce a short-lived but invariable sclerokeratitis at 6–12 weeks after surgery. Accordingly, it has been superseded by newer materials and is no longer considered to be suitable as a corneal suture.
2. Braided silk is produced from virgin silk, and has the natural gums extracted. This reduces the volume of the silk to about 30 per cent, and it is then braided for use. It is classified as non-absorbable, but is in fact slowly absorbable; 50 per cent of its strength is lost by 1 year, and all of it by 2 years. It is relatively inflammatory. Its most noteworthy characteristic is that it has exceptional handling, and this makes braided silk the 'gold standard' against which the handling characteristics of other sutures are compared. It is the suture material of choice for situations where it can be readily removed (e.g. skin closure and traction sutures).

Monofilament polyamide (nylon, Ethilon™)

This is a synthetic, non-absorbable suture, and it comes in two forms. Polyamide 6 is formed by polymerization of E-caprolactam, while polyamide 66 is formed from hexamethylenediamine and adipic acid; both types are produced by extrusion and have similar physical properties. Its smooth surface makes it particularly inert, but also gives relatively poor handling and knot security. It is useful for subcuticular closure, as its smooth surface allows it to slip past tissue with little resistance, allowing relatively easy removal. The smooth surface resists bacterial colonization.

The concept that this suture is completely non-absorbable is false, and in fact the amide links undergo slow hydrolysis. Monofilament nylon (10/0) is commonly used for corneal wound closure and, when used at this location, broken sutures can be found in 90 per cent of cases, half of which are symptomatic[3]. In these cases, most clinician's would recommend routine removal within the first year[4]. The suture absorbs more quickly in the uvea[5], and it is thus not recommended for such procedures as sutured intraocular lens implants and iris fixation sutures[6] – both polypropylene (Prolene®) and polyester (Mersilene®) are less absorbable and preferable for this indication. Anecdotal observation indicates that the speed of nylon suture resorption also depends on how close the stitch is to the limbus, with the suture lasting longer in the central cornea (as after corneal graft surgery) compared to peripherally located sutures (as after cataract surgery). The rate of hydrolysis may also be accelerated by tension on the material[7].

It should be noted that broken nylon sutures in the cornea are a cause of significant complications. They can cause giant papillary conjunctivitis[4], and they have a high incidence of microbial contamination (most commonly *S. epidermidis*[8]) that can result in serious ocular infection.

Polypropylene (Prolene®)

This is a synthetic non-absorbable suture that is relatively elastic compared to nylon. It has been used for corneal sutures with the idea that the elasticity may compensate for variable tension in suturing and allow less postoperative astigmatism in extracapsular cataract surgery. In one study the results were no different with regard to astigmatism, but there was a four-fold higher incidence of iris prolapses[9]. This suggests that the elasticity makes it unsuitable when watertight and tissue-tight wounds are required.

Prolene® is the most hydrophobic of the synthetic plastics and absorbs less than 0.1 per cent water; accordingly it is less absorbable, with no clinically detectable resorption of 9/0 corneal sutures at 30 months[10]. A second advantage is that although it has a low coefficient of friction it will also mould with pressure, thus giving it surprisingly good knot security.

Polyester (Ethibond®, Tecron®, Mersilene® and Dacron®)

Polyester polyethylene terephthalate appears under a number of commercial names (Ethibond®, Tecron®, Mersilene® and Dacron®). It is another synthetic non-absorbable suture, and is superior to nylon in many ways. It is the strongest of the monofilaments – 11/0 Mersilene® is equivalent in strength to 10/0 nylon. It has a high coefficient of friction, which results in good knot security[11] but makes the suture harder to remove; this may be an issue in cataract surgery, where it may be desirable to remove sutures to control postoperative astigmatism. It also absorbs very little moisture, and as a result is less absorbable than nylon. For example, one study looking at corneal sections sutured with 11/0 Mersilene® found no clinically determined degradation and minimal microscopic degradation at 2 years[12], and there would appear to be no requirement for routine removal[13].

A problem with this material is its poor handling properties and knot security.

NEEDLES

Needles can be classified according to their cross-sectional profile, radius, degree of curvature, chord length and whether they are swaged or eyed (Figure 4.1). The length of a needle refers to the length if it was straightened, but more important features are the chord length and the radius of curvature, which determine the width and depth of the bite respectively.

Most sewing needles are eyed, but it is extremely hard to thread fine suture material and there is the added disadvantage that the needle has to be of greater diameter than the thread and so makes a larger than necessary hole. Both of these problems are solved by swaged needles. As the diameter of the needle is close to the diameter of the thread, swaged needles are also known as atraumatic.

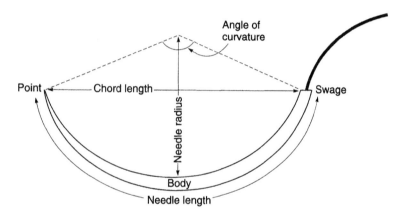

Figure 4.1 Needle anatomy.

Needle cross-section
There are four basic types of needle cross-section (Figure 4.2); round-bodied, conventional cutting, reverse cutting and spatulate.

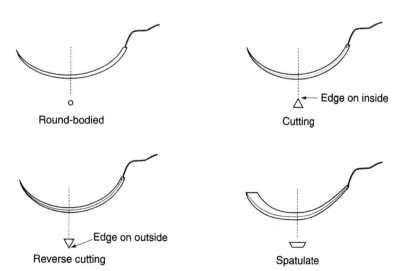

Figure 4.2 Cross-sections of different types of needles.

A round-bodied needle simply has a sharp point and a round shaft. The major advantage of this needle is that the needle track is of the same diameter as the suture, and this reduces any tendency for microleaks from the suture track. However, the 'cutting edge' is limited to the point, which is very easily blunted, and thus its use is mainly limited to suturing the conjunctiva when a watertight wound is desirable (e.g. following a trabeculectomy). In most situations a more robust needle is required, and the needles in general surgery are mainly 'cutting' – that is, they have a sharp edge that runs along either the top (cutting), the bottom (reverse cutting) or the side (spatulate) of the needle.

Conventional cutting needles have the sharp edge along the top or inside edge, thereby minimizing the risk of accidental damage to deep structures and making them relatively safe to use, but they do tend to cut out. The opposite occurs with reverse cutting needles, which resist cutting out and are ideal when there is no danger of accidental damage to deep tissues (e.g. suturing skin). Reverse cutting needles are not ideal for suturing within the wall of a viscus, and *should not be used for suturing cornea or sclera.*

Spatulate or side-cutting needles are designed to stay within a layer. They have a broad, flat cross-section, and this is the ideal shape when suturing within a structure such as the cornea, the sclera or the tarsal plate. These needles are indicated with strabismus or conventional retinal detachment surgery. However, the broad cross-section of a spatulate needle makes a passage that is larger than the suture, and there is therefore a risk of microleaks from the suture tracks – especially when suturing cornea.

There are a number of 'composite' needles available with the intention of combining the advantages of more than one needle type. These include the tapercut needle, which is a round-bodied needle with a reverse cutting tip, and the micropoint needle, which is a round-bodied needle with a spatulate tip. The tapercut is the needle often used for suturing the mucosal flaps in a DCR, and the micropoint (or a variant thereof) is often used for suturing corneal sections and grafts.

Needle length and curvature
Apart from straight needles, a number of different curvatures are available, including quarter-circle, three-eighths circle, half circle, five-eighths circle and compound curvature. Most needles are on a three-eighths circle, which is ideal for most applications. A straight needle is used most commonly for subcuticular stitching, where alternate bites require the needle curve to be in the opposite direction, and a straight needle is a compromise that prevents having to remount the needle after each stitch.

The degree of curvature is a major determinant of the depth of bite. In sequence, the depth of bite from shallow to deep is straight, quarter circle, three-eighths circle, half circle, five-eighths circle and compound curvature.

A five-eighths circle needle is used for stitching down a hole where there is limited room, and is most often used when suturing the posterior flaps of a DCR.

Holding needles
It is important to use the appropriate-sized needle holder to avoid damage to either the holder or the needle. The tips of the needle holder can be either straight or curved.

Needles should generally be held two-thirds of the way along their shaft from their tip. Holding the needle too close to the tip will result in damage and blunting, whereas holding it too near the suture end will result in an unstable grip with a tendency to rotate laterally and loss of control. A common mistake is to blunt the tip by grabbing it when trying to pull the needle through tissue; for this reason, good suturing technique requires that the needle is pushed as far through the tissue as possible before pulling it out. A tip for fast suturing is to pick the needle up with the needle holder held in the correct manner for the next bite (i.e. with the hand supinated and not pronated, even though the latter feels more lateral) to save the need for altering the grip or remounting the needle between bites.

The technique for suturing is to pass the needle in a course reflecting its shape – usually a circular course. A rotary action can be generated in several different ways. For large needles and needle holders it is done with the wrist and forearm, aided by having the needle-holder jaws curved towards the surgeon. For small needles and needle holders it is done by rotating the needle holder with the fingers and thumb, and is helped by an 'away' curve to the needle-holder jaws.

SUTURE FORCEPS

The suture material is very fine and therefore can only be grasped by blocked forceps (Figure 4.3). These are easily damaged and must be handled with care.

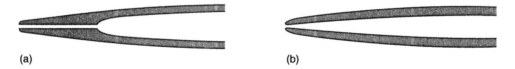

(a)   (b)

Figure 4.3 (a) Blocked forceps; (b) plain-tipped forceps.

KNOTS

THE SURGICAL KNOT

The basic knot used in surgery is the surgical or 2–1–1 knot, and classically it is two throws, then one and one single throws. The purpose of the double initial throw is to prevent slackening of the first throw while performing the second or locking throw, and the third is to provide adequate security. Some of the synthetic suture materials used routinely in ophthalmology (e.g. 10/0 nylon) have poor knot security, and accordingly the surgical knot is adapted to be 3–1–1 for these materials (Figure 4.4). Given the nature of ophthalmic surgery and the fine gauge of the suture used, it is invariably tied with instruments.

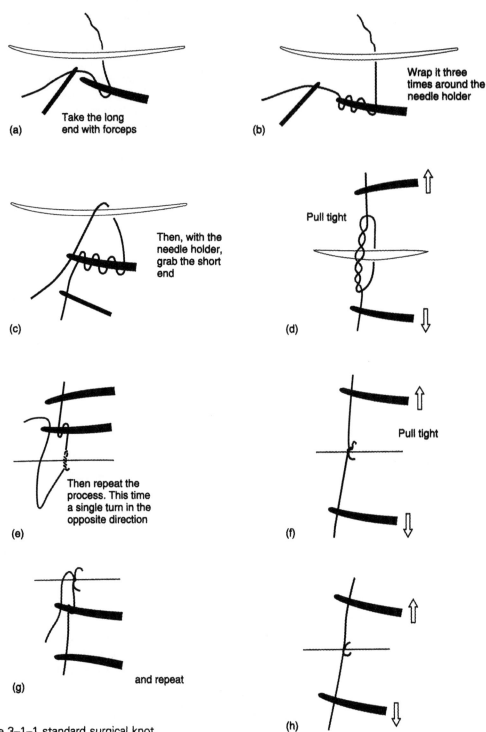

(a) Take the long end with forceps

(b) Wrap it three times around the needle holder

(c) Then, with the needle holder, grab the short end

(d) Pull tight

(e) Then repeat the process. This time a single turn in the opposite direction

(f) Pull tight

(g) and repeat

(h)

Figure 4.4   The 3–1–1 standard surgical knot.

It is important that the knot is laid correctly, otherwise it is very possible to generate a succession of half-hitches, which can slip. This is achieved by placing equal tension on both ends of the suture and making sure that the direction of pull is in the direction in which the knot wants to bed down. This means reversing the direction of pull on the ends between each throw.

THE SLIPKNOT

The purpose of the slipknot is to be able to adjust the tension in the suture before locking it. Its major use is for suturing corneal wounds, where tension in the sutures can have a marked effect on the post-operative astigmatism. Several types of slipknot have been described, including the single ('Terry tie') and double slipknots.

There are two ways of tying the single slipknot; the parallel suture (Figure 4.5) and the crossed suture technique (Figure 4.6). These knots can be tightened by pulling on the long end and loosened by pulling on the short end. The advantage of a slipknot is that it can be adjusted to the required tension, but once adjusted it must be secured by tying at least two square throws or a full surgical knot over it. This technique is favoured by some surgeons in situations where correct suture tension is all-important, as in suturing a corneal wound after extracapsular cataract surgery.

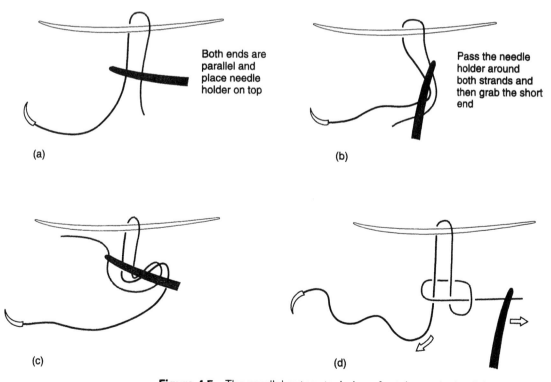

Figure 4.5 The parallel suture technique for tying a single slipknot.

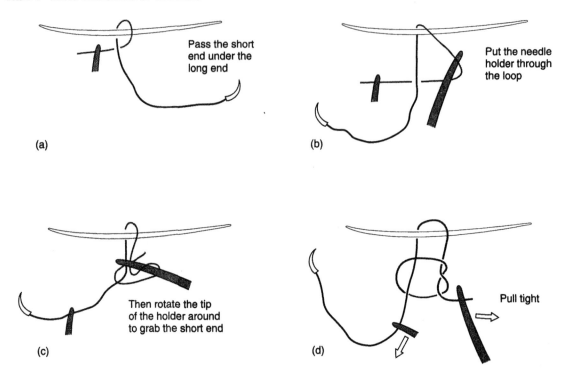

(a) Pass the short end under the long end

(b) Put the needle holder through the loop

(c) Then rotate the tip of the holder around to grab the short end

(d) Pull tight

Figure 4.6   The crossed-suture single slipknot.

OTHER METHODS

SKIN TAPES OR 'CUTANEOUS SUTURES'

The idea of closing cutaneous wounds by the use of adhesive tapes is recorded as early as 1600 BC, when Ancient Egyptians used flour and water as an adhesive for wound closure. Tapes have a number of potential advantages: there is no suture track infection; no foreign body reactions in the skin; and no risk of suture track epithelialization. However, they must be correctly applied so that they stick properly and support the wound, and they are relatively time-consuming to apply.

There are two basic types of adhesive tape; reinforced and elasticated. Elasticated tapes should be used if wound swelling or oedema is anticipated.

For successful use of tapes, the skin surface must be clean and dry. Adhesion is aided by cleaning the skin with a tincture (alcoholic solution) of benzoin (Friar's balsam), which acts as a degreasing agent, prior to application. Tapes should not be applied with transverse tension, as this may cause mechanical injury to the skin; this applies especially to non-distensible reinforced strips (e.g. Steri-strips[TM]) and in situations where distension can be expected, when elasticated tapes should be used. As most adhesives are pressure-dependent, simply applying the tape may not result in good adhesion. Once applied, the tape should be massaged or rubbed for a few seconds.

There are a number of complications reported with their use:

1. Mechanical injury from excessive transverse tension can result in blisters (often at both ends of the applied tapes).
2. Non-tension mechanical injury can occur, particularly at removal. Tapes should be removed gently and in the direction of the wound so as to prevent wound dehiscence, supporting the skin all the time.
3. Occlusive tapes can cause skin maceration, although this is unlikely to happen with thin strips.
4. Allergic reactions are surprisingly uncommon, but have been described.
5. A number of rare complications can occur, such as skin stripping, folliculitis, chemical injury and problems due to residual adhesive.

TISSUE ADHESIVES

Tissue adhesives are used to glue wounds back together as a substitute for stitches. Their use in cutaneous wounds has so far been restricted to superficial closure.

Tissue adhesives have a number of potential advantages in that they do not require removal or form tracks. The only synthetic adhesive currently available is butyl-2-cyanoacrylate (enbucrilate), a clear substance which is dyed blue to help visualization (Histoacryl®) and polymerizes on contact with a trace of water. Care must be taken with its use, as if it gets between the wound edges it will inhibit healing by forming an impervious barrier and, once it has set (in 20 s to 2 minutes, depending on the amount of moisture present), any mistakes in tissue alignment cannot be corrected. Care must also be taken to ensure that none gets on the conjunctiva or cornea (which can be protected by a liberal coat of an ointment e.g. oc. chloramphenicol). It is used by drying the skin and pinching the edges firmly together, and then applying it to the surface of the wound and holding the edges together for 2 minutes while it sets.

Many of the skin wounds in ophthalmic surgery are suitable for closure in this manner.

Closure of microperforations
Enbucrilate has found a clear niche in routine ophthalmic practice for the closure of small corneal perforations, particularly those following trauma. It is only suitable for small or 'microperforations', and the area of leakage needs to be dry to allow the glue to bond.

1. Prepare the eye as for intraocular surgery.
2. If the anterior chamber is shallow or flat, then reform it using a viscoelastic injected through a paracentesis to prevent gluing the iris or the lens to the cornea[14]. In these cases the paracentesis requires particular care, as it is very easy to damage the anterior lens capsule accidentally; this can be avoided by entering very obliquely with an MVR blade (Figure 4.7).

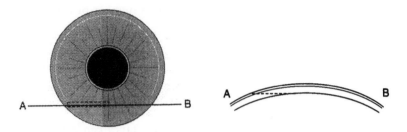

Figure 4.7 A paracentesis when the eye is flat is best done with a very oblique passage in the mid-periphery.

3. Dry the cornea at the site of the microperforation with a small swab just before application as, although a trace of moisture helps the adhesive to set, it will not bind to a frankly wet surface. As it will not stay dry for long, it is helpful to have an assistant to do the drying while the surgeon is ready to apply the glue immediately. It is also sensible to debride frankly necrotic tissue and epithelium from around the perforation or the glue will simply slough off with it.

4. To apply the glue neatly to the perforation without getting excess glue on the adjacent tissue, cut out a small piece of the plastic drape and use K-Y jelly to attach it to the top of a dressed orange stick[15]. Put a drop of glue on the plastic drape, and it can then be positioned on the perforation with some precision. The glue sets very quickly, and the plastic drape can be left attached to the glue.

5. Apply a soft bandage contact lens, otherwise the rough surface will cause a giant papillary conjunctivitis-like reaction[16].

Close follow-up is required as the symptoms and signs of microbial keratitis may be masked by the presence of glue[17], which normally falls off after 6–8 weeks.

Other ophthalmic applications have included securing orbital implants[18] and securing scleral explants in retinal detachment surgery in the presence of thin sclera[19]. One group has experimented with its use intraocularly to close retinal breaks directly[20].

Fibrin glue

There is a second adhesive, fibrin glue, which has more limited applications. It is prepared from homologous blood and it comes in two syringes, one with fibrinogen and Factor XIII and the other with thrombin and calcium chloride. Like enbucrilate it requires a dry surface, but its setting time is much slower (at least 2 minutes, and 30–90 minutes for maximum strength). Although it has been used for sealing corneal perforations[21], it is not as suitable as enbucrilate. Its advantage is that it is absorbable[22].

WOUND CLOSURE AT SPECIFIC SITES

The ophthalmic surgeon has to close wounds involving a number of different tissues, including the cornea, conjunctiva and skin. The principles at these sites are markedly different.

THE CORNEA

The key issue here is that the wound must be watertight. Large leaks of aqueous fluids put the eye at risk by causing collapse of the globe and hypotony, but even small leaks can give rise to intraocular infection. The cornea is also the major refracting surface of the eye, and sutures (particularly if over-tightened) are a major cause of postoperative astigmatism. The need for sutures to close corneal wounds can be greatly reduced by proper wound design, and the technique of wound formation is therefore of great importance.

Various types of sutures can be used to close corneal wounds – virgin silk, nylon or Mersilene®.

THE CONJUNCTIVA

Conjunctival wounds heal particularly well by secondary intention, and would appear to be a sanctuary site for keloid scar formation. In fact, simple conjunctival lacerations need not be sutured.

The major cosmetic defect that results from poor conjunctival closure is when Tenon's capsule is incorporated in the closure, which tends to occur particularly after squint surgery. It is an avascular structure, and appears pearly white against the slight pink of the vascular conjunctiva.

Suturing conjunctiva to provide a watertight closure is of major importance after glaucoma drainage surgery (see Chapter 23).

It is often stated that sutures in the conjunctiva tend to fall out after a few days and hence the suture material chosen is not critical, but this is not true and sutures can persist for many weeks or longer. Nylon knots need to be buried so they do not give rise to a foreign body sensation; Vicryl® sutures avoid this, but they do dissolve and in the process can cause a degree of tissue reaction – 'vicrylitis'.

THE SKIN

The aim of skin wound closure is to minimize scar formation. The principles involved are:

- Good deep closure to eliminate dead space in order to prevent haematoma formation and subsequent risk of infection and to prevent a depressed scar
- To evert the edges to avoid a depressed scar
- To avoid dog-ear formation.

Deep closure

This serves two functions: the elimination of dead space and removal of tension from the skin suture line. The skin closure cannot take tension because skin stitches are routinely removed at 5–7 days to prevent epithelialization of the suture tracks, and at this stage the wound is only 5 per cent of its final strength.

The suture material should be of suitable strength and dissolvable – for example, Dexon®, Vicryl® or PDS®. For good closure, the edges of the wound must be well approximated and the knot buried.

Wound edge eversion

The second factor that needs to be addressed to prevent formation of a depressed wound is that the wound's edges must be everted by ensuring that the skin suture incorporates more deep than superficial tissue. This is achieved by everting the edges when suturing so that the needle enters the skin at an angle of less than 90°. Eversion of skin edges can be achieved in three ways:

1. By the use of forceps or skin hooks to evert the edge; this is best for the initial edge (Figure 4.8).

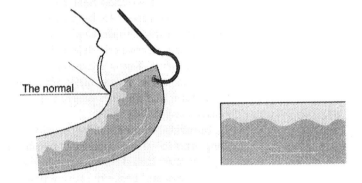

The normal

Figure 4.8 Evert the edge by 90°, and a deep bite can be achieved with the three-eighths needle in a vertical position.

2. By using an object to provide counter-pressure which, along with the needle, will act to evert the edge (Figure 4.9). Some textbooks suggest using the other thumb to provide this counter-pressure, but this is a risk factor for needle stick injury[23] and the use of an inanimate object such as a pair of forceps is safer.
3. By using a mattress suture (Figure 4.10).

Deep closure is particularly important on the face due to the presence of the muscles of facial expression. These muscles insert into the skin and can therefore put skin wounds under significant tension.

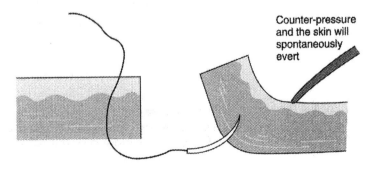

Counter-pressure and the skin will spontaneously evert

Figure 4.9 Completing the passage using counter-pressure.

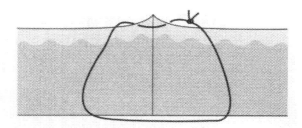

Figure 4.10 The mattress suture.

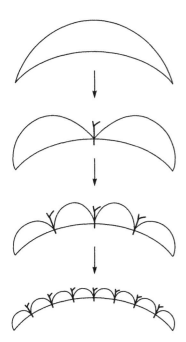

Figure 4.11 Close by halving and halving again to create many small dog ears.

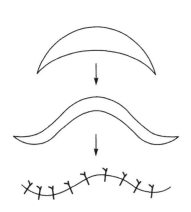

Figure 4.13 Extend the excision with a reverse curve.

Prevention of dog ears

Dog ears arise when the wound edges being sutured are of unequal length, and the problem classically arises when excising a crescent of material as in a blepharoplasty or a brow lift. The following techniques have been described to address this problem:

1. Halving, in which the first suture is placed in the centre of the wound, thereby halving the size of the defect. The next two sutures are placed in the centre of the two remaining defects, and so on. This creates a number of much smaller dog ears that may flatten with time (Figure 4.11).
2. Bürow's triangle, where a wedge is excised from the longer edge to shorten its contour. It can be placed anywhere along the longer edge (Figure 4.12).

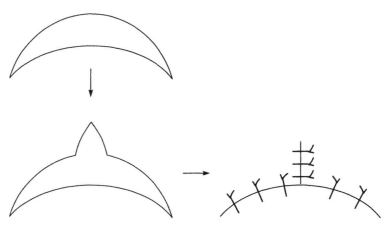

Figure 4.12 Use of Bürow's triangle.

3. Extending the wound with a reverse curvature, which is the technique of choice for a brow lift (Figure 4.13).
4. Using Z-plasties, which are uncommon due to the complexity of wound design. Z-plasties have the potential advantage of breaking up the scar into shorter segments.

Subcuticular sutures

Subcuticular stitches may be used as an alternative to interrupted sutures for closing the skin. Absorbable sutures such as undyed

Vicryl® can be used and the stitch left in place, or a non-absorbable suture can be used which, as it does not result in suture track epithelialization, can be left in longer than interrupted stitches (up to 12 days). These stitches often heal as a fine line and therefore give an excellent final cosmetic result.

When placing a subcuticular stitch that needs removal, it is important to use one that has minimal tissue drag (e.g. Prolene®). Subcuticular stitching is most easily done with a straight needle, using a running stitch and avoiding doubling back. There is no need to pull the stitch through after each bite.

Long subcuticular sutures can be difficult to remove, depending upon the gauge of the material. For this reason the suture should periodically be brought to the surface to take a standard bite (Figure 4.14) so that it can be cut and removed in segments. For large gauge material this should be at least every 10 cm, and for fine gauges every 5 cm. Subcuticular stitches are also not as good as interrupted sutures when accurate tissue alignment is needed and, if used, the deep closure must be meticulous.

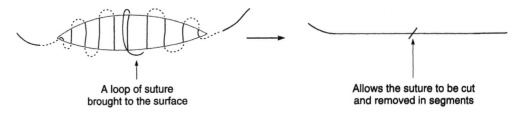

A loop of suture brought to the surface

Allows the suture to be cut and removed in segments

Figure 4.14   Subcuticular sutures.

The ends of the suture can be secured either by taking a bite of skin and tying a knot or by tying the two ends together across the wound (Figure 4.15).

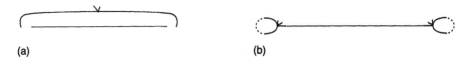

(a)

(b)

Figure 4.15   Two ways of securing the ends of a subcuticular stitch.

DRESSINGS

Dressings help to prevent haematoma formation and infection, to protect the wound from mechanical trauma during the early stages and to provide a hospitable environment for wound healing.

For different operations, different features are more important – for example, after extracapsular cataract extraction the single most important function is protection from accidental mechanical trauma, which may cause section rupture. Prevention of haematoma is the major aim after most forms of lid surgery, while for healing by secondary intention the key feature is provision of an optimal environment.

Dressings must not adhere to the surgical wound, and this is particularly important if a discharge is expected. For intraocular surgery, this is achieved effectively by having the eye closed.

The two most commonly used non-adherent dressings are tulle gras and Melolin™. Tulle gras is gauze impregnated with soft paraffin so that the threads are coated but the mesh pores remain open; it should not be folded or it will loose its porous character. Melolin™ is a wound dressing pad with a non-adherent layer to face the wound, and the bulk of the dressing is placed over this.

Pressure dressings

'Pressure' here means vertical pressure downwards, and this is desirable to prevent bleeding – particularly low pressure ooze from small blood vessels. This is particularly important for lid surgery, as tissue turgor in the lids is lower than for other parts of the body and fluid can readily collect there. In order to achieve pressure it is necessary for the point of action of the tape to be raised off the surface, and this is achieved with the use of padding. The tape used must also be elasticated. Finally, this type of dressing does cause much greater transverse than vertical tension, and this means that adhesion of the tape is a problem; this is helped by ensuring a clean and dry surface to adhere to (e.g. by cleaning with benzoin tinc.). This type of dressing clearly has the same potential problems as skin tapes, particularly with respect to mechanical skin trauma.

BANDAGES

These are used when it is important to generate maximum pressure. As they can be wrapped around the head, downward pressure can be achieved without transverse pressure and thus greater pressure can be achieved than with elastic tape. The standard bandage is the crepe bandage.

BOLSTERS

These are used in the application of skin grafts to allow continuous pressure over the graft to help it to 'take'. They are rarely used in routine ophthalmic surgery.

SHIELDS

Shields are used to protect the eye from accidental mechanical injury. This is particularly important when there are large corneal or scleral wounds held together by fine sutures (as occurs after extracapsular cataract surgery). Mild blunt trauma that results in a sudden rise in intraocular pressure may result in these stitches being broken, with devastating consequences. Accordingly a shield should be worn at night for the first month following extracapsular cataract surgery, and during the day as well if there is a tendency for the patient to rub the eye.

DRAINS

Lister gets the credit for first using surgical drains in Britain, when draining an abscess under the axilla of Queen Victoria. Drains form a passage to prevent haematoma formation. They do carry a risk of infection, and this can be reduced (at the same time as enhancing the draining function) by placing them under suction. If a drain is used, it must be removed when it has stopped draining. This may be on the first postoperative day or after 2 weeks. The use of drains in ophthalmology is restricted to some of the larger oculoplastic procedures.

REFERENCES

1. Duprez, K., Bilweis, J., Duprez, A. and Merle, M. (1988). Experimental and clinical study of fast absorption cutaneous suture material. *Ann. Chir. Main*, 7, 91–6.
2. Tandon, S. C., Kelly, J., Turtle, M. and Irwin, S. T. (1995). Irradiated polyglactin 910: a new synthetic absorbably suture. *J. R. Coll. Surg. Edinb.*, 40, 185–7.
3. Jackson, H. and Bosanquet, R. (1991). Should nylon corneal sutures be routinely removed? *Br. J. Ophthalmol.*, 75, 663–4.
4. Acheson, J. F. and Lyons, C. J. (1991). Ocular morbidity due to monofilament nylon corneal sutures. *Eye*, 5, 106–12.
5. Hayasaka, S., Ishiguro, S. I., Shiono, T. *et al.* (1982). A scanning electron microscopic study of nylon degradation by ocular tissue extracts. *Am. J. Ophthalmol.*, 93, 111–17.
6. Cohan, B. E., Pearch, A. C. and Schwatz, S. (1979). Broken nylon iris fixation sutures. *Am. J. Ophthalmol.*, 88, 982–9.
7. Blanksma, L. J. and Siertsema, J. V. (1977). Changes in the structure of intraocular nylon. *Doc. Ophthalmol.*, 44, 223–9.
8. Heaven, C. J., Davison, C. R. N. and Cockcroft, P. M. (1995). Bacterial contamination of nylon corneal sutures. *Eye*, 9, 116–18.
9. O'Driscoll, A. M., Goble, R. R., Hallack, G. N. and Andrew, N. C. (1994). A prospective, controlled study of a 9/0 elastic polypropylene suture for cataract surgery; refractive results and complications. *Eye*, 8, 538–42.
10. O'Driscoll, A. M., Quraishy, M. M. and Andrew, N. C. (1996). Elastic polypropylene suture in cataract surgery: long-term follow-up. *Eye*, 10, 99–102.
11. Herrmann, J. B. (1971). Tensile strength and knot security of surgical suture materials. *Am. Surgeon*, 37, 209–17.
12. King, A. J., Deane, J. and Sandford-Smith, J. (1994). *In situ* degradation of 11/0 polyester (Mersilene®) suture material following cataract surgery. *Eye*, 8, 676–9.
13. Hollick, E. J., Moosa, M. and Casswell, A. G. (1996). Do Mersilene® sutures need to be removed after cataract surgery? *Eye*, 10, 555–7.
14. Weiss, J. L., Williams, P., Lindstrom, R. L. and Doughman, D. J. (1983). The use of tissue adhesion in corneal perforations. *Ophthalmology*, 90, 610–15.
15. Choong, Y. Y., Daya, S. M. and Dua, H. S. (1998). How to do it – corneal gluing. *Con. Med. Ed. J. Ophthalmol.*, 2, 63–5.
16. Carlson, A. H. and Wilhelmis, K. R. (1982). Giant papillary conjunctivitis associated with cyanoacrylate glue. *Am. J. Ophthalmol.*, 104, 437.
17. Cavanaugh, T. B. and Gottsch, J. D. (1991). Infectious keratitis and cyanoacrylate adhesive. *Am. J. Ophthalmol.*, 111, 466–72.
18. Tse, D. T. (1986). Cyanoacrylate tissue adhesion in securing orbital implants. *Ophthalmic Surg.*, 17, 577–80.

19. Follk, J. C. and Dreyer, R. F. (1986). Cyanoacrylate adhesive in retinal detachment surgery. *Am. J. Ophthalmol.*, **101**, 486–7.
20. McCuen, B. W. 2nd, Hida, T. and Sheta, S. M. (1987). Transvitreal cyanoacrylate retinopexy in the management of complicated retinal detachment surgery. *Am. J. Ophthalmol.*, **104**, 127–32.
21. Lagoutte, F. M., Gauthier, L. and Comte, P. R. M. (1989). A fibrin sealant for perforated and preperforated corneal ulcers. *Br. J. Ophthalmol.*, **73**, 757–61.
22. Bartley, G. B. and MacCaffrey, T. V. (1990). Cryoprecipitated fibrinogen (fibrin glue) in orbital surgery. *Am. J. Ophthalmol.*, **109**, 227–8.
23. Brookes, A. (1994). Infection control. Surgical glove perforation. *Nursing Times*, **90**, 60–62.

5

WOUND HEALING AND AFTERCARE

Wound healing is classified into healing by primary and by secondary intention. The distinction between the two types of healing applies predominantly to full-thickness wounds; in the former there is no tissue deficit to be made good, while in the latter there is loss of tissue between the wound edges that has to be made good during the healing.

The major difference from a surgical viewpoint is that wounds that heal by primary intention usually leave a much smaller scar compared to those that heal by secondary intention. For this reason, most surgical wounds are designed to be closed with apposition and no gaping. There are rare situations when full-thickness healing by secondary intention occurs without significant scar formation.

Partial-thickness wounds heal extremely well by secondary intention without scarring.

HEALING BY PRIMARY INTENTION

The key event in healing by primary intention is the development of tensile strength in the wound. Re-epithelialization is not an issue, except for the requirement for early suture removal to prevent epithelialization along the suture tracks. For this reason skin suture removal is recommended at 1 week, or as early as day five for particularly susceptible sites such as the forehead. At this time the wound strength is only 5 per cent of normal, which is why supporting deep sutures are required to prevent wound dehiscence, and strapping (e.g. Steri-strips™) is often used routinely for the next 2–3 weeks.

SUTURE REMOVAL

The first step is to cut the suture. For corneal stitches the cutting edge of a hypodermic needle works well; for skin stitches either scissors or a blade can be used. A no. 11 blade can be used, being sure to cut with the point away from the skin, but the sickle blade (no. 12) is designed for suture removal. This blade has the cutting edge on the inside of the curve, so there is minimal risk of accidentally cutting the skin.

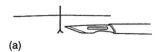

(a)

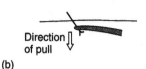

Direction
of pull

(b)

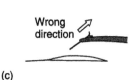

Wrong
direction

(c)

Figure 5.1   (a) Cut the suture and (b) pull it out towards the wound. (c) Pulling it away from the wound runs the risk of wound dehiscence.

The key point on removing the suture is to pull it *towards* the wound (Figure 5.1); this minimizes the risk of wound dehiscence.

DERMAL HEALING

The best-studied model of wound healing is the dermis, but although many tissues show similarities in their healing there are also important differences. However, skin healing will be discussed in detail here because it is the tissue in which healing is best understood.

Dermal wound healing is divided into three phases:

1. Inflammatory, which occurs during the first week
2. Cellular, which occurs over the next 2–3 weeks and merges imperceptibly with the final stage
3. Contracture and remodelling, which starts from around the third to fourth weeks and proceeds over many months; there may still be some activity a year later.

The inflammatory phase

The earliest cells that appear in wounds are lymphocytes, at 6–12 hours. However, lymphopenic animals heal normally, and the key cell is the monocyte, which starts to accumulate from the fourth day. Animals that lack monocytes do not heal normally.

At the end of the inflammatory phase, the wound is essentially held together by fibrin and similar proteins and is only 5 per cent of the strength of normal skin. It can be considered as a 'stop-gap' repair, and is designed for speed of closure only – probably with the aim of preventing infection.

The cellular phase

A key process in the cellular phase of repair is removal of the fibrin and the attendant temporary protein matrix. Plasmin is an important enzyme in this process, and animals deficient in the components of the plasmin system show a marked deficit in this phase of wound healing[1,2]. This molecular understanding is confirmed in the clinical situation, where 'wet is best' – wounds that are left to heal by secondary intention do so more quickly if they are kept moist, which inhibits the formation of a scab (essentially composed of fibrin). It also suggests that fibrin may be a barrier to cell migration. The key cellular players in this phase are the fibroblast and the endothelial cell.

The contracture and remodelling phase

The cellular and contracture phases overlap, with wound contracture beginning around day seven but not usually becoming noticeable until about day 14. The contracture phase continues for months and is not usually complete until 1 year; it is characterized by reorganization of the laid down collagen fibres. The final wound strength usually stabilizes at around 70–80 per cent of the original tissue strength.

WOUND-MODIFYING AGENTS

As yet there are no agents in routine use that are used for the purpose of accelerating normal wound healing, although a number exist in theory (e.g. Epidermal Growth Factor). However, there are a number of agents in use to slow wound healing, and these are used in fistulizing surgery (e.g. trabeculectomy for glaucoma) and for prevention of keloid formation.

The first agents to be used were corticosteroids, which clearly inhibit the inflammatory stage of wound healing. The antimetabolite 5-fluorouracil (5-FU) and the cytotoxic agent mitomycin C (MMC) are also used, and they act predominantly on the fibroblast, inhibiting the cellular phase of wound healing. Radiotherapy is another option, and this inhibits both the inflammatory and the cellular phases. Although wound modification agents are most commonly used in glaucoma surgery, 5-FU has been used in conjunction with cicatricial lid abnormalities and both 5-FU and MMC in lacrimal surgery[3], and these areas are set to expand.

HEALING BY SECONDARY INTENTION

Healing by secondary intention depends upon whether the wound is partial or full-thickness. Re-epithelialization for partial-thickness wounds comes from the reservoirs of epithelial tissues (the transected adnexal structures), and the speed of re-epithelialization depends upon the density of these structures. Partial-thickness wounds heal extremely well by secondary intention.

In full-thickness wounds, all re-epithelialization must come from the edges. There is a lag phase of about 1 week, and then closure occurs in an exponential manner – thus wounds four times as large only take twice the time to close. The lag phase corresponds to the inflammatory phase of wound healing.

In secondary intention healing, capillary loops form at the base of the wound within a few days and appear as red granules – granulation tissue. The key practical points regarding healing by secondary intention are:

1. Wet is best – wounds should be kept moist because cells cannot migrate when desiccated
2. The time to closure is determined by the *smallest* wound dimension, and this should be taken into account when designing wounds (Figure 5.2)
3. Partial-thickness wounds heal extremely well by secondary intention
4. The amount of scarring following full-thickness secondary intention healing depends upon the contour of the surface; wounds in concavities heal well by this technique (e.g. the medial canthus), while the results are much worse on convex surfaces (e.g. the forehead).

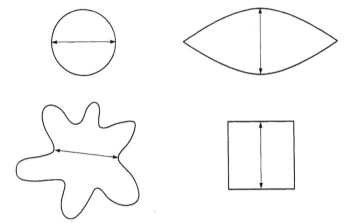

Figure 5.2   Healing by secondary intention. The smallest dimension (marked) for each of these four shapes is the same, and therefore they will all heal in approximately the same time.

5. Speed of healing is dependent upon location, with wounds on the face healing the most quickly.

CARE OF WOUNDS HEALING BY SECONDARY INTENTION

These wounds heal best in a moist environment, and should be gently washed twice a day to remove any scabs. A thin layer of Vaseline under a semi-occlusive dressing (e.g. elastoplast) will keep them moist.

Mucous membranes are naturally moist and so heal particularly well by secondary intention, but these wounds can still form crusts composed of dried mucus (e.g. in the nose following a DCR), and these crusts can become sites for infection. The crusts can be removed by nasal douching (i.e. sniffing up and snorting out), using half a teaspoon of salt, half a teaspoon of sugar and half a teaspoon of bicarbonate in 0.5 l of cooled boiled water. If nasal drops are prescribed, they should be used just after douching. A standard regime would be to perform douching on the side of DCR surgery twice a day for a fortnight afterwards.

COMPLICATIONS OF WOUND HEALING

EARLY COMPLICATIONS

Early complications of wound healing include dehiscence and inflammation.

Dehiscence
A number of factors can predispose to wound breakdown, but probably the two most important are wound closure under tension, and movement. Skin, conjunctival, corneal and scleral wound closure should all be without tension, and the basic principle is that a graft

should be used if closure will require excessive tension. Examples of this principle in action include:

- Skin grafts, when there is a lack of skin for direct closure
- Amniotic membrane grafts, used for persisting leaking blebs in trabeculectomies (when subconjunctival scarring and contracture results in a shortage of available tissue)
- Corneal grafts, which are usually deliberately oversized to prevent closure under tension.

Another alternative is to allow healing by secondary intention, and most conjunctival wounds and many skin defects will heal well in this way. Clearly corneal and scleral defects will not, and grafting ('tectonic grafts') is obligatory in these cases.

Movement is the second major cause of dehiscence, and immobility is a particular problem for the upper lid. In such cases (e.g. a graft in a lid reconstruction), manoeuvres such as paralysing lid movement with botulinum toxin should be considered.

Other factors that may lead to wound dehiscence are wound infection, which can cause sutures to loosen, and poor suturing technique, which may result in stitches cutting out or knots unravelling.

Wound inflammation

All wounds go through an inflammatory phase as a normal part of wound healing, but excessive inflammation is a cause for concern because it may lead to wound breakdown. The three commonest causes of this are wound infection, seborrheic dermatitis and contact or allergic dermatitis.

Wound infection

This is the most important complication as, unchecked, it may even threaten life. The excellent blood supply to the face means that generally wounds heal quickly and flaps do well; however, the reason for the potentially life-threatening nature of wounds is that the 'danger' area of the face drains via the cavernous sinus. Thrombosis of the cavernous sinus is a recognized complication of infection in these locations.

Seborrheic dermatitis

This is the least recognized but one of the commonest causes of widespread erythema following surgery, and may even be accompanied by superficial erosions. The clinical picture may resemble contact dermatitis, but patch testing is negative[4]. In contrast to infection, it is not painful and there is no suppuration.

People with pre-existing seborrheic dermatitis are predisposed to this complication. The aetiology of this condition is unknown, but it is becoming less frequent – possibly due to improved diet and personal hygiene. It predominantly affects males and occurs at any age, but must be clearly distinguished from infantile seborrheic dermatitis (cradle cap), which is a separate entity. The condition is characterized by erythema, scaling and mild irritation, and it particularly affects the scalp, behind the ears, the nasolabial folds, the presternal area, the axillae, the submammary folds and the groin, and inspection of these areas may help in cases of diagnostic doubt. It also affects the eyelids and is a cause of blepharitis. Wounds in these areas are particularly susceptible.

The treatment for acute exacerbations is topical ketoconazole to which a steroid can be added. A typical regime would be ketoconazole 2% (Nisoral®) shampoo for the scalp, to be used twice a week for a month, and either ketoconazole 2% cream b.d. or a combination of hydrocortisone 1% and miconazole nitrate (Daktacort®) b.d. for the skin while the rash lasts.

LATE COMPLICATIONS

Late complications of wound healing include wound depression, suture marks, altered pigmentation, keloid and contracture.

Wound depression
A depressed scar can be attributed to poor closure technique (i.e. failure to close the deep layers or failure to cause wound eversion of the margins of the skin layer).

Suture marks
Suture marks are caused by epithelialization of the suture tracks, and hence skin sutures should be removed at 1 week for most areas, and on day five in susceptible areas such as the forehead. As the wound strength is only 5 per cent at this stage, it is usual to support the wound for a further 2 weeks with strapping.

If the skin stitches need to remain *in situ* for longer than 1 week, then consideration should be given to using the subcuticular closure technique (when removal is typically at 10–14 days).

Altered colour and pigmentation
Wounds undergo a number of colour changes, and it is often the colour change rather than any other feature that is cosmetically the most disturbing. All wounds are initially vascular and appear pink, and this can take up to 9 months to fade. A mature wound is relatively avascular and will end up whiter than the surrounding tissue.

A further problem is secondary pigmentation; this can be a particular issue in dark-skinned races and can be exacerbated by sun exposure during the healing phase (which patients should be counselled to avoid).

Keloid
Keloid formation (excessive collagen deposition in the dermis) is influenced by site and race. The eyelids are a 'sanctuary' site for this problem due to the very thin dermal layer and absence of subcutaneous fat but, by contrast, keloid readily forms on the forehead. It is influenced by factors that include race and site. Afro-Caribbean races are predis-

posed to keloid formation, where there is a suggestion that the predisposition follows an autosomal dominant pattern.

Contractures

Contractures can progress up to a year after the wound. For this reason, revisionary surgery should be delayed for at least 6 months and preferably a year. This complication is not seen in corneal or scleral injuries. It can occur after conjunctival injuries, where it can cause a restriction of oculomotility and skin injuries affecting the eyelids.

Skin contractures can lead to two morphologies: linear wounds give rise to linear contraction lines, while circular wounds can give rise to pin-cushion deformities. The basic surgical principle used to correct these is the Z-plasty, and it is the simplest of a number of techniques used to redistribute tissue. The principle is explained in Figure 5.3.

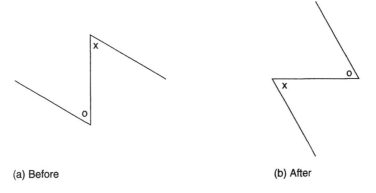

Figure 5.3 The Z-plasty. Essentially, two equilateral triangles are constructed; (a), which then transposes (b). The central limb is the one that is lengthened by the procedure. A feature of equilateral triangles is that each side is the same length, and so it can be rapidly marked out with a pair of calipers.

(a) Before   (b) After

REFERENCES

1. Romer, J., Bugge, T. H., Pyke, C. *et al.* (1996). Impaired wound healing in mice with a disrupted plasminogen gene. *Nat. Med.*, **2**, 287–92.
2. Vassalli, J. D. and Saurat, J. H. (1996). Cuts and scrapes? Plasmin heals! (editorial). *Nat. Med.*, **2**, 284–5.
3. Kao, S. C. S., Liao, C. L., Tseng, J. H. S. *et al.* (1997). Dacrocystorhinostomy with intraoperative mitomycin C. *Ophthalmology*, **104**, 86–91.
4. Zitelli, J. A. (1996). Wound healing by first and second intention. In: *Dermatological Surgery. Principles and Practice*, 2nd edn (R. K. Roenigk and H. H. Roenigk Jr, eds), pp. 10–130. Marcel Dekker Inc.

6

CONTROLLED TISSUE DESTRUCTION

Controlled tissue destruction can be performed in a number of different ways, including cryotherapy, diathermy, lash electrolysis, radiotherapy and chemotherapy.

CRYOTHERAPY

This has been widely used in ophthalmology, although in some areas (such as cataract surgery and refractory glaucoma) it has been superseded by more modern techniques. It is still used:

- To kill lash follicles in cases of districhiasis
- To destroy tumours, including some lid tumours such as small basal cell carcinomas and conjunctival lesions; in particular, as adjunctive treatment for conjunctival melanoma or squamous cell carcinoma
- In retinal surgery, where it is still the technique of choice for treating retinal breaks during conventional surgery.

HOW CRYOPROBES WORK

There are a number of ways of achieving cooling, and these can be subdivided into two classes; the first class consists of those using pre-cooled applicators (e.g. a probe cooled by liquid nitrogen before use), and the second class consists of those in which there is continuous cooling. The latter work on one of two physical principles – phase transition or the Joule–Thomson effect.

A phase transition is when a substance undergoes a change in physical state (e.g. from solid to liquid or liquid to gas). This takes up heat and therefore results in cooling, and a clinical example of this is the use of liquid nitrogen as a spray.

The Joule–Thomson effect is how most clinical cryoprobes work, and it works on the principle that as a gas expands it cools. It is achieved by having gas compressed in a cylinder under considerable pressure, and the gas is then allowed to escape through a small hole at the tip of the cryoprobe. As it passes through this hole it goes from an area of high pressure to an area of low pressure and accordingly expands and cools.

TISSUE RESPONSE TO CRYOTHERAPY

The rationale behind many of the applications of cryotherapy is that there is a differential sensitivity of cell types to cold, and hence it is possible to cause differential destruction of particular cell types. In situations where the lesion is small and differential destruction is not an issue, it is a simple and clean way of tissue destruction that is usually accompanied by minimal or no bleeding.

The mechanism of cell death is by intracellular ice crystal formation, which ruptures the lipid membranes of intracellular organelles. Refreezing a cell that has just being thawed causes disproportionately more damage (as can be seen by refreezing thawed chicken), and thus it is standard practice to perform at least two cycles of freezing and thawing (the double freeze–thaw technique).

The problem with cryotherapy is that there is little recognition or control of factors such as speed of freezing. The temperature for killing a particular cell type does not take into account the number of freeze–thaw cycles, but clearly varies as the technique is potentiated by multiple cycles. Cryotherapy is thus a relatively uncontrolled technique.

TWO EXAMPLES OF CLINICAL USE OF CRYOTHERAPY

Districhiasis

It is important to make a clear distinction between misdirected eyelashes and districhiasis. Misdirected eyelashes occur when the lashes that are irritating the ocular surface are the normal lashes turning in (i.e. all the lashes arise from the anterior lamella and in front of the grey line). This situation implies a lid malposition, and the solution is therefore surgical correction of the malposition. Districhiasis occurs when lashes emerge from the meibomian gland orifices, and is therefore a case of transdifferentiation; it often causes very little damage to the ocular surface (e.g. no corneal neovascularization and minimal corneal staining) and very variable symptoms. In this situation there is often co-existent blepharitis and this, rather than the districhiasis, may be the cause of the patient's symptoms.

Thus cryotherapy should not be undertaken without careful consideration, as it is potentially destructive. A key point is that a temperature of −20°C will cause death of the follicles, but −30°C will cause damage to the lid margin and tissue necrosis. There is therefore only a limited margin for safety, and lash cryotherapy should only be performed under thermocouple control. Given the unpredictable penetration of the ice ball, the thermocouple should be placed in the lid 2 mm from the lid margin, as this is where the follicles reside. A double freeze–thaw technique is standard. It normally takes 30–60 seconds for this temperature to be reached.

Retinal cryotherapy

Cryotherapy is a particularly effective treatment for flat retinal breaks. It causes localized tissue destruction, and the ensuing inflammatory response results in localized scar tissue formation with obliteration of the subretinal space, thereby greatly reducing the risk of a retinal detachment from that particular site. This is an example of cryotherapy being used to cause non-specific destruction.

It should be noted that the aim of the treatment is to provoke inflammation rather than tissue destruction *per se*. Very heavy cryotherapy is unnecessary, and can lead to the rare complication of cryonecrosis, when the retina basically disintegrates at the treatment site. The endpoint of treatment is when the retina over the tip of the cryoprobe turns white, and a double freeze–thaw technique is again standard.

DIATHERMY

Tissue can also be destroyed by electrosurgery, particularly the technique of fulguration (see Chapter 4).

LASH ELECTROLYSIS

This is an excellent technique if there are only one or two aberrant lashes. It is not acceptable if there is extensive districhiasis, as it can result in extensive damage.

RADIOTHERAPY

Radiotherapy is a technique of controlled cell destruction, and it preferentially kills dividing cells and/or lymphocytes. For most tissues there is a clear relationship between mitotic activity and radiosensitivity, but lymphocytes do not fit into this pattern – they are postmitotic cells, and yet are exquisitely radiosensitive. Accordingly radiotherapy has been used to treat inflammatory processes, the inflammatory and cellular phases of wound healing, and neoplasms.

Radiation treatment requires a special licence. The main indication for use is the treatment of malignant ocular tumours, which is highly specialized; however, radiotherapy is currently being assessed as a wound-modifying agent for high-risk trabeculectomies. It may eventually find a role in routine ophthalmic practice, but to date it remains in the province of the subspecialist.

CHEMOTHERAPY

Controlled tissue destruction can be achieved by local chemotherapy, and this is a serious option for patients with surface neoplasia. It is probably the treatment of choice for squamous cell carcinoma-*in-situ* on the eyelid skin, where fluorouracil 5% cream (Efudix®) is applied twice on the same day, 1 day per week for 12 weeks. Areas of dysplastic skin (including those that are not clinically apparent) become red, peel and then heal.

Topical chemotherapy has also being showing some promise for conjunctival malignancy. There have been initial reports of successful use of topical mitomycin C[1], retinoic acid[2] and interferon-α2[3] for conjunctival squamous cell carcinoma, and agents have also been tried for conjunctival malignancy. The exact role of such agents in conjunctival surface malignancy has not yet been fully established, but the promise is unquestioned.

REFERENCES

1. Frucht-Pery, J. and Rozenman, Y. (1994). Mitomycin C therapy for corneal intra-epithelial neoplasia. *Am. J. Ophthalmol.*, **117**, 164–8.
2. Herbort, C. P., Zografos, L., Zwingli, M. *et al.* (1988). Topical retinoic acid in dysplastic and metaplastic keratinization of corneo-conjunctival epithelium. *Graf. Arch. Clin. Exp. Ophthalmol.*, **226**, 22–6.
3. Maskin, S. L. (1994). Regression of limbal epithelial dysplasia with topical interferon. *Arch. Ophthalmol.*, **112**, 1145–6.

7

FLUIDS

BASIC PROPERTIES OF FLUIDS

VISCOSITY

A liquid is a substance with fixed volume but no fixed form. A liquid will flow if it is under any pressure differential, and the rate of flow is related to its viscosity. There are two basic flow patterns; laminar and turbulent. Laminar flow occurs when all the individual molecules are moving in the same direction as each other (and therefore in the same direction as the flow of the liquid), while turbulent flow occurs when all the molecules are moving in a chaotic fashion with only an overall drift in the direction of flow.

The laminar flow of many liquids is relatively well understood and modelled mathematically, and the key concepts are shear rate and viscosity. As always in mathematical modelling, a number of simplifying assumptions are made and it is hoped that the model is still close enough to reality to be useful. The standard model of fluid flow assumes laminar flow, which has the fluid stationary at the boundary with a solid wall and a constant velocity gradient across the fluid (Figure 7.1). Under these conditions the shear rate is constant, and this corresponds to the viscosity of the liquid being constant and independent of the shear rate. Such a fluid is called a Newtonian fluid, and many liquids closely follow this model, including water and most infusion fluids.

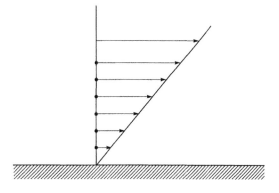

Figure 7.1 The conditions of Newtonian flow. There is a constant velocity gradient across the flow.

Some fluids do not follow this model. The viscosity may increase with shear rate, in which case the fluid is called dilatant (e.g. sand in water), or the viscosity may decrease with increasing shear rate, in which case the fluid is called pseudoplastic (e.g. tomato ketchup). Ophthalmologists call pseudoplastics viscoelastics.

WETABILITY (COATABILITY)

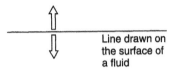

Line drawn on the surface of a fluid

Figure 7.2   Surface tension.

The ability to wet depends upon the surface tension and the contact angle. The surface tension is the force on the surface of the fluid; it is proportional to the length of line drawn on the surface of the fluid and acts in a direction perpendicular to it (Figure 7.2). The surface tension is dependent on temperature and on the medium on the other side of the fluid.

A contact angle occurs when the other medium of the interface is solid, and the lower the contact angle the greater the wetability. The surface tension and wetability are related to the ratio of the attractiveness of the molecules of the fluid to each other versus the attractiveness these molecules have to those in the other medium. Accordingly, it is not surprising that there is a positive correlation between the angle of contact and the surface tension.

OSMOTIC AND ONCOTIC PRESSURE

Osmotic pressure determines the distribution of fluid between the intra- and extracellular spaces, and is predominantly determined by sodium. The oncotic pressure determines the distribution of fluid between the vascular and extravascular compartments and is predominantly determined by protein (particularly albumen). To be compatible a fluid must be of the correct osmotic pressure, while the oncotic pressure will affect its distribution. It is the osmotic pressure that is important for ocular solutions.

PHYSIOLOGICAL SOLUTIONS AND INFUSION FLUIDS

Research into physiological solutions originated with the work of physiologists on isolated organs and tissues. These tissues need to be bathed in a fluid that should, ideally, cause minimal disruption of their normal function. Infusion solutions in surgery need essentially similar properties as, like the 'physiological salines', they are replacing the interstitial fluid that surrounds cells.

The importance of infusion fluids has increased with modern surgical techniques. The trend in modern intraocular surgery is towards closed surgical techniques, which are characterized by maintenance of the intraocular pressure (IOP) during surgery. The IOP is maintained by the use of infusion solutions, and it is not uncommon for half a litre to be infused through the eye during an operation.

The single most important requirement for any physiological solution is that it is isotonic. A hypotonic solution has a dramatic effect on red blood cells and will simply lyse them; hypotonic solutions will kill most cells. The early work on physiological salines concerned the beating heart of a frog, which will survive in an isotonic glucose solution but will not beat. The heart will beat in isotonic sodium chloride for a short while, but will then cease in diastole (or relaxed state). If at this point calcium chloride is added, it will start to beat again for a little while longer until it stops again, this time in systole (a contracted state). A further addition of potassium chloride will allow the heart to beat for several hours. It was Ringer who investigated this and determined the optimum proportions of sodium, calcium and potassium chlorides, now known as Ringer's solution.

The next most important criteria is for the solution to be buffered. Normal saline has been used as an intraocular irrigant, but with an unpredictable pH of 4.5–7.2 it is potentially toxic and can cause severe corneal endothelial cell damage after 1 hour[1]. Cells will only survive in a fairly limited pH range of 6.5–8.5, with a pH of 7.4 being optimal. The most important physiological buffer is the bicarbonate buffering system, of which one of the key components is carbonic acid. This is in equilibrium with carbon dioxide and accordingly is a 'volatile acid'; it is therefore not stable and other buffers, while non-physiological, are more practical. Lactate is used in Hartman's solution (lactate Ringer's solution), as it can be metabolized by cardiac tissue, but it is not a major substrate for ocular tissue, while balanced salt solution (BSS) uses acetate and citrate and BSS Plus (modified glutathione bicarbonate Ringer's) uses bicarbonate. A buffering system will only work over a limited pH range of about 2 units centred on the pKa value (the pH value when 50 per cent of the buffer is present in the dissociated form and 50 per cent in the associated form), and Table 7.1 shows why lactate is the least satisfactory buffer, with the lowest pKa value.

Table 7.1 The pKa values of the most commonly used buffers

Acid–base pair	pKa
Acetic acid	4.76
Carbonic acid	6.1
Citratic acid (three carboxyl groups and so three pKa values)	3.14, 4.77, 5.40
Lactic acid	3.9

BSS Plus is unstable because of the bicarbonate buffer. It has to be mixed and, once mixed, is only stable for around 6 hours. However, bicarbonate is a physiological buffer and the other modifications in BSS Plus are aimed to make it more physiological. The addition of dextrose is to provide an energy source while the addition of glutathione was suggested by experiments mainly looking at clearing of

Table 7.2 Composition of the most commonly used irrigation solutions (adapted from McDermott et al.[1])

Ingredient	Normal saline	Lactated Ringer's (Hartman's)	BSS	BSS Plus
Electrolytes (mmol/l)				
Sodium chloride	154	102	110	122.3
Potassium chloride		4	10	5.08
Calcium chloride		3	3	1.05
Magnesium chloride			1.5	0.98
Buffers (mmol/l)				
Sodium lactate		28		
Sodium acetate			29	
Sodium citrate			6	
Disodium phosphate				3
Sodium bicarbonate				26.9
Additives (mmol/l)				
Dextrose				5.11
Glutathione (oxidized)				0.30
Physical properties				
pH	4.5–7.2	6.0–7.2	7.4	7.4
Osmolality (mOsm)	290	277	305	305

BSS and BSS Plus are both manufactured by Alcon Laboratories, Inc., Fort Worth, Texas, USA.

the rabbit cornea[2]. Glutathionine exists predominantly in the reduced form and is thought to act to protect tissues from oxidative stress, but reduced glutathione is not stable and it is therefore provided in the oxidized form in BSS Plus. It is not clear that the addition of oxidized glutathione offers any advantage[3].

Most trials have shown that Hartman's solution (lactate Ringer's) does not perform as well as BSS Plus. BSS lacks an energy source and accordingly it is not surprising that intraoperative tissue function is better preserved with BSS Plus; however, it has been much harder to demonstrate any significant differences in outcome between the two infusion solutions at 1 week after surgery. Most units therefore use BSS, as it is the more stable and cheaper.

ADDITIVES TO INFUSION SOLUTIONS

Most infusion solutions are classified as medical aids and not as pharmaceuticals, and as such require significantly less testing. By adding a drug to an infusion solution it stops being a medical aid and becomes a pharmaceutical, and accordingly most companies officially state that no drug should be added to the infusion solution. If anything is added, then it must be the surgeon's responsibility. Despite this, nearly 95 per cent of surgeons will routinely have adrenaline added to the infusion solutions, and 10 per cent in England (more in the USA) will also add antibiotics for cataract surgery.

Adrenaline (epinephrine)
Adrenaline is added to the infusion solution to prevent perioperative miosis, as a large pupil is essential for most intraocular surgery. The usual concentration of adrenaline in intraocular infusion solutions is 1 : 1 000 000; it has been shown to have a beneficial effect in maintaining mydriasis and is free from local and systemic side effects[2]. There have been problems with adrenaline at concentrations of 1 : 1000 and 1 : 10 000 being toxic to the corneal endothelium, but these problems appear to be due to associated preservatives and/or antioxidants in the preparations[4].

Intracameral antibiotics
Antibiotics have been added to the infusion solution as endophthalmitis prophylaxis. As with most postoperative infection, the majority of cases of endophthalmitis occur as a result of inoculation at the time of surgery. The organisms are those that might be expected from surface commensals or from airborne contamination (i.e. dust)[5], and they enter the eye either by instrumentation or on the surface of the intraocular lens[6]. It has been demonstrated that the commonest organism found on conjunctival swabs is coagulase-negative Staphylococcus, and that anterior chamber aspirates taken at the end of cataract surgery grow bacteria in the region of 20–30 per cent with coagulase-negative Staphylococcus again being the most common[7,8]. This organism is one of the most common cultured in postoperative endophthalmitis, and it is hard to avoid the conclusion that the association is causal. It is perhaps surprising that endophthalmitis occurs in less than 1 per cent of cases, given the much higher rate of positive cultures at the end of surgery and the presence of an implant, and this indicates significant ocular resistance to infection. It is therefore logical to consider two intracameral antibiotics, and the most commonly used are vancomycin (2–5 mg/ 100 ml) and gentamicin (0.4–0.8 mg/100 ml).

Vancomycin at a dose of 2 mg/100 ml and gentamicin at a dose of 0.8 mg/100 ml has been shown to reduce the rate of positive cultures from anterior chamber aspirates from 20 per cent to 2.7 per cent[7]. Two large series[9,10] from centres routinely using intracameral vancomycin and/or gentamicin have reported endophthalmitis rates of 0.003 per cent, which are more than a hundredfold lower than other series with rates of 0.3–0.7 per cent[11,12].

The use of vancomycin and gentamicin has been shown to be safe, with no adverse effects on the corneal endothelium and no reports of macular infarcts (a recognized side effect of subconjunctival gentamicin)[10]. There has been one randomized control trial suggesting that vancomycin may cause postoperative cystoid macular oedema[13], but this is hard to evaluate because of the relatively low numbers, poor outcome ascertainment (fluorescein angiography available on 70 per cent at 1 month and 50 per cent at 4 months; clinical assessment on

100 per cent at 1 month and 75 per cent at 4 months) and poor randomization procedure (the exclusion criteria were applied after rather than before randomization). The vancomycin group had three more diabetics and, if there were three patients less with cystoid macular oedema in the vancomycin group and using the Yates corrected Chi-squared, the p-value rises to 0.09 (non-significant). The anterior chamber has a volume of about 0.4 ml and the total dose of vancomycin left in the anterior chamber at the end of surgery for this study group would be 4 μg, which is 250 times lower than the dose of 1000 μg of vancomycin used in the endophthalmitis vitrectomy study (where no vancomycin toxicity was reported)[14]. There has been considerable clinical experience with vancomycin with no other reports suggesting that it causes macular oedema, and it is likely that further studies will follow in the near future to help resolve this issue of safety.

There is the other issue regarding whether the routine use of intracameral antibiotics causes an increase in resistance. Vancomycin is still the mainstay of treatment for methicillin-resistant *S. aureus* (MRSA), and accordingly anything that could potentially exacerbate this problem is subject to controversy. This concern is shared by the Royal College of Ophthalmologists, who have stated that: 'The use of antibiotics in irrigating solutions has been widely condemned and the choice of vancomycin can be especially criticized from a public health stance because vancomycin resistance has been encountered in MRSA'[15]. However, there is active controversy over this, and the arguments are outlined below:

1. Low-dose exposure of organisms to vancomycin will lead to resistance. However, there should be no organisms in the anterior chamber; any present should be considered pathogens.
2. Should the infusion solution leak out of the eye, it will expose skin, conjunctival and possibly gut and nasal (due to drainage via the nasolacrimal duct) commensals. However, the exposure will be very low due to the very low initial dose and the degree of dilution, and is a one-off.
3. It is argued that this is precisely the scenario that may lead to resistance. However, vancomycin was isolated from soil and is a naturally occurring compound; hence low-dose exposure occasionally occurs normally.
4. The time that these antibiotics take to kill bacteria *in vitro* is measured in hours[16], while the exposure time *in vivo* may be as short as 15 minutes for the experienced cataract surgeon. However, there is very poor correlation between the times required for an antibiotic to be efficacious in *in vivo* and *in vitro* settings, and the limited available evidence suggests that it is effective[17,18].
5. Given the concern over vancomycin, why not use another antibiotic instead? The counter to this is that *S. epidermidis* has a similar resistance profile to MRSA and, as this is the most common cause of endophthalmitis, vancomycin is the logical choice.

6. If a patient suffers endophthalmitis after vancomycin and genta-
mician prophylaxis, it will be much harder to treat. This is best
countered by a thought experiment. Imagine a series of 2000 cases
with a potential of 15 cases of endophthalmitis, of which one is
resistant to vancomycin and gentimicin. Without prophylaxis
there will be 15 cases of endophthalmitis and 14 will respond to
standard treatment with no clue as to which will be the non-
responsive one. With prophylaxis there will be only one case,
and there will already be the indication that it may not respond
to first line treatment of vancomycin and gentamicin – surely this
is preferable to the first scenario?

Filters

There is a concern that the introduction of any additive will compromise the sterility of the infusion solution by accidental inoculation of
micro-organisms. The original distinction between bacteria and viruses
was that bacteria could be removed by filters and viruses could not,
and therefore a fine filter could be expected to remove any accidentally
introduced bacteria; accordingly, some have suggested their routine
use[9]. However, this is probably a rare source of contamination and
the routine use of intracameral antibiotics could reasonably be
expected to provide adequate cover.

VISCOELASTICS

A liquid has fixed volume but no form, while a solid has both volume
and form. There are a number of substances that show behaviour
intermediate between these two extremes. A plastic is something that
when static behaves as a solid, but dynamically behaves as a liquid and
requires a force to start moving (e.g. tomato ketchup); these substances
are termed viscoelastics by ophthalmologists.

Elasticity refers to the ability of a body to recover after deformation.
A viscous substance will maintain the anterior chamber by resisting the
deforming force, but will not reform it should the anterior chamber
collapse. An elastic substance, by contrast, will let the anterior chamber deform under pressure but will reform it when the pressure is
released. Both these properties are useful and can be combined to
different extents.

It is the elastic property that allows viscoelastics to be injected
through a small cannula; purely viscous substances need a large cannula.

HYDROXYPROPYLMETHYL-CELLULOSE

Hydroxypropylmethyl-cellulose (HPMC) is a highly viscous material
with poor viscoelastic properties. It is derived from methylcellulose
(Methocel®), and a 1% solution was the first 'viscoelastic' used,
being described as an agent to coat intraocular lenses prior to

implantation[19]. The 1% solution does not maintain the anterior chamber well, but a 2% solution does. HPMC is purified from methylcellulose, and differs from the other substances by being a plant derivative rather than a natural body product. It is cleared from the anterior chamber within 24 hours, but it is not known how it is metabolized and eliminated. It is cheap, can be purified by autoclaving (although the purification procedure itself can be expensive), and it has excellent coatability or wetability due to its low surface tension and low angle of contact. Thus it readily coats lenses and the cornea. However, it is a poor viscoelastic and does not retain shape well; it is therefore less suitable for complex surgery.

SODIUM HYALURONATE AND CHONDROITIN SULPHATE

Sodium hyaluronate was introduced in the 1970s, and can be produced from either rooster combs (e.g. Healon®) or by bacterial fermentation (e.g. Provisc®, which comes from *Streptococcus zooepidemicus*). It is used at a concentration of 10 mg/ml (Healon®, Amvisc®, Provisc®), 14 mg/ml (Healon GV®) and 16 mg/ml (Amvisc plus®). It has a relatively high surface tension and large contact angle, so it coats poorly.

Chondroitin sulphate is found in Visocoat® in a 1:3 ratio of 4% chondroitin sulphate and 3% hyaluronate. Chondroitin sulphate is a much smaller molecule than hyaluronate and has a much smaller chain length, and a suitably concentrated solution to be a useful viscoelastic would be too hyperosmotic and therefore toxic to the eye. The mixture has a higher viscosity than each component alone when measured separately.

The advantages of chondroitin sulphate are its wetability and coating properties, and the combination with hyaluronate is intended to combine the advantages of each. Chondroitin sulphate is also a coagulant[20].

REFERENCES

1. McDermott, M. L., Edelhauser, H. F., Hack, H. M. and Langston, R. H. (1988). Ophthalmic irrigants: a current review and update. (Review) *Ophthal. Surg.*,19(10), 724–33.
2. Abdel-Latif, A. A. (1997). Iris–ciliary body, aqueous humor and trabecular meshwork. In: *Biochemistry of the Eye*, 1st edn (J. J. Harding, ed.), pp. 52–93. Chapman and Hall.
3. Puckett, T. R., Peele, K. A., Howard, R. S. and Kramer, K. K. (1995). Intraocular irrigating solutions: a randomized clinical trial of balanced salt solution plus and dextrose bicarbonate lactated Ringer's solution. *Ophthalmology*, 102, 291–6.
4. Edelhauser, H. F., Hyndiuk, R. A., Zeeb, A. and Schultz, R. O. (1982). Corneal edema and the intraocular use of epinephrine. *Am. J. Ophthalmol.*, 93, 327–33.
5. Sherwood, D. R., Rich, W. J., Jacob, J. S. *et al.* (1989). Bacterial contamination of intraocular and extraocular fluids during extracapsular cataract extraction. *Eye*, 3, 308–12.
6. Doyle, A., Beigi, B., Early, A. *et al.* (1995). Adherence of bacteria to intraocular lenses: a prospective study. *Br. J. Ophthalmol.*, 79, 347–9.

7. Beigi, B., Westlake, W., Chang, B. *et al.* (1998). The effect of intracameral per-operative antibiotics on microbial contamination of anterior chamber aspirates during phakoemulsification. *Eye*, **12**, 390–94.
8. Vafidis, G. C., Marsh, R. J. and Stacey, A. R. (1984). Bacterial contamination of intraocular lens surgery. *Br. J. Ophthalmol.*, **68**, 520–23.
9. Gills, J. P. (1991). Filters and antibiotics in irrigation solutions for cataract surgery. *J. Cataract. Refract. Surg.*, **17**, 385.
10. Gimbel, H. V., Sun, R. and De Brof, B. M. (1994). Prophylactic intracameral antibiotics during cataract surgery: the incidence of endophthalmitis and corneal endothelial cell loss. *Eur. J. Implant Refract. Surg.*, **6**, 280–85.
11. Kattan, H. M., Flynn, H. W. Jnr, Pflugfelder, S. C. *et al.* (1991). Nosocomial endophthalmitis survey: current incidence of infection after intraocular surgery. *Ophthalmology*, **98**, 227–38.
12. Verbracken, H. (1995). Treatment of postoperative endophthalmitis. *Ophthalmological*, **209**, 165–71.
13. Axer-Siegel, R., Stiebel-Kalish, H., Rosenblatt, I. *et al.* (1999). Cystoid macular edema after cataract surgery with intraocular vancomycin. *Ophthalmology*, **106**, 1660–64.
14. Endophthalmitis Study Group (1995). Results of the endophthalmitis vitrectomy study. A randomized trial at immediate vitrectomy and of intravenous antibiotics for the treatment of postoperative bacterial endophthalmitis. *Arch. Ophthalmol.*, **113**, 1479–96.
15. Royal College of Ophthalmologists (1996). Management of endophthalmitis. *Focus*, **1**, 1–2.
16. Gritz, D. C., Cevallos, A. V., Smolin, G. and Whitcher, J. P. J. (1996). Antibiotic supplementation of intraocular irrigating solutions. An *in-vitro* model of antibacterial action. *Ophthalmology*, **103**, 1204–8.
17. Masket, S. (1997). Endophthalmitis: state of the prophylactic art. *Eye World*, **8**, 42–3.
18. Schmitz, S., Dick, H. B., Krummenauer, F. and Pfeiffer, N. (1999). Endophthalmitis in cataract surgery. Results of a German survey. *Ophthalmology*, **106**, 1869–77.
19. Fechner, P. U. (1977). Methylcellulose in lens implantation. *J. Am. Intraocul. Soc.*, **3**, 180–81.
20. Pandolfi, M. and Hedner, U. (1984). The effect of sodium hyaluronate and sodium chondroitin sulphate on the coagulation system *in vitro*. *Ophthalmology*, **91**, 864–6.

PART 2

OCULAR ANAESTHESIA

8

ANAESTHESIA

If the first major problem of surgery was sepsis, the second was how to make the patient tolerate the operation. Before anaesthesia, procedures could only last a few minutes.

The majority of ophthalmic surgery can be performed under local anaesthesia, and this chapter describes the various forms of local anaesthesia that have been developed for this. In discussing blocks, there are four variables that need to be considered; the choice of agent(s), the volume, the site, and the use of an adjunctive block.

AGENTS

COCAINE

Cocaine was first isolated in 1860. Its use as a local anaesthetic followed the observation of Carl Koller that his mouth went numb when he took it (he was helping Sigmund Freud with his research), and he was the first to use it as a local anaesthetic for an enucleation procedure in 1884. Cocaine is also a sympathomimetic agent, as it blocks the re-uptake of catecholamines into the nerve terminals (the uptake 1 mechanism); thus it is also a powerful vasoconstrictor. The combination of local anaesthesia and vasoconstriction explains why it is still used for dacrocystorhinostomies. Due to its local and systemic toxic side effects, it must never be given by injection. The maximum recommended application is 1.5 mg/kg.

Its use in clinical practice is limited by its toxicity. It is the most toxic of the local agents for the corneal epithelium, causing the appearance of grey pits that resolve spontaneously; however, this makes it unsuitable for intraocular surgery. Nasal ulceration is well described in those who abuse the drug by sniffing, and this may be a consequence of its vasoconstrictor action. It is a central nervous system stimulant, and for this reason is a controlled drug.

LOCAL ANAESTHETICS

After the discovery of the local anaesthetic effect of cocaine, there was a search for derivatives that had this action without its other effects. A number of agents have been discovered, and the most widely used are lignocaine (Lidocaine® or Xylocaine®) and bupivacaine (Marcain®). They all act by essentially the same mechanism, blocking sodium channels intracellularly and thereby causing conduction block. Vascular absorption is not necessary for their main effect, but their termination of action and toxic side effects are dependent upon this, with maximum plasma concentrations tending to occur 20–30 minutes after administration. The patient should therefore be observed for this period. The toxic reactions to local anaesthesia may be mild, moderate or severe.

Features of a mild reaction include talkativeness, a metallic taste in the mouth, excitability, dysarthria, tremor, rapid pulse, rapid respiration, tremor, twitching and raised blood pressure. The management of this is to stop injecting and monitor.

A moderate reaction may include reduced blood pressure, reduced pulse rate, lethargy and tonic–clonic seizures. Management of fitting is with i.v. diazepam, and of low blood pressure is by intravenous volume expansion. The patient requires careful monitoring.

A severe reaction is characterized by cardiovascular collapse and respiratory arrest. This requires full resuscitation, including intubation and ventilation and such drugs as atropine and adrenaline as required, and transfer to an intensive care unit.

The maximum safe dose is 3 mg/kg of lignocaine and 2 mg/kg of bupivacaine (which equates, for a 70-kg man, to 21 ml of 1% lignocaine and 28 ml of 0.5% bupivacaine). Most ocular blocks use volumes of less than 10 ml, but care must be used if more concentrated solutions (e.g. lignocaine 2%) are used in small people.

Hypersensitivity reactions are also well described. They are commonest for the ester-type anaesthetics (amethocaine, procaine, cocaine) and rarer for the amide types (bupivacaine and lignocaine).

The most commonly used agent is lignocaine, which is usually used in conjunction with adrenaline. Its duration of action is 40–60 minutes, but with adrenaline it is increased to approximately 1.5 h. The standard concentration for infiltration is 1%, though many ophthalmic surgeons use 2%.

Bupivacaine is frequently combined with lignocaine as it has a much longer duration of action (5–12 hours, depending upon the concentration), and it is sensible to add this to any procedure that is expected to take longer than 1 hour. However, in day case surgery the block will still be working at the time of discharge, causing possible blurred and double vision.

Pain from the injection of local anaesthetic has several components, the first of which is from the needle. A second consideration is temperature, and warming the solution to body temperature reduces discomfort[1]. The third source is from pH imbalance – acidic solution stings in its own right and also slows the onset of anaesthesia, and this is why inflamed tissues (which are often acidic) are harder to anaesthetize than non-inflamed tissues. Commercial local anaesthetic solutions are usually buffered to a neutral pH, but there is an important interaction with added adrenaline that can make the resulting solution acidic.

ADRENALINE

Adrenaline is often combined with local anaesthetics. It has two major advantages; it reduces bleeding and it slows absorption of the local anaesthetic. A disadvantage of combining adrenaline with lignocaine is that, while both drugs are close to pH neutral, the combination is acidic, and it is this acidity that is one of the causes of the stinging that occurs with infiltration. Lignocaine 1% with adrenaline 1 : 200 000 can be returned to pH 7.0 by adding sodium bicarbonate (e.g. 2.2 ml of 8.4% sodium bicarbonate to 17.8 ml of lignocaine with adrenaline to give a final volume of 20 ml). The resulting solution is not stable and should be prepared just before use. This interaction of lignocaine with adrenaline is particularly important when using intra-cameral lignocaine, as the infusion solution for cataract surgery usually has added adrenaline.

Adrenaline is a potentially toxic drug. It induces vasoconstriction and therefore should not be used at all for digits or appendages. The total dose should not exceed 500 μg, and the concentration is usually 1 : 200 000 (5 μg/ml).

HYALURONIDASE

Hyaluronidase increases the diffusion of local anaesthetic agent by breaking down some of the extracellular matrix. Hyaluronic acid is a normal constituent of tissue interstitial spaces, but it is not found in the walls of capillaries and is therefore non-inflammatory and does not affect capillary permeability. The permeability of tissues returns to normal within 48 hours due to formation of new hyaluronic acid.

It improves the effectiveness of both retro- and peribulbar anaesthesia[2], and is not associated with toxic side effects. A standard ampoule contains 1500 units, and this is dissolved in 1 ml of water or normal saline for use before being further diluted with local anaesthetic to give a typical final concentration of 15–i.u./ml.

It has been suggested that hyaluronidase may increase the risk of muscle toxicity and brainstem anaesthesia.

TOPICAL AGENTS

The most commonly used topical anaesthetics are lignocaine, proparacaine (Ophthaine®), benoxinate and amethocaine.

TRANSCUTANEOUS AGENTS

These are the cutaneous variants of the topical agents. However, while the mucous membranes are relatively permeable to many local anaesthetics, skin is much more of a barrier. This can be overcome by mixing lignocaine with prilocaine; the mixture is liquid at room temperature and the permeability of skin can be increased by adding an oil in water emulsion, resulting in a 'eutectic mixture of local anaesthetics' (EMLA). EMLA contains 2.5% lignocaine and 2.5% prilocaine and its effect is enhanced by occlusion, but even so absorption is relatively slow and it takes over an hour to achieve good surface anaesthesia.

Its major role is to allow the insertion of needles without pain, and this is particularly relevant for children.

REGIONAL BLOCKS

There are four distinct mechanisms by which regional anaesthesia can be achieved:

1. Topical or transcutaneous
2. Infiltration (tumescent technique is a variant of this)
3. Regional nerve block
4. Intravenous regional block (the Bier block), which is not used in ophthalmic practice.

TISSUE INFILTRATION

Lignocaine and bupivacaine (Marcain®) are the standard agents used for infiltration. The idea is to infiltrate the tissue that is to be operated on, and the infiltrate can be combined with adrenaline and hyaluronidase. The hyaluronidase helps the anaesthetic diffuse evenly through the tissue, while the adrenaline is a vasoconstrictor and helps to reduce bleeding.

TUMESCENT ANAESTHESIA

This technique is not used much by ophthalmologists, and was first described by cosmetic surgeons performing liposuction under local anaesthesia. In essence, the technique involves large volumes of very dilute agents. The concentration of lignocaine is 0.1–0.05% and of adrenaline is 1 : 1–2 000 000, using over a litre of the agent. Although the total dose is well into the toxic range, plasma toxic levels are not achieved. The advantages of this technique are that profound and long lasting anaesthesia can be achieved over a large area, and that within this area there is a near bloodless field.

REGIONAL NERVE BLOCK

The peri- and retrobulbar techniques can also be considered to be regional nerve blocks, but they are described separately in the next section.

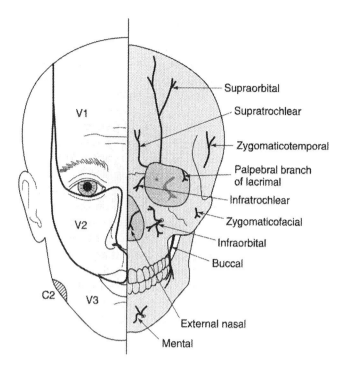

Figure 8.1 The cutaneous branches of the trigeminal nerve. All these are amenable to a local block by direct infiltration.

INTRAOCULAR SURGERY

There are a number of sites of blocks used for intraocular surgery; retrobulbar, peribulbar, sub-Tenon's, topical and intracameral. The choice of which block depends upon the requirements, of which there are three; anaesthesia, paralysis of ocular movements (akinesia), and paralysis of the orbicularis oculi to prevent squeezing during the operation.

Retrobulbar block

The retrobulbar block produces excellent anaesthesia and akinesia with a very small volume of anaesthetic; a good block can often be achieved with as little as 2 ml of agent. The orbit is enclosed by bone on four out of five surfaces, and injection of large volumes can cause a marked increase in orbital pressure and proptosis.

The aim is to place the local anaesthetic behind the globe inside the intraconal space close to the ciliary ganglion, which is located 7 mm anterior to the orbital apex[3]. The major risk of this form of anaesthesia, although rare, is brainstem anaesthesia, which will cause respiratory arrest. This is the most major complication of local anaesthesia. The presumed route of access is via the subarachnoid space, and is assumed to occur when the retrobulbar needle penetrates the optic nerve sheath. The nerve is most at risk where it is fixed at the optic nerve foramen, which is 42–54 mm from the orbital rim[3], and it is at risk if the needle approaches within 1 cm. It has been estimated that a standard 38-mm retrobulbar needle would encroach on this danger area in 11 per cent of the population, and accordingly it is recommended that the maximum safe length for a needle is 31 mm[3]. Another problem in approaching the apex of the orbit too closely is that this is one of its most vascular areas, and there is therefore an increased risk of causing a retrobulbar haemorrhage.

Traditional teaching is to have the patient look away from the line of attack, i.e. up and in when performing an inferotemporal injection. In this position of gaze the macula and optic nerve are rotated so as to be closer to the proposed path of the needle, and a compromise position is to have the patient keep the eye in the primary position of gaze or to look down and in[4].

There was a vogue for using semi-blunt needles for retro- and peri-bulbar anaesthetics on the assumption that a semi-blunt needle could not penetrate sclera or the optic nerve sheath; however, this is erroneous[5] they can cause severe damage. Blunt needles also cause more pain than sharp ones, and the whole idea contravenes the basic principle that the greater the force required, the less the control.

There are a large number of variants on the technique. The needle can be inserted through the conjunctiva (which may be less painful) or through the lid skin (in which case some anaesthetic can be deposited in the orbicularis oculi). The landmarks are:

- The junction of the outer and middle thirds of the orbital rim. By placing a finger just above the orbital rim, the eye can be pushed up while feeling for the equator of the globe, thereby minimizing the risk of inadvertently perforating it.
- When directing the needle up and backwards, the anatomical landmark to aim for is the back of the occiput; do not angle up before passing the equator of the globe so as to minimize risk of perforating it.

If the globe appears to be perforated, the needle must be withdrawn without either aspirating or injecting because frequently damage is a consequence of injecting the anaesthetic agent rather than from the needle track. Needle track injuries without apparent injection of agent into the eye are compatible with a good outcome without further intervention[6,7]. If there is any uncertainty, the needle should be left in place and the patient asked to look from left to right; if the needle does not move, then its tip cannot be in the globe. However, this manoeuvre may increase the risk of a retrobulbar haemorrhage[8,9], and should be used judiciously.

The retrobulbar technique does not paralyse the orbicularis oculi muscle, and this is important for many types of intraocular surgery and essential for extracapsular cataract surgery.

Peribulbar block

Many ophthalmologists prefer the peribulbar block, as there is a much reduced risk of the two serious complications of brainstem anaesthesia and eye perforation. This is because:

1. A shorter needle can be used.

2. Since the needle is not aiming behind the globe, the need to angle it up from below is reduced.
3. The technique can be combined with paralysing the orbicularis oculi muscle without the need for a separate facial nerve block.

As always the advantages are obtained at a price; in this case as the anaesthetic is not placed in the optimal position and more than one injection is usually needed with greater volume of agent – typically 6–8 ml. The injections may be:

1. Inferotemporal (described above).
2. Superior. This injection can be given through the conjunctiva in the superior fornix. The patient is asked to look down and the needle passes the globe at a tangent; since the point of closest approach can be directly visualized and a tangential course will take the tip of the needle away from the globe, this is extremely safe. It very effectively blocks the orbicularis muscle in the upper lid and when combined with a transcutaneous inferotemporal injection there is no need for a separate facial block. It is also targeted at the superior rectus muscle, and so blocks any tendency to a Bell's phenomenon.
3. Medial. The needle is pushed straight back through the caruncle and the medial canthal tendon and, presumably, the fundus of the lacrimal sac, which never seems to come to any harm. This is again a safe injection site, as there is a reasonable space between the globe equator and the medial orbital wall of 4–10 mm. It is also a relatively avascular site, with the nearest big vessels being the anterior ethmoidal artery and vein, which should be superior to the needle track. This injection site seems to result in good spread of the local anaesthetic, making it an excellent adjunct.

Further injections can be given if akinesia is required, although the need for akinesia for modern cataract surgery can be questioned. The only area that should not be directly injected is the superio-nasal quadrant, due to its vascularity.

The increased volume of agent can cause elevation in the ocular pressure following administration of the block. To overcome this rise in pressure, two precautions can be taken. First, a pressure device should be used. A Honan's balloon is a device that can be used to elevate the pressure over the orbit to a predetermined level (usually 30–50 mm Hg) to facilitate diffusion of the agent and disperse the excess volume. There have been no reports of ocular ischaemic events associated with the use of such devices[10]. Secondly, it is good practice to allow a time delay between the block and the start of surgery to allow it to work. Pressure spikes following intraorbital injections decay over 15 minutes, and this is reduced to 10 minutes with pressure lowering devices.

Complications of retro- and peribulbar injections
Although retro- and peribulbar blocks are described as separate techniques, the distinction is often blurred in practice. Reported complica-

tions include brainstem anaesthesia, perforation of the globe, optic atrophy, oculomotility defect, ptosis, and retrobulbar haemorrhage.

Brainstem anaesthesia is life threatening. The accepted mechanism is that it is a result of injection into the optic nerve sheath and that this space is in direct continuity with the subarachnoid space[6]. It has a rapid onset, with time to first symptom of around 2 minutes and maximum effect at 10–20 minutes. The exact manifestations vary considerably and presumably depend upon the exact intracranial distribution of the local anaesthetic. Confusion, cranial nerve palsies, convulsions, hemiplegia, quadriplegia, cardiovascular instability and a few cases of respiratory arrest have all been reported, and this is why an anaesthetist must be available when a peri- or retrobulbar block is being given. It is not clear how the anaesthetic agent reaches the intrasheath space, and thus whether hyaluronidase would be a risk factor or if the closeness of the injection sites to the optic nerve is important, or whether this complication reflects a rare anatomical variant with deficient nerve sheaths.

The National Survey of Local Anaesthesia for Ocular Surgery conducted by the Royal College of Ophthalmologists, reported an incidence of severe systemic reaction (death, life threatening requiring transfer to ITU, or seizure) of 0.034 per cent, but they suspected a degree of under-reporting[11]. Interestingly, all the local techniques seemed to have equal complication rates, although this is higher in other series (Table 8.1).

It was the perceived risk of globe perforation with retrobulbar anaesthesia that led to peribulbar blocks, but globe perforations are well described with both approaches (Table 8.2).

The impression that globe perforations are less likely with a peribulbar technique may be erroneous and a survey in the United Kingdom suggested that the rate for retro- and peribulbar blocks may be very similar at 0.1 per cent[21]. Like many complications, it is experience related; one centre reported an initial rate of 0.75 per cent when their departmental policy switched from general to local anaesthesia[6]. A second well-recognized risk factor is increased axial length, and it has been suggested that the incidence may be as high as 0.7 per cent for such eyes[22] (an increased relative risk of greater than 20).

Table 8.1 Reported severe systemic or brainstem reactions to local anaesthesia

Type of local block	Size of series	Incidence (%)	Agents	Author
Retrobulbar block	3123	0.79	4% lignocaine	Wittpenn et al.[12]
		0.09	2% lignocaine	
	6000	0.13	2% lignocaine/ 0.5% bupivacaine/ hyaluronidase	Nicholl et al.[13]
Retrobulbar block	5235	0.15		Davies and Mandel[14]
	16244	0.006		Hamilton et al.[15]
Sub-Tenon's	3000	0	2% lignocaine	Fuksaku and Marron[16]

Table 8.2 The reported incidence of globe perforation with local anaesthetic techniques

Series	Incidence (%)
Retrobulbar	
Cibis[17]	0.1
Ramsay and Knoblach[18]	0.07
Peribulbar	
Davies and Mandel[14]	0.006
Kimble et al.[19]	0.025
Arnold[20]	Nil
Mixture of peribulbar and retrobulbar	
Hamilton et al.[15]	0.008
Eke and Thompson[11]	0.035

Much of the damage probably comes from the intraocular injection, so this should not be performed if perforation is suspected. The clinical features of perforation include hypotony, loss of red reflex and pain. However, it may only be diagnosed as an incidental postoperative finding on routine fundoscopy.

The prognosis varies with the degree of damage. Perforation that simply involves the sclera and choroid and results in a linear equatorial scar has a good prognosis[6], but this worsens if there is a traumatic retinal tear and probably with increasing number of breaks[21]. Injecting fluid worsens the prognosis as it increases the intraocular pressure and will strip off the retina or choroid if the injection is into the suprachoroidal or subretinal spaces, and any additives may be directly toxic. Management depends upon the degree of damage and varies from simple observation to complex vitreoretinal surgery.

Direct optic nerve injury is described and the retinal vasculature is also at risk with these injuries. A Putscher-type retinopathy (associated with sudden raising of the ocular venous pressure) is another described manifestation[23]. Imaging by CT or MRI may demonstrate intrasheath haematoma[24-26]. It should be noted that haemorrhage occurs at sites of injury, and it is likely that most of the complications that occur are as a result of the direct injury and removal of the associated haematoma may have little effect on the outcome.

The common causes of oculomotility problems following cataract surgery are pre-existing oculomotility defects, loss of binocular status secondary to sensory deprivation in cases of longstanding cataract, and anisometropia. Local anaesthesia will invariably cause transient diplopia as a consequence of deliberately causing akinesia, and this should resolve as the anaesthetic wears off over a matter of hours to 1 day. Local anaesthetics can occasionally cause long-term oculomotility problems and, although these are very rare and the mechanism uncertain, they are well described. There is some evidence that local anaesthetics may be myotoxic and that higher concentrations of agent[27], use of hyaluronidase or use of adrenaline[28] may make the solution more myotoxic. However, it is more likely to occur as a result of direct muscle trauma and the most commonly implicated muscle is the inferior rectus. At least one author has suggested that this complication is technique-related[5].

Postoperative ptosis is well described after procedures such as cataract surgery, but only a few cases are directly attributable to the local anaesthetic. While the incidence appears to be greater after procedures under local rather than general anaesthetic, this may simply reflect selection bias because the elderly are more likely to have a local anaesthetic. Most of the patients who develop a postoperative ptosis may have been predisposed towards this. Like cataract, ptosis secondary to aponeurosis insufficiency is a normal ageing change, and it is reported as being present in over half of cataract patients preoperatively (defined as the upper lid margin being 2 mm or more below the superior limbus)[29]. The treatment, if it develops, is lid surgery.

Retrobulbar haemorrhage is the least severe and most common complication. Like all injection techniques, it is done 'blind' and will occasionally perforate an orbital blood vessel. The chances of this complication are minimized by aiming for the relatively avascular part of the orbit, which is the anterior orbit with the exception of the supero-nasal quadrant. Bleeding into the orbit will cause proptosis and raised intraocular pressure. The reported incidence of 'severe' retrobulbar haemorrhage varies from 0–3 per cent. The correct management is to do nothing. The management of loss of vision in association with a retrobulbar haemorrhage is uncertain; the problem is whether the loss of vision is due to direct action of the local anaesthetic or to compression of the optic nerve. Pressure itself will cause a conduction block in nerves, even in the absence of any disruption of the blood supply. There has been a case report of central retinal artery occlusion secondary to a retrobulbar haemorrhage[30], but this is an extremely rare occurrence. If it is thought appropriate to decompress the orbit, then the simplest procedure is a lateral canthotomy.

Finally, it should be noted that not all cases of postoperative optic atrophy have an explanation[31].

The key points for safe anaesthesia can be summarized as follows[5]:

1. Choose appropriate agent(s) – e.g. lignocaine with adrenaline is suitable for most cataract operations
2. Check axial length and be aware of increased risk of perforation in eyes with increased axial length
3. Avoid the eye looking up when injecting inferiorly, as this increases the risk to the optic nerve
4. Use a sharp needle
5. Do not use needles longer than 31 mm
6. Avoid direct injection into extraocular muscles
7. Avoid excessive volumes (more than 8 ml) of anaesthetic
8. Use decompression devices if large volumes are used
9. Ensure patient is observed/monitored by an anaesthetist for 20 minutes following the injection.

The following two techniques are free of the above complications, and the questions over them are solely related to efficacy of the block.

Subconjunctival and sub-Tenon's blocks

The only ways to avoid the complications described above are to be able to visualize the needle tip at all times (subconjunctival anaesthesia), or to avoid using a needle altogether (sub-Tenon's block).

Subconjunctival block is simply injection of local anaesthetic under the conjunctiva at the superior limbus, but despite being able to observe the needle tip at all times, accidental ocular perforation has been reported[32]. Injection at this location often weakens the superior rectus muscle and so inhibits the Bell's phenomenon, but needs to be augmented by a facial block for extracapsular surgery. This technique was never widely accepted for extracapsular cataract surgery as the reduction in anaesthetic risk is probably more than offset by increased operative risks due to lack of akinesia[33], but would be very suitable for phakoemulsification.

Sub-Tenon's anaesthesia was first described by Swan in 1956[34], but was developed and popularized by Stevens[35-39]. The Stevens' technique uses a blunt cannula and so there is no risk of accidentally impaling sensitive structures. Topical anaesthesia is first applied, then the conjunctiva and Tenon's button-holed with spring scissors and forceps 4 mm from the limbus. It can be done in either the inferonasal or the inferotemporal quadrant, but the former may be preferable as the inferior oblique muscle is present in the latter. A blunt-tipped cannula is then passed into the sub-Tenon's space, and resistance is felt at the equator due to folds of Tenon's in the sub-Tenon's space arising from the muscle insertions. The cannula can be pushed through this. Resistance is also caused by the needle lifting off the globe and catching and being snagged by Tenon's capsule, but this can be avoided by ensuring that the tip of the cannula is kept abutting the globe. Once past the equator, anaesthetic can be injected and a wave of solution passed around the globe. The sensory nerves to the globe have to cross the sub-Tenon's space, so rapid onset anaesthesia is achieved. A feature of the technique is that, if the cannula is in the correct place, the globe proptoses forward as the surgeon injects. Tenon's capsule is incomplete posteriorly and so anaesthetic solution will diffuse into the intraconal space and it will also cause akinesia.

The disadvantages are that it is technically more demanding than the other blocks, and that, if poorly performed, it will cause the conjunctiva to balloon forward, causing chemosis. This can make cataract surgery difficult.

With the development of closed surgical techniques such as phakoemulsification, akinesia or orbicularis oculi paralysis is no longer necessary and corneal anaesthesia, which can be achieved by topical medication, is often sufficient.

Cataract surgery under topical anaesthesia

The cornea has pain sensation only, and is relatively easily anaesthetized. Classically amethocaine is used, but there is a randomized control trial showing that proxymetacaine is just as effective and stings less[40]. Three drops of amethocaine or proxymetacaine given a few minutes before starting surgery is sufficient. Even for such a simple technique it is possible to go astray. Amethocaine will cause corneal epithelial toxicity if too much is used, and the consequence is a cloudy or opaque corneal epithelium.

The iris is a structure with acute pain sensation, and care must be taken not to touch it. For this reason, intracameral block has been developed as an adjunct to topical anaesthesia[41]. Non-preserved[42] lignocaine 2% is used, diluted to 1% with balanced salt solution without adrenaline. Plain lignocaine has a pH of 6.0 with a range of 5.0–7.0, while the cornea can withstand a pH range of 6.5–8.5, but it has a weak buffering capacity. Neutral pH can easily be achieved by dilution with BSS and BSS Plus[43]. Half a millilitre of the 1% lignocaine is then used to irrigate the anterior chamber after an initial stab incision, and this reduces the frequency of any intraocular sensation from 26 per cent to 3 per cent and extends the technique for use on patients who may require iris manipulation[41,44]. It is certainly possible to do a full anterior vitrectomy under topical anaesthesia augmented by intracameral lignocaine. It appears to be a safe technique, with a washout time in the region of 5 minutes and no observed toxic effects[43].

LACRIMAL SURGERY

Conventional dacrocystorhinostomy can be performed under local anaesthetic, but general anaesthetic is preferable. The major problem for patients is that they are expected to swallow any bleeding. A 150-ml blood loss (equal to a cupful) is not uncommon, and this is unpleasnt to swallow and can induce vomiting. It is this that makes the technique of DCR under local anaesthetic problematic.

An advantage of endoscopic lacrimal surgery is that bleeding is not a major problem and it can be routinely performed under local anaesthesia.

FACIAL NERVE BLOCKS

Facial nerve block is an important adjunct to regional anaesthesia for intraocular procedures. Spasm of the orbicularis oculi muscle can generate very high intraocular pressures, causing expulsion of the intraocular contents in the case of an open ocular wound (e.g. in extracapsular cataract surgery). This is one of the reasons for modern surgical techniques favouring a 'closed' approach.

A number of different techniques have been described and these are, in anatomical order from proximal to distal, Nadbath and Rehman, Spaeth, O'Brien, Wright/Atkinson and van Lint.

NADBATH AND REHMAN BLOCK

The Nadbath and Rehman technique exploits the fact that the facial nerve's most constant location is at the point that it leaves the stylomastoid foramen and a correctly given block can generate a complete facial nerve palsy on 'the end of the needle'. Disadvantages are that it requires a good knowledge of the regional anatomy, and because the complete side of the face is affected and at this site the vagal and glossopharyngeal nerves are nearby, it can temporarily affect speech, eating, drinking and swallowing. It must never be given bilaterally[45]. There have been four reports of permanent facial nerve damage by this block[46], and accordingly this block failed to achieve widespread acceptance over the O'Brien and the Van Lint techniques.

O'BRIEN BLOCK

The O'Brien (or antetragus) block is designed to intercept the facial nerve as it crosses the neck of the mandible *en route* to entering the parotid gland. The aim is to give 2–4 ml of anaesthetic down to the periosteum at the junction of the upper third and the lower two-thirds of the distance from the zygomatic arch to the angle of the jaw. The block can affect the lower as well as the upper branches of the facial nerve, and there has been one reported of permanent facial nerve damage from this block[47].

VAN LINT BLOCK

The Van Lint block is the easiest to understand and perform, and is essentially direct infiltration of the orbicularis with the needle entering just lateral to the lateral canthus. The nerve fibres innervate the orbicularis muscle from its deep surface and so, for the block to be maximally effective, the injection must be deep to the muscle and close to the bone. In this manner, it will 'catch' all the branches of the facial nerve entering the orbicularis muscle. Being the most distal of the blocks, its action is the most localized. The only disadvantage is that it is also the closest to the operation site, and so the occasional haematoma that will occur with any injection can potentially interfere with the surgery.

GENERAL ANAESTHESIA

General anaesthesia gives not only analgesia and akinesia, but also amnesia. However, it can depress the cardiovascular and respiratory systems. While ophthalmologists and anaesthetists may dispute who should be giving local ocular anaesthetics, general anaesthesia is unequivocally the province of the anaesthetist and is outside the remit of this book.

REFERENCES

1. Bell, R. W. D., Butt, Z. A. and Gardner, R. F. M. (1996). Warming lignocaine reduces the pain of injection during local anaesthetic eyelid surgery. *Eye*, 10, 558–60.
2. Morsman, C. D. and Holden, R. (1992). The effects of adrenaline, hyaluronidase and age on peribulbar anaesthesia. *Eye*, 6, 290–92.
3. Katsev, D. A., Drews, R. C. and Rose, B. T. (1989). An anatomic study of retrobulbar needle path length. *Ophthalmology*, 96, 1221–4.
4. Liu, C., Youl, B. and Moseley, I. (1992). Magnetic resonance imaging of the optic nerve in extremes of gaze: implications for the positioning of the globe for retrobulbar anaesthesia. *Br. J. Ophthalmol.*, 76, 728–33.
5. Grizzard, W. S., Kirk, N. M., Pavan, P. R. *et al.* (1991). Perforating ocular injuries caused by anaesthesia personnel. *Ophthalmology*, 98, 1011–16.
6. Hamilton, R. C. (1996). The complications of orbital regional anaesthesia. In: *Ophthalmic Anaesthesia. A Practical Handbook*, 2nd edn (G. B. Smith, R. C. Hamilton and C. A. Carr, eds), pp. 148–89. Arnold.
7. Mount, A. M. and Seward, H. C. (1993). Scleral perforations during peribulbar anaesthesia. *Eye*, 7, 766–7.
8. Edge, K. R. and Nicoll, J. M. V. (1993). Retrobulbar haemorrhage after 12 500 retrobulbar blocks. *Anesth. Analg.*, 76, 1019–22.
9. Morgan, C. M., Schatz, H., Vine, A. K. *et al.* (1988). Ocular complications associated with retrobulbar injections. *Ophthalmology*, 95, 660–5.
10. Zabel, R. W., Clarke, W. N., Shirley, S. Y. and Rock, W. (1988). Intraocular pressure reduction prior to retrobulbar injection of anaesthetic. *Ophthalmic Surg.*, 19, 868–71.
11. Eke, T. and Thompson, J. R. (1999). The National Survey of Local Anaesthesia for Ocular Surgery. II. Safety profiles of local anaesthesia techniques. *Eye*, 13, 196–204.
12. Wittpenn, J. R., Rapoza, P., Sternberg, P. Jr *et al.* (1986). Respiratory arrest following retrobulbar anaesthesia. *Ophthalmology*, 93, 867–70.
13. Nicoll, J. M. V., Acharya, P. A., Ahlen, K. *et al.* (1987). Central nervous system complications after 6000 retrobulbar blocks. *Anesth. Analg.*, 66, 1298–1302.
14. Davies, D. B. and Mandel, M. R. (1994). Efficacy and complication rate of 16 224 peribulbar anaesthesia: a prospective multicenter study. *J. Cataract Refract. Surg.*, 20, 327–37.
15. Hamilton, R. C., Gimbel, H. V. and Strunin, L. (1988). Regional anaesthesia for 12 000 cataract extraction and intraocular lens implantation procedures. *Can. J. Anaesth.*, 35, 615–23.
16. Fukasaku, H. and Marron, J. A. (1994). Sub-Tenon's pinpoint anesthesia. *J. Cataract Refract. Surg.*, 20, 673.
17. Cibis, P. A. (1965). General discussion: opening remarks. In: *Controversial Aspects of the Management of Retinal Detachments*, 1st edn (C. L. Schepens and C. D. J. Regan, eds), p. 22. Little Brown.
18. Ramsay, R. C. and Knobloch, W. H. (1978). Ocular perforation following retrobulbar anaesthesia for retinal detachment surgery. *Am. J. Ophthalmol.*, 86, 61–4.
19. Kimble, J. A., Morris, R. E., Witherspoon, C. D. and Feist, R. M. (1987). Globe perforation from peribulbar injection. *Arch. Ophthalmol.*, 105, 749.
20. Arnold, P. N. (1992). Prospective study of a single-injection peribulbar technique. *J. Cataract Refract. Surg.*, 18, 157–61.
21. Gillow, J. T., Aggarwal, R. K. and Kirkby, G. R. (1996). A survey of ocular perforation during ophthalmic local anaesthesia in the United Kingdom. *Eye*, 10, 537–8.
22. Duker, J. S., Belmont, J. B., Benson, W. E. *et al.* (1991). Inadvertent globe perforation during retrobulbar and peribulbar anesthesia. Patient characteristics, surgical management and visual outcome. *Ophthalmology*, 98, 519–26.
23. Lemagne, J. M., Michiels, X., Van Causenbroeck *et al.* (1990). Putscher-like retinopathy after retrobulbar anaesthesia. *Ophthalmology*, 97, 859–61.
24. Hersch, M., Baer, G., Dieckert, J. P. *et al.* (1989). Optic nerve enlargement and central retinal artery occlusion secondary to retrobulbar anaesthesia. *Ann. Ophthalmol.*, 21, 195–7.
25. Pautler, S. E., Grizzard, W. S., Thompson, L. N. and Wing, G. L. (1986). Blindness from retrobulbar injection into the optic nerve. *Ophthalmic Surg.*, 17, 334–7.
26. Sullivan, K. L., Brown, C. G., Forman, A. R. *et al.* (1983). Retrobulbar anesthesia and retinal vascular obstruction. *Ophthalmology*, 90, 373–7.
27. McLoon, L. K. and Wirstschafter, J. (1993). Regional differences in the subacute response of rabbit orbicularis oculi to bupivacaine-induced myotoxicity as quanti-

fied with a neural cell adhesion molecule immunohistochemical marker. *Invest. Ophthalmol. Vis. Sci.*, **34**, 3450–8.

28. Yagiela, J. A., Benoit, P. W., Buocristiani, R. D. *et al.* (1981). Comparison of myotoxic effects of Lidocaine® with epinephrine in rats and humans. *Anesth. Analg.*, **60**, 471–8.

29. Kaplan, L. J., Jaffe, N. S. and Clayman, H. M. (1985). Ptosis and cataract surgery. A multivariant computer analysis of a prospective study. *Ophthalmology*, **92**, 237–42.

30. Goldsmith, M. O. (1967). Occlusion of the central retinal artery following retrobulbar anaesthesia. *Ophthalmologica.*, **153**, 191–6.

31. Carroll, F. D. (1973). Optic nerve complications of cataract extraction. *Trans. Am. Acad. Ophth. Otolaryngol.*, **77**, 623–9.

32. Yanoff, M. and Redovan, E. G. (1990). Anterior eyewall perforation during subconjunctival cataract block. *Ophthalmic Surg.*, **21**, 362–3.

33. Aquavella, J. V. (1990). Limbal anesthesia for cataract surgery (commentary). *Ophthalmic Surg.*, **21**, 26.

34. Swan, K. C. (1956). New drugs and techniques for ocular anesthesia. *Trans. Am. Acad. Ophth. Otolaryngol.*, **60**, 368.

35. Stevens, J., Giubilei, M., Lanigan, L. and Hykin, P. (1993). Sub-Tenon, retrobulbar and peribulbar anaesthesia for cataract surgery. *Eur. J. Implant Refract. Surg.*, **5**, 25.

36. Stevens, J. D. (1992). A new local anaesthesia technique for cataract extraction by one quadrant sub-Tenon's infiltration. *Br. J. Ophthalmol.*, **76**, 670–4.

37. Stevens, J. D. (1993). Curved, sub-Tenon cannula for local anaesthesia. *Ophthalmic Surg.*, **24**, 121–2.

38. Stevens, J. D., Foss, A. J. E. and Hamilton, A. M. P. (1993). No-needle one-quadrant sub-Tenon's local anaesthesia for panretinal photocoagulation. *Eye*, **7**, 768–71.

39. Stevens, J. D. and Restiori, M. (1993). Ultrasound imaging of no-needle one-quadrant sub-Tenon's infiltration. *Eur. J. Implant Refract. Surg.*, **5**, 35.

40. Hamilton, R. and Claoue, C. (1998). Topical anesthesia: proxymetacaine versus amethocaine for clear corneal phacoemulsification. *J. Cataract Refract. Surg.*, **24**, 1382–4.

41. Gills, J. P., Cherchio, M. and Raanan, M. G. (1997). Unpreserved Lidocaine® to control discomfort during cataract surgery using topical anesthesia. *J. Cataract Refract. Surg.*, **23**, 545–50.

42. Fry, L. L. (1997). Intracameral preserved Lidocaine® (letter). *J. Cataract Refract. Surg.*, **23**, 10.

43. Anderson, N. J., Woods, W. D., Kim, T. *et al.* (1999). Intracameral anesthesia. *In vitro* iris and corneal uptake and washout of 1% Lidocaine® hydrochloride. *Arch. Ophthalmol.*, **117**, 225–32.

44. Koch, P. S. (1997). Anterior chamber irrigation with unpreserved Lidocaine® 1% for anesthesia during cataract surgery. *J. Cataract Refract. Surg.*, **23**, 551–4.

45. Rabinowitz, I., Livingston, M., Schneider, H. and Hall, A. (1986). Respiratory obstruction following the Nadbath facial nerve block (letter). *Arch. Ophthalmol.*, **104**, 1115.

46. Wright, J. E. (1926). Blocking of the main trunk of the facial nerve in cataract operations. *Arch. Ophthalmol.*, **55**, 555.

47. O'Brien, C. S. (1934). Local anesthesia. *Arch. Ophthalmol.*, **12**, 240.

PART 3

SURGICAL TECHNIQUES

The right operation done badly does better than the wrong operation done well

9

TEMPORAL ARTERY BIOPSY

INDICATIONS

Temporal artery biopsy is indicated when temporal arteritis is suspected. A firm diagnosis is desirable as the patient will require long-term treatment with prednisolone, and long-term corticosteroid therapy is associated with marked morbidity in the elderly.

Temporal arteritis, like many of the vasculitides, is characterized by 'skip' lesions. A small biopsy specimen therefore increases the risk of a false negative result, and thus 3 cm of artery should be removed. False negative rates run at 9–61 per cent[1,2], and histopathological examination of multiple levels along this length reduces the risk to the lower end of the range.

The second issue is timing of the biopsy. Treatment with steroids results in resolution of the diagnostic pathological features, but they appear to resolve quite slowly[3]. Most departments aim to have the biopsy performed within a week of commencing treatment.

ANATOMY

The superficial temporal artery is a branch of the external carotid artery, which itself runs through the parotid gland and terminates by dividing into the maxillary artery and the superficial temporal artery (Figure 9.1).

The superficial temporal artery emerges above the gland and towards the skin by piercing the deep fascia, and crosses the root of the zygomatic arch just in front of the auriculotemporal nerve and the antetragus of the ear. It then runs forward about 2 cm before dividing into frontal and parietal branches to supply the scalp over these bones. The artery runs on the surface of the deep fascia.

The key to understanding where to look for the vessel is to understand the differences between the superficial and the deep fascia (Figure 9.2). 'Fascia' comes from the Latin meaning sash or bandage, and was used by anatomists to simply mean layer; when not qualified this is potentially misleading, but is usually intended to mean the deep fascia. The superficial fascia is the layer just below the dermis; in most

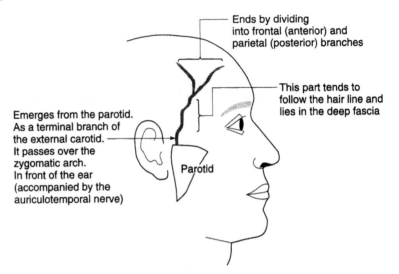

Ends by dividing into frontal (anterior) and parietal (posterior) branches

This part tends to follow the hair line and lies in the deep fascia

Emerges from the parotid. As a terminal branch of the external carotid. It passes over the zygomatic arch. In front of the ear (accompanied by the auriculotemporal nerve)

Parotid

Figure 9.1 Course of the superficial temporal artery.

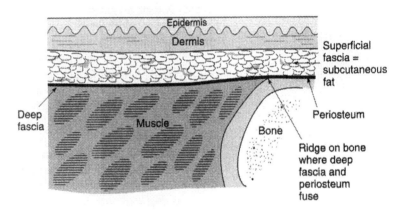

Epidermis

Dermis

Superficial fascia = subcutaneous fat

Deep fascia

Muscle

Periosteum

Bone

Ridge on bone where deep fascia and periosteum fuse

Figure 9.2 The superficial and deep fascia.

mammals this is a thin layer of loose connective tissue and is the plane entered when skinning an animal. In mammals with very little hair, such as pigs and humans, this layer is greatly thickened and contains the subcutaneous fat (panniculus adiposus), which is used as the alternative to hair for insulation. This layer may also contain muscle (panniculus carnosus), and the muscles of facial expression are derived from this.

The deep fascia is a layer of tough connective tissue that overlies the muscles. Where there are no underlying muscles but only bone, there is periosteum instead. Where underlying muscle gives way to bone, the deep fascia fuses with the periosteum and there is often a mark on the bone at this site (e.g. at the inferior temporal line on the side of the skull).

The scalp has a very generous blood supply and the superficial temporal artery can usually be removed without problems. However, in patients with temporal arteritis there has been the occasional case report of vascular problems following its removal. These problems have not been confined to the territory of the external carotid artery, and the occasional stroke has been reported.

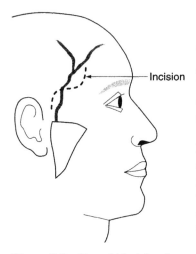

Figure 9.3 Sigmoid incision for temporal artery biopsy.

PROCEDURE

The first step is to mark out the vessel and shave off any hair that covers the incision site. If the vessel cannot be felt, then its position can be estimated as it roughly follows the hairline. The incision should overlie the vessel, but if it cannot be felt, a sigmoid incision located along the hairline is probably optimal (Figure 9.3).

If the vessel has been occluded by the disease process, then it can be hard to locate. The key point in finding the vessel is to look in the correct plane; it lies in the deep fascia on the surface of the temporalis muscle, just deep to the subcutaneous fat. On cutting the skin, lift the wound edges up to undermine in the potential space beneath the subcutaneous fat (i.e. within the superficial fascia) and extend. By doing this, there should be minimal chance of inadvertently cutting it. Retract the sides of the wound, and the vessel should then be visible on the surface of the temporalis muscle within the deep fascia.

First occlude the proximal end of the vessel and take a second to check that the patient can wriggle the fingers and toes and can still speak (i.e. no stroke has been precipitated). Assuming no problems, proceed to ligate it. Dissect the vessel for a length of 3 cm if possible. The vessel anastomoses with other arteries of the scalp, so the distal end also needs to be tied off before cutting. Vicryl® (4/0) can be used for the ligature.

Close the wound in the standard manner. Use an absorbable suture such as Vicryl® for deep closure, and interrupted 6/0 silk sutures or 6/0 nylon subcuticular stitches to close the skin.

PRECAUTIONS

There are a number of sites of potential anastomoses between the internal and external carotid circulations. One such site is the forehead, which is supplied by both the superficial temporal artery (branch of the external carotid) and the supraorbital and supratemporal arteries (derived from the internal carotid artery via the ophthalmic artery). Occasionally the temporal artery provide a significant blood supply to the intracranial circulation. Strokes following temporal artery biopsy have been reported, but are extremely rare; it is possible that the described strokes were incidental rather than causal and it should be noted that temporal arteritis itself is a recognized predisposing factor for a stroke.

AFTERCARE

Remove the stitches at 7 days. Otherwise, aftercare is care of the underlying condition.

REFERENCES

1. Hedges, T. R. 3rd, Gieger, G. L. and Albert, D. M. (1983). The clinical value of negative temporal artery biopsy specimens. *Arch. Ophthalmol.*, **101**, 1251–4.
2. Roth, A. M., Milsow, L. and Keltner, J. L. (1984). The ultimate diagnosis of patients undergoing temporal artery biopsies. *Arch. Ophthalmol.*, **102**, 901–3.
3. McDonnell, P. J., Moore, G. W., Miller, N. R. *et al.* (1986). Temporal arteritis: a clinicopathological study. *Ophthalmology*, **93**, 518–30.

10

TEMPORARY TARSORRHAPHY

INDICATIONS

The major indication for temporary tarsorrhaphy is if the ocular surface is at risk of damage from exposure, although it can be employed in principle for any ocular surface disorder. There is a general principle that the larger the palpebral aperture the more uncomfortable the eye and *vice versa*. The classic situation is with a facial nerve palsy and poor lid closure.

A second indication is to disguise proptosis (e.g. in patients with thyroid eye disease). However, it is arguable whether this is appropriate; the underlying pathology in thyroid eye disease is usually a combination of lid retraction and proptosis, and it may be better if these underlying problems are more directly addressed.

PROCEDURE

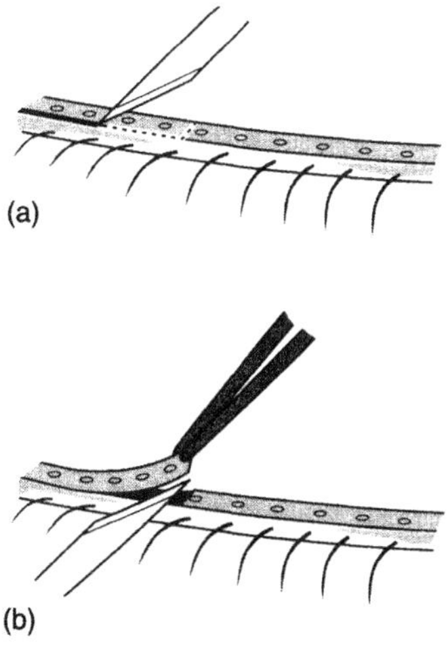

'Temporary' tarsorrhaphy, if done correctly, will last permanently; however, it has the advantage of being easily reversed.

First, remove the posterior part of the outer third of both upper and lower lid margins. This is most easily done with a no. 11 blade, which is run along the grey line before making a transverse cut (Figure 10.1). Grasp the end of the strip to be removed and free it using the no. 11 blade.

Next, stitch with a 6/0 black silk or a similar suture, taking care that the bites of the suture take in the tarsal plates. The stitches need to be tied tightly, and a bolster or tubing should be used to reduce the risk of cheese-wiring the skin and loosening. Small pieces of rubber tubing (tarsorrhaphy tubing) are threaded onto the suture like beads on a string (Figure 10.2). The stitches need to stay in for 3 weeks.

(a)

(b)

Figure 10.1 (a) First mark out the strip to be excised with the point of a no. 11 scalpel blade, then (b) lift the end and cut the strip off.

AFTERCARE AND COMPLICATIONS

Aftercare is really no more than care of the underlying condition.

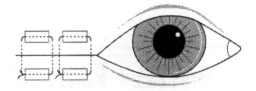

Figure 10.2 Two box sutures tied on tarsorrhaphy tubing to prevent cheese-wiring.

The major complication is that the tarsorrhaphy does not hold when a permanent tarsorrhaphy is required[1].

REFERENCES

1. Collin, J. R. O. (1989). *A Manual of Systematic Eyelid Surgery*, 2nd edn. Churchill Livingstone.

11

LOWER LID ENTROPION REPAIR

Entropions can be classified as congenital or acquired, and acquired can be further subdivided into involutional, cicatricial and consecutive. By far the most common cause of entropion is acquired involutional entropion in the elderly, and this is the condition discussed here.

PATHOGENESIS

A number of factors act in concert to cause involutional entropion, but all the factors share a common theme of loss of tissue substance with concomitant increased tissue laxity. They include:

1. Increased horizontal lid laxity. This is a well-recognized feature, and Neuhaus suggested that the majority of this laxity occurred at or around the lateral canthal tendon[1]. There is no clear consensus of what constitutes horizontal lid laxity. Dortzbach and McGetrick[2] suggested the ability to distract a lid by 6 mm meant that it required shortening, but the median distraction value in normals was 8 mm in the over 50 years age group.

2. Orbicularis spasm. This is assumed by many to be secondary to ocular irritation and not part of the primary pathology[3]. A tendency to orbicularis oculi (O.O.) hypertrophy in patients with entropion as compared to ectropion has been reported[4]. Paralysing orbicularis does not result in curing entropion[5] according to some, but others report excellent short-term palliation with botulinum toxin[6].

3. Disinsertion of the inferior lid retractors. This was emphasized by Dryden and colleagues[7] and supported by Wesley and Collins, who stated that it was invariably present[8], and Schaefer, who found it in half of his patients[9]. They suggest two clinical features: the first is a 'distraction test', whereby when the lower lid skin is retracted, the tarsus fails to evert but remains vertical; the second is a change in colour of the lateral inferior fornix, which appears pinker due to the absence of underlying connective tissue. The current author would anticipate a third sign of loss of the inferior skin crease on down-gaze, but not even this is specific for entropion[10]. Wesley[11] and Putterman[12] have proposed that entropion occurs if Muller's remains attached and ectropion occurs if Muller's detaches.

4. Enophthalmos. Bick[13] postulated that entropion was caused by loss of pressure between the orbital contents and the lid, and showed that entropion could be reversed by injecting 2–4 ml of saline into the muscle cone of the orbit.

TREATMENT

Over 100 procedures have been described for the surgical correction of involutional entropion, although these are no more than permutations of a limited number of components, but there has not been one randomized control trial. Table 11.1 summarizes some of the aetiological factors and the proposed ways of correcting them.

EVERTING SUTURES

INDICATION

Everting sutures give a temporary solution to lower lid entropion. Their major advantage is that they are very quick to perform, but they only provide temporary relief and are no substitute for a definitive repair.

Table 11.1 Indications and procedures for treatment of entropion

Indication	Procedure	Examples
Horizontal lid shortening		
Full thickness	Pentagonal wedge excision	Quickert's[14,15] and Rainin[16] procedures
	Triangular wedge excision	Bicks procedure[13,17]
	Lateral canthal sling	Corin[18], Caroll and Allen[19], Hurwitz et al.[20], Schimek[21] procedures
Posterior lamella	Removal of tarso-conjunctiva	Fox's[22], Bowlegs[23] and corncribs[24] procedures
Preventing orbicularis override	Lid sutures	Quickert's sutures, Wies and Quickert's procedures
	Horizontal lid split	Wies and Quickert's[14,15], Nowinski[25]
	Attaching preseptal O.O. to orbital rim	Wheeler 1 operation[26]
	Plication of pretarsal O.O.	Hsu and Liu[27]
	Removal of O.O.	Nowinski's modification[25], Dresner and Karesh[28], Corin[18], Lessa[29]
	Thermocautery	Ziegler[30,31]
Inferior retractors	Plication	Jones et al.[32], Dresner and Karesh[28], Dryden[7]
	Reattachment/redirection	Wies and Quickert's and Jones procedures
Anterior lamella shortening	Removal of skin (blepharoplasty)	Brackup[33], Rainin[16]
Posterior lamellar lengthening	Posterior lamella graft	Siegel[34]

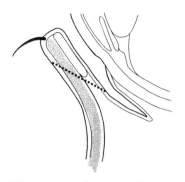

Figure 11.1 Passage of an everting suture. The conjunctival end is inferior to the dermal end so that when it is tightened the lid margin will evert.

PROCEDURE

Most absorbable sutures (e.g Vicryl®) can be used and the needle type is not particularly important, but the procedure is easier and safer with a double-armed needle. Pass the suture from the conjunctival surface towards the skin, entering the conjunctiva at an inferior point to where it leaves so that when it is tightened it will generate a torque that will cause the lid margin to evert (Figure 11.1).

AFTERCARE

Minimal aftercare is required. If there is gross overcorrection the sutures can be removed at 1 week; otherwise, let the sutures dissolve.

THE WIES PROCEDURE

INDICATION

A Wies procedure is indicated for correction of involutional entropion where there is little or no horizontal lid laxity. The use of this procedure in cases where there is horizontal lid laxity is associated with a high recurrence rate[35].

PROCEDURE

The operation is essentially composed of two components; a horizontal lid split so that when it heals there will be a barrier of scar tissue preventing orbicularis oculi override, and everting sutures.

1. Anaesthetize the ocular surface with amethocaine and the eyelid with lignocaine 2% and adrenaline. It is often worthwhile injecting subconjunctivally as well as subdermally to ensure good anaesthesia. Prepare the skin in the standard manner.
2. Use an eyeguard and make a horizontal full-thickness incision with a no. 15 scalpel blade 4 mm below the lid margin and parallel to it so that it is at the lower border of the tarsus (Figure 11.2). Complete the incision with sharp, pointed straight scissors; the sharp points can be pushed through the conjunctiva if the initial incision was not quite full thickness.
3. Pass the everting sutures, which is most easily done with double-ended sutures. The aim is to alter the direction of pull of the lower lid retractors more anteriorly. Pick up the conjunctiva and the associated underlying connective tissue with a pair of toothed forceps, and this will invariably include the lower lid retractor complex. Pass both needles from the conjunctival surface through this layer.

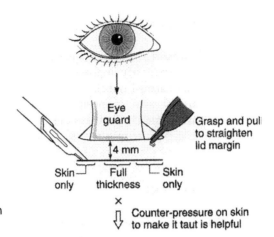

Figure 11.2   The initial incision for the Wies procedure.

4. Use this suture as a traction suture to hold the tissue up and then pass another pair of needles from a double-armed suture either side of the first (Figure 11.3).

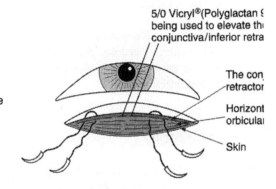

Figure 11.3   The central 5/0 Vicryl® (Polyglactan 910) suture can be used to elevate the conjunctiva/inferior retractor complex, and this will facilitate passage of the other two everting sutures.

5. Pass all the needles through the orbicularis and skin to emerge 2 mm below the lash line.
6. Close the skin (6/0 black silk on a reverse cutting needle is suggested).
7. Finally, tie the catgut everting sutures, starting laterally and ending medially (Figure 11.4). It is very easy to over-tighten the lid and cause a consecutive ectropion, so position the lid with just a minimal amount of overcorrection, which will reverse when the local anaesthetic wears off and the orbicularis muscle regains its function. The reason for tying the medial suture last is to avoid punctal ectropion and a watery eye.

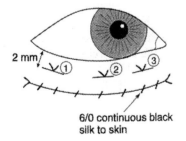

Figure 11.4   Closure. First close the skin with a continuous 6/0 black silk, and then tie the Vicryl® sutures in the numbered order. The medial suture is tied last to avoid a punctal ectropion.

AFTERCARE AND COMPLICATIONS

The aftercare for most lid procedures is the same. Apply a pressure dressing for 24–48 hours. Swelling after lower lid surgery is usually less of a problem than with upper lid surgery, but the use of icepacks can still be considered.

It is usual to prescribe a short course of topical antibiotics such as chloramphenicol for 1 week. Review the patient at 1 week for removal of the skin suture and the everting sutures if there is overcorrection.

The only complication of significant note is lid overcorrection or undercorrection. In either case, persisting lid malposition is usually a consequence of unrecognized horizontal lid laxity and therefore a lid-shortening procedure is generally indicated. For consecutive ectropion, this can be combined with an undermining of the original horizontal lid split to break down the scar tissue and allow the lid to take up the correct position. Rare complications include lid fistula and infection.

THE QUICKERT PROCEDURE

INDICATION

This is for the correction of involutional entropion in the presence of horizontal lid laxity. The procedure addresses both horizontal and vertical components, and is simple to perform.

PROCEDURE

This has been described as a four-snip procedure[14] (Figure 11.5):

1. Snip one is placed at the site where the lid closure will be; it is at right angles to the lid margin and located at the junction of the lateral third and medial two-thirds. The cut is the full height of the tarsus (i.e. about 4 mm).
2. Snip two is at right angles to the first cut. It is parallel to the lid margin going medially and is just below the border of the tarsus. It extends to the point beneath the inferior punctum.
3. Snip three is at the same horizontal location as snip two, but this time heading laterally rather than medially.
4. Snip four removes part of the lid. As for wedge resection, overlap the two parts of the lid to judge how much to remove and then remove the desired amount from the medial portion by making a single cut at right angles to the lid margin.

Figure 11.5 The four-snip procedure. The cuts are made with straight scissors, in the numbered sequence. The position of the fourth cut is determined by overlap of the two ends.

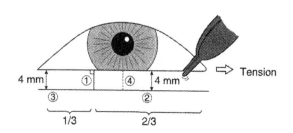

Next recreate the lid margin, avoiding a lid margin notch at the point of closure. A notch is the equivalent of a depressed scar on the skin and can usually be avoided with good closure technique:

1. Use an absorbable suture (e.g. 5/0 Vicryl®) for deep closure of the tarsus. Good alignment of the lid margin is essential (Figure 11.6). Two or three horizontal sutures can be used to close the tarsal plate, but to ensure that the lid margin is correctly aligned the top posterior corner of the tarsus must also be correctly aligned, and this can be done by passing the suture obliquely (Figure 11.6). One well-placed suture is often sufficient to ensure good closure of the tarsus.

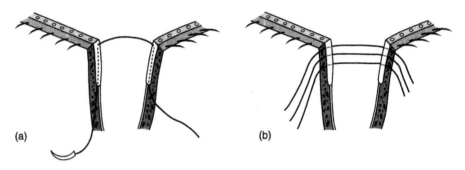

Figure 11.6 Two different ways of suturing the tarsus. Both are equally effective; the key point is to make sure that the lid margin is correctly aligned.

2. Insert a grey line suture and be careful not to pass the stitch through the tarsus as the needle may cut the tarsal stitch. As the lid margin is firmly adherent to the tarsus, the only way to evert the wound margin in this position is with a mattress stitch. The ends should be left long (Figure 11.7).
3. Insert a lash line suture – either a simple stitch or a mattress stitch – again, leave the ends long.
4. Close the skin with interrupted stitches. After tying the knot of one of the interrupted sutures, place the long ends of the grey line and lash line sutures across it and tie a second knot (Figure 11.8) to keep the ends out of the eye.

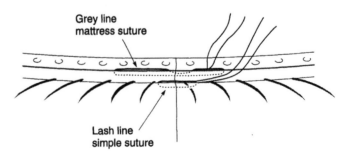

Grey line mattress suture

Lash line simple suture

Figure 11.7   The lid margin sutures.

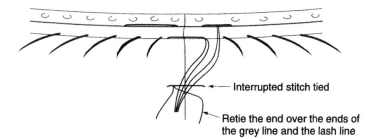

Figure 11.8 Method for securing the loose ends of the lid margin sutures so that they do not irritate the ocular surface.

There is now only a horizontal lid split. Place everting sutures and close the horizontal split as for a Wies procedure.

AFTERCARE

Aftercare is similar to that of a Wies procedure, but the lid margin sutures need removing after 2 weeks.

THE JONES PROCEDURE

INDICATION

This is a powerful technique for correcting involutional ectropion without significant horizontal lid laxity. It corrects the vertical component by plicating the inferior lid retractor and redirecting its pull towards the anterior lamella. If the inferior retractors are dehisced, then it will clearly result in their reattachment. Its advantage over the Wies procedure is that the inferior retractors are positively identified. While the Jones procedure is the logical procedure if the aetiology is inferior retractor dehiscence, there is no reliable way to diagnose this. The procedure is frequently used if there is no significant horizontal lid laxity and a Wies procedure has already failed.

It appears that there is a greater incidence of overcorrection than with the Wies procedure. However, there has been no controlled trial comparing the two procedures. The Jones procedure can be combined with a lid-shortening procedure, which reduces the chance of consecutive ectropion.

SURGICAL ANATOMY

The lower lid anatomy bears a strong resemblance to that of the upper lid.

The lower lid retractors lie just deep to the conjunctiva, separated by a layer of smooth muscle (i.e. Muller's muscle) although this is less well defined than in the upper lid. The retractors lie just deep to the inferior fat pad, which is the key landmark.

PROCEDURE

This is similar to that for ptosis surgery:

1. Using a no. 15 blade, make the skin incision 4 mm from the lid margin, through the skin only.
2. Lift the orbicularis muscle on either side of the incision with toothed forceps. The aim is to buttonhole the full thickness of the muscle to expose either the tarsus or inferior retractors. This is surprisingly hard to do, as the muscle tends to form 'pseudo-layers'. The buttonhole is best made by blunt dissection with blunt-tipped scissors, as all muscle bleeds when cut.
3. Once the muscle has been buttonholed, there should be a potential space that can be opened by blunt dissection. Diathermy the full thickness of the muscle and cut in line with the skin incision (Figure 11.9).

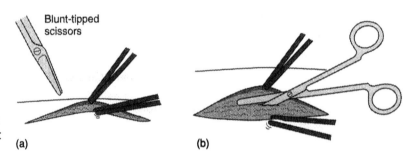

Figure 11.9 Negotiating the orbicularis oculi muscle by blunt dissection. (a) Insert blunt-tipped scissors and spread; (b) then, preferably after diathermy, insert one blade of the scissors and cut in line with the skin incision.

4. Reflect the lower skin-muscle flap to expose the septum. It is often translucent and fat can be seen behind it to confirm the anatomy (Figure 11.10); failing that, gentle pressure on the upper lid will cause the fat and hence the septum to bulge forward. Open it up at the site of maximum bulging. Note that the orbital septum and the inferior lid retractors are fused from just below the inferior tarsal border, so to find them as distinct layers requires looking at least 5 mm below the inferior tarsal border.
5. Once the septum is open, the inferior fat pad will be exposed. Push this backwards by blunt dissection or using spring scissors to

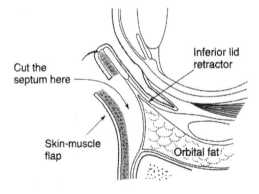

Figure 11.10 Finding the lower lid retractors. Note the orbital fat lies just in front of the lower lid retractors.

nibble at connective tissue strands that prevent it being retracted. Insert a Desmarres retractor to hold the fat back.

6. The inferior retractors are a white layer and move on up-and-down gaze. Use a 4/0 or 5/0 suture, starting with skin, taking a bite of the retractor, a bite of the tarsus and out through the skin of the upper border of the wound (Figure 11.11). Three to six such sutures can be passed. When these sutures are tied, they will plicate the retractors, reattach them if dehisced, redirect their action anteriorly and close the wound. As always, tie them starting laterally and finishing medially so as to prevent punctal ectropion. Further skin stitches can be added if necessary.

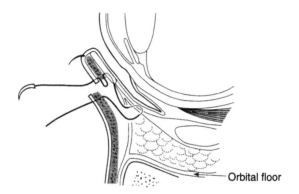

Figure 11.11   The stitch required for lower lid retractor application.

Orbital floor

AFTERCARE

This is as for the Wies procedure except that, as the orbital septum has been opened, it is sensible to give a short course of a systemic antibiotic (e.g. augmentin 375 mg t.d.s. for 5 days).

REFERENCES

1. Neuhaus, R. W. (1985). Anatomical basis of 'senile' ectropion. *Ophthalmic Plast. Reconstr. Surg.*, **1**, 87–9.
2. Dortzbach, R. K. and McGetrick, J. J. (1983). Involutional entropion of the lower eyelid. *Adv. Ophthalmol. Plast. Reconstr. Surg.*, **2**, 257–67.
3. Tyers, A. G. (1982). Aging and the ocular adnexa: a review. *J. R. Soc. Med.*, **75**, 900–902.
4. Sisler, H. A., Lebay, G. R. and Finlay, J. R. (1976). Senile ectropion and entropion: a compared histopathological study. *Ann. Ophthalmol.*, **8**, 319–22.
5. Fox, S. A. (1959). The etiology of senile entropion. *Am. J. Ophthalmol.*, **48**, 607.
6. Lingua, R. W. (1985). Sequelae of botulinum toxin injection. *Am. J. Ophthalmol.*, **100**, 305–7.
7. Dryden, R. M., Leibsohn, J. and Wobig, J. (1978). Senile entropion. Pathogenesis and treatment. *Arch. Ophthalmol.*, **96**, 1883–5.
8. Wesley, R. E. and Collins, J. W. (1983). Combined procedure for senile entropion. *Ophthalmic Surg.*, **14**, 401–5.
9. Schaefer, A. J. (1983). Variation in the pathophysiology of involutional entropion and its treatment. *Ophthalmic Surg.*, **14**, 653–5.
10. Tse, D. T., Kronish, J. W. and Buus, D. (1991). Surgical correction of lower-eyelid tarsal ectropion by reinsertion of the retractors. *Arch. Ophthalmol.*, **109**, 427–31.
11. Wesley, R. (1982). Tarsal ectropion from detachment of the lower eyelid retractors. *Am. J. Ophthalmol.*, **93**, 491–5.

12. Putterman, A. M. (1978). Ectropion of the lower eyelid secondary to Muller's muscle–capsulopalpebral fascia detachment. *Am. J. Ophthalmol.*, **85**, 814–17.
13. Bick, M. W. (1966). Surgical management of orbital tarsal disparity. *Arch. Ophthalmol.*, **75**, 386–9.
14. Allen, L. H. (1991). Four-snip procedure for involutional lower lid entropion: modification of the Quickert and Jones procedures. *Can. J. Ophthalmol.*, **26**, 139–43.
15. Markovits, A. S. (1980). Variations on the theme of involutional entropion and the Quickert repair. *Ann. Ophthalmol.*, **12**, 1028–30.
16. Rainin, E. A. (1979). Senile entropion. *Arch. Ophthalmol.*, **97**, 928–30.
17. Weene, L. E. (1977). Bick procedure for correction of senile entropion and ectropion. *Ophthalmic Surg.*, **8**, 40–41.
18. Corin, S., Veloudios, A. and Harvey, J. T. (1991). A modification of the lateral tarsal strip procedure with resection of orbicularis muscle for entropion repair. *Ophthalmic Surg.*, **22**, 606–8.
19. Carroll, R. P. and Allen, S. E. (1991). Combined procedure for repair of involutional entropion. *Ophthalmic Plast. Reconstr. Surg.*, **7**, 123–7.
20. Hurwitz, J. J., Mishkin, S. K. and Rodgers, K. J. A. (1987). Modification of Bick's procedure for treatment of eyelid laxity. *Can. J.Ophthalmol.*, **22**, 262–5.
21. Scheie, H. G., Crandall, A. S. and Karp, L. A. (1978). Senile entropion: a modified Schimek operation. *Ann. Ophthalmol.*, **10**, 95–9.
22. Fox, S. A. (1976). Senile (atonic) entropion. *Ann. Ophthalmol.*, **8**, 167–72.
23. Hecht, S. D. (1981). Bowlegs procedure for recurrent and primary senile entropion. *Ann. Ophthalmol.*, **13**, 119–21.
24. Saunders, D. H., Shannon, G. M. and Nicolitz, E. (1980). The corncrib repair of senile entropion. *Ophthalmic Surg.*, **11**, 128–30.
25. Nowinski, T. S. (1991). Orbicularis oculi muscle extirpation in a combined procedure for involutional entropion. *Ophthalmology*, **98**, 1250–56.
26. Leber, D. C. and Cramer, L. M. (1977). Correction of entropion in the elderly. A muscle flap procedure. *Plast. Reconstr. Surg.*, **5**, 704–8.
27. Van der Meulen, J. C. (1983). Radical correction of senile entropion and ectropion. *Plast. Reconstr. Surg.*, **71**, 318–25.
28. Dresner, S. C. and Karesh, J. W. (1993). Transconjunctival entropion repair. *Arch. Ophthalmol.*, **111**, 1144–8.
29. Lessa, S. and Carreira, S. (1980). A simple method for the correction of senile entropion. *Ann. Plast. Surg.*, **4**, 7–13.
30. el-Kasaby, H. T. (1992). Cautery for lower lid entropion. *Br. J. Ophthalmol.*, **76**, 532–3.
31. Ziegler, S. L. (1909). Galvanocautery puncture in ectropion and entropion. *J. Am. Med. Assoc.*, **53**, 183.
32. Jones, L. T., Reeh, M. J. and Wobig, J. L. (1972). Senile entropion – a new concept for correction. *Am. J. Ophthal.*, **74**, 327–9.
33. Brackup, A. H. (1979). Modified Wheeler orbicularis overlap procedure for senile entropion. *Ophthalmic Surg.*, **10**, 35–47.
34. Siegel, R. J. (1988). Involutional entropion: a simple and stable repair. *Plast. Reconstr. Surg.*, **82**, 42–6.
35. Hoh, H. B. and Harrad, R. A. (1998). Factors affecting the success rate of the Quickert and Wies procedures for lower lid entropion. *Orbit*, **17**, 169–72.

12

LOWER LID ECTROPION REPAIR

Ectropion is an out-turning of the lid. It can be classified into congenital and acquired, and acquired ectropion can be further subdivided into primary (or involutional) and secondary. The causes of secondary acquired ectropion are mechanical, cicatricial and paralytic (i.e. secondary to facial nerve palsy). The majority of ectropions seen clinically are primary acquired in origin, and it is the correction of this subgroup that is described here.

AETIOLOGY

The exact aetiology of involutional ectropion is not clear, but a key feature, as with entropion, is increased tissue laxity[1]. The described changes are:

1. Horizontal lid laxity. In entropion, discussion is centred on lateral canthal laxity, whereas in ectropion, laxity is often most marked medially. This can be tested for by pulling the lid laterally and seeing how far the lacrimal punctum can be displaced. In lax lids, it can be displaced as far as the pupil.
2. Inferior lid retractor laxity.
3. Reduced tone in the orbicularis oculi. The significance of this in the absence of a facial nerve palsy is not clear.
4. Vertical skin tightness. This can be a secondary change of long-standing ectropion due to chronic blepharo-dermato-conjunctivitis, and be an exacerbating factor. When this is the primary cause, the ectropion is classified as cicatricial.

As in the upper lid, these changes tend to be most pronounced medially. Clinically, involutional ectropion can be subdivided into medial (i.e. only affecting the medial portion of the lid) and generalized.

ASSESSMENT

The symptoms of mild ectropion are epiphora (due to displacement of the lacrimal punctum) and recurrent conjunctivitis. More severe displacement can lead to a cosmetic defect. It is rare for the cornea to be damaged or compromised by lower lid ectropion in the absence of other pathology, and the indication for correction is based on the patient's symptoms. Asymptomatic ectropions may not need to be corrected.

First, assess the following to exclude secondary causes:

- Facial nerve function
- Mechanical causes (i.e. lower lid tumours)
- Cicatricial causes – a localized contracted scar, or secondary following skin shrinkage.

Next, assess which part of the lid is most affected and whether the ectropion is medial or generalized. With both subtypes, look for the presence of excessive medial canthal laxity. Horizontal lid laxity is easier to assess and is more common. Involutional ectropion due to posterior lamella laxity has been termed tarsal ectropion[2], and is characterized by almost complete tarsal eversion with little lid laxity; the presumed aetiology is capsulo-palpebral dehiscence. Four clinical features have been suggested that may point to this aetiology: deep inferior fornix, raised lid margin, reduced lid excursion and altered colour at base.

It should be noted that all four signs are subtle, and in practice capsulo-palpebral dehiscence and horizontal lid laxity usually coexist to varying degrees; accordingly, the basic treatment is horizontal lid shortening. This can be either by wedge resection or by a lateral canthal sling (tarsal strip procedure), which is essentially a shortening of the lateral canthal tendon. Either is acceptable for diffuse lid laxity, but when the lid laxity is focal, as in medial ectropion, it seems logical that the abnormal part should be excised by an appropriately placed wedge resection.

The presence of gross medial canthal laxity when combined with a lid-shortening procedure will result in the lacrimal punctum being displaced laterally and, although small degrees of displacement are insignificant, large amounts result in an odd cosmetic result. Excessive laxity is defined as the ability to displace the punctum to the level of the pupil with the eye in the primary position of gaze, and there are two solutions for this:

1. Medial canthal plication, where the anterior limb of the medial canthus is reinforced by a non-absorbable suture. This can be combined with a lateral canthal sling or lateral wedge resection.
2. Medial canthal resection, which involves scarifying much of the lower canaliculus and marsupializing the remnant into the conjunctival sac[3,4].

Full descriptions of these procedures can be found in more specialized texts[4,5].

Another approach is to turn the lower lid in by either shortening the posterior lamella or lengthening the anterior lamella (Figure 12.1). Posterior lamella shortening is achieved either by causing scarring (as with retropunctal cautery) or by inverting sutures (as in the lazy-T procedure). Anterior lamella lengthening requires skin grafting and is the approach used for cicatricial ectropion.

Figure 12.1 Two ways to correct the vertical components in ectropion. The problem is that the posterior lamella is longer than the anterior lamella (a). The anterior lamella can be lengthened with a graft (b), or the posterior lamella can be shortened (c).

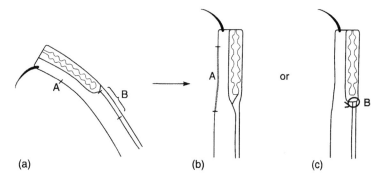

(a)   (b)   (c)

WEDGE RESECTION

INDICATION

Wedge resection is indicated for lower lid malposition in association with horizontal lid laxity. It can be used on its own or in combination with other procedures; in entropion it is usually combined with everting sutures (Quickert's procedure), whereas in medial ectropion it is combined with inverting suture(s) (Lazy-T procedure). For generalized ectropion the indication is the same as for a lateral canthal sling, which has supplanted wedge resection for many surgeons, although there has never been any controlled trial comparing the two methods.

PROCEDURE

Excise the wedge as a pentagon:

1. The site of the wedge excision is usually at the join of the lateral third and the medial two-thirds of the lid. Make the first cut at this site and at right angles to the lid margin.
2. Overlap the cut ends to assess the degree of shortening required, then make the second cut from the medial end, again at right angles to the lid margin.
3. Make two further cuts to form the excised portion into a pentagon (Figure 12.2).
4. Reconstruct the tarsus and lid margin as in Quickert's procedure, and close the skin with interrupted 6/0 silk sutures.

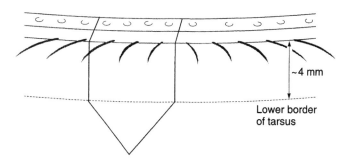

~4 mm

Lower border of tarsus

Figure 12.2 Wedge resection of the lower lid. The excised portion should be pentagonal.

AFTERCARE

This is similar to that for any of the entropion repairs; a short course of topical antibiotics, skin sutures out at 1 week and lid margin sutures out at 2 weeks.

The major problem for all ectropion surgery is late recurrence, and this should be assessed and treated on its merits. Poor closure can cause lid margin notching.

LATERAL CANTHAL SLING

INDICATION

This is a lid-shortening procedure also known as the tarsal strip procedure, and is indicated for the correction of generalized lid laxity. It has three advantages over wedge resection for lid shortening: first, laxity of the lateral canthal tendon is considered by many to be the major site of horizontal lid laxity; second, the procedure does not cause horizontal narrowing of the palpebral aperture; and third, it avoids notching of the lid margin, which is a potential complication of wedge resection.

The aim of the operation is to recreate a new lateral canthal ligament and attach this to the orbital margin under the appropriate tension. The operation was first described by Kirby in 1953[6], and since then a number of variants that mainly differ on the exact point of reattachment of the tarsal strip have been described[7].

PROCEDURE

1. Expose the lateral canthus. Make an incision from the lateral canthus to the orbital margin (Figure 12.3), and cut through the lateral raphe of the orbicularis muscle, which is immediately underlying the skin. It is inevitable the supply to the marginal arterial arcade will be cut.

2. Identify the lateral canthal tendon by pulling on the lid medially and making it taut, then cut it (Figure 12.4). There is commonly a small pocket of orbital fat, and occasionally the tip of the lacrimal gland will enter into the potential space between the orbicularis

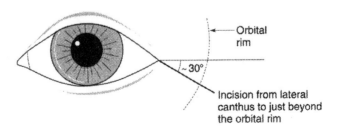

Figure 12.3 The incision for a lateral canthus sling procedure.

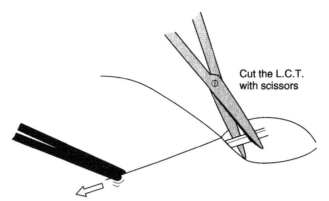

Figure 12.4 Single cut using scissors. Pull the lid taut, and this puts the lateral canthal tendon on stretch so it can be felt as a taut band.

raphe and the lateral canthal tendon. It is worth avoiding damaging the lacrimal gland, as it is very vascular.

3. Mobilize the lower lid by using scissors to cut through the orbital septum for the lateral two-fifths of the lower lid to allow it to be pulled laterally. Pulling the lid up makes the orbital septum taut, allowing it to be identified by feel alone.

4. Make a new tendon from tarsus. Cutting along the grey line with scissors effectively removes the skin surface from the tarsus and generates a triangle, which must be trimmed (Figure 12.5). Remove the lid margin with either scissors or a scalpel, and remove the conjunctival surface by scraping it off with a scalpel blade. This is easier if it has been partially de-epithelialized with bipolar cautery.

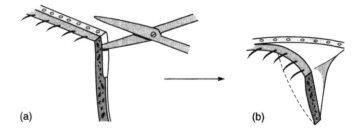

Figure 12.5 (a) Cutting along the grey line with scissors effectively removes the skin surface from the tarsus and generates a triangle (b), which has to be trimmed.

(a)   (b)

5. Use a 5/0 non-absorbable suture to reattach the new tendon to the orbital wall. Use a double-ended suture and pass both needles through the new tendon, emerging on the anterior surface, and then pass both needles through the loop of the suture (Figure 12.6).

6. Reinsert the new tendon. Most anatomical textbooks suggest that this structure inserts on the lateral tubercle just inside the orbital rim, but at surgery it seems to insert directly onto the orbital rim. It probably does not matter which insertion is used, as the difference in direction of pull is small and the action of the orbicularis muscle is to pull it into apposition to the eye anyway (Figure 12.7). Kirby described passing the lateral tarsal strip through a periosteal

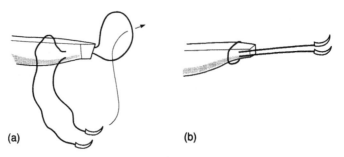

(a)   (b)

Figure 12.6 To attach the suture to the new lateral canthal tendon, pass both needles through it (a) and back through the loop of suture to lock it (b).

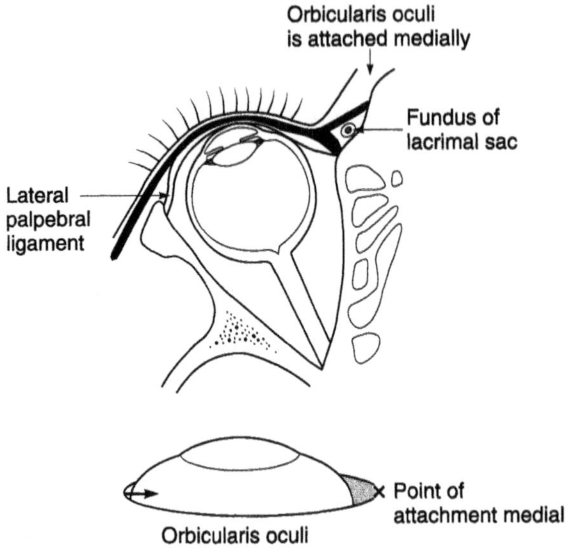

Orbicularis oculi
is attached medially

Fundus of
lacrimal sac

Lateral
palpebral
ligament

Orbicularis oculi

Point of
attachment medial

Figure 12.7 Contraction of the orbicularis will cause the lateral canthus to be applied to the globe.

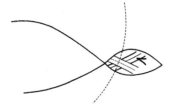

Figure 12.8 The new lateral canthal tendon passes through the upper lateral canthal tendon and is sutured to the periosteum.

tunnel at the orbital margin. Tenzel described passing the strip through a buttonhole in the upper lateral canthal tendon[8], while Anderson and Gordy suggested simply suturing it to the periosteum at the orbital rim[9]. The first two variants are described as lateral tarsal slings and the later as a lateral tarsal strip procedure[7]; the distinction is probably not significant. It can certainly be sutured to the periosteum just inside the orbital rim, but this is not an easy place to suture and care must be taken not to break the needle in the bone. It can be sutured to the orbital rim, or it can be passed through the limb of the upper lid's lateral canthal tendon (Figure 12.8), and this manoeuvre will result in redirection of the pull of the tarsal strip in a more posterior (and therefore physiological) direction.

7. The lateral canthal angle is reformed using a 6/0 Vicryl® stitch. This stitch uses small bites along the grey line of the upper and lower lids, and its aim is to reform the lateral angle and prevent either lid from overriding the other.

8. Use 5/0 Vicryl® to close the orbicularis in layers so as to ensure that the non-absorbable suture holding the lateral tarsal strip will not erode through; use 6/0 silk for skin closure.

AFTERCARE AND COMPLICATIONS

Aftercare is the same as for wedge resection, the only difference being that the orbital septum has been breached; therefore consider giving a short course of systemic antibiotics. Advise the patient not to retract the lower lid if instilling ointment or drops, as this will increase the risk of dehiscence.

Reported complications include:

- Dehiscence of the lateral tarsal strip; a stitch to reform the lateral canthal angle may be sufficient to support the lid even if the lateral tarsal strip dehisces
- Granuloma formation; this can be minimized by making sure that the sutures are properly buried
- Orbital rim tenderness, which is self-limiting
- Infection and haemorrhage.

RETROPUNCTAL CAUTERY

Scarring of the posterior lamella was one of the earliest methods used to correct ectropion. Its use is for minimal, or punctal, ectropion. The procedure is, following a local anaesthetic, to place two rows of three burns on the conjunctival surface of the lid 4–5 mm below the inferior punctum.

INVERTING SUTURES

The methods discussed so far have been mainly directed at correcting horizontal lid laxity, but the second major component in ectropion is vertical lid laxity affecting the posterior lamella. The presumed cause of this is inferior lid retractor weakness or dehiscence, and the process tends to start and be more severe in the medial part of the lid. Thus it seems logical that when trying to shorten the posterior lamella with sutures, a simultaneous attempt should be made to strengthen the lower lid retractors. This is most commonly done as part of the lazy-T procedure, when it is combined with lid shortening; however, it can be performed alone.

LAZY-T PROCEDURE

INDICATION

This is a combination of lid shortening by wedge resection and inverting sutures, and is designed for correction of medial involutional ectropion and normal facial nerve function. There have been no controlled trials, and any combination of an inverting procedure with a lid-shortening procedure will probably give broadly equivalent results.

Gross medial ectropion is a feature of longstanding facial nerve palsy. The standard surgical approach is lid shortening by a lateral canthal sling combined with a medial canthoplasty[5].

PROCEDURE

The operation consists of lid shortening by wedge excision combined with lid-everting sutures.

1. Perform a wedge resection (described above). It should not get closer than 3 mm to the inferior punctum so as to have room to pass the lid margin sutures without risk of damaging the inferior canaliculus.
2. As in any procedure performed near a canaliculus, insert a lacrimal probe to protect it. On the conjunctival surface, mark out a diamond with a no. 11 blade (Figure 12.9a), placing the apex of the diamond under the inferior punctum and 2 mm from it so as to prevent accidental damage. Undermine the space between the two cuts with a pair of spring scissors, then make the cuts in the other two sides of the diamond.
3. Use 5/0 Vicryl® for the everting suture and close the diamond (Figure 12.9b), being sure to bury the knot.
4. Close the lid defect as previously described.

AFTERCARE

The aftercare is as for a wedge excision of the lid.

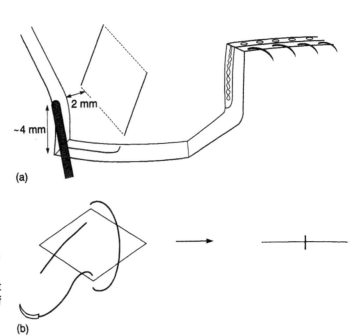

Figure 12.9 (a) Marking out the diamond. Cut two sides with no. 11 blade, then undermine and cut the other two sides with a pair of spring scissors. (b) Close the diamond and bury the knot.

REFERENCES

1. Tyers, A. G. (1982). Aging and the ocular adnexa: a review. *J. R. Soc. Med.*, **75**, 900–902.
2. Tse, D. T., Kronish, J. W. and Buus, D. (1991). Surgical correction of lower eyelid tarsal ectropion by reinsertion of the retractors. *Arch. Ophthalmol.*, **109**, 427–31.
3. Crawford, G. J., Collin, J. R. O. and Moriarty, P. A. J. (1984). The correction of paralytic medial ectropion. *Br. J. Ophthalmol.*, **68**, 639–41.
4. Sullivan, T. J. and Collin, J. R. O. (1991). Medial canthal resection: an effective long-term cure for medial ectropion. *Br. J. Ophthalmol.*, **75**, 288–91.
5. Collin, J. R. O. (1989). *A Manual of Systematic Eyelid Surgery*, 2nd edn. Churchill Livingstone.
6. Kirby, D. B. (1953). Surgical correction of spastic senile entropion: a new method. *Am. J. Ophthalmol.*, **36**, 1372–80.
7. Olver, J. M. (1998). Surgical tips on the lateral tarsal strip. *Eye*, **12**, 1007–12.
8. Tenzel, R. R., Buffam, F. V. and Miller, G. R. (1977). The use of the 'lateral canthal sling' in ectropion repair. *Can. J. Ophthalmol.*, **12**, 199–202.
9. Anderson, R. L. and Gordy, D. D. (1979). The tarsal strip procedure. *Arch. Ophthalmol.*, **97**, 2192–6.

13

PTOSIS SURGERY

Ptosis refers to a drooping of the upper lid. There is a long list of causes, but the two commonest are addressed here – congenital ptosis due to levator muscle dystrophy, and acquired ptosis in the adult due to aponeurosis deficiency. Together, these account for the majority of cases.

Other causes include:

- Mechanical, usually due to a lid tumour pulling the lid down.
- Neurogenic, of which there are two types. The first is due to Horner's syndrome (the combination of 1–2 mm of ptosis, raised skin crease, lower lid raised by 1–2 mm, pupil miosis and possibly heterochromia of the iris if congenital). Surgical correction is purely cosmetic as the ptosis is only small, and this is one of the few indications for the Fasanella–Servat procedure. The second neurogenic cause is a third nerve palsy, and there is usually an associated severe oculomotility deficit. In this case, the ptosis may be helpful by preventing diplopia.
- Myogenic, due to either disease of the neuromuscular junction (e.g. myasthenia gravis) or myopathy (e.g. chronic external ophthalmoplegia), where a characteristic finding is the combination of both poor lid opening and poor lid closure.

ASSESSMENT

For both congenital and acquired ptosis, exclude underlying corneal disease and assess the risk of postoperative exposure (e.g. fifth or seventh cranial nerve problems), which are relative contra-indications to raising the lid. The presence of ocular discomfort should be noted since, as a general principle, the wider the palpebral aperture the greater the ocular discomfort and *vice versa*.

It is essential that the distinction between these two types of ptosis is clear, due to differences in the surgical technique.

CONGENITAL PTOSIS

Congenital ptosis is present from birth, and the features include:

1. Lid ptosis. The normal palpebral aperture is around 10 mm, and the key feature is that this is reduced. Congenital ptosis is often unilateral and therefore these cases will also have an asymmetry in upper lid position.
2. Reduced depth of the skin crease, reflecting reduced levator function.
3. Reduced levator function. This is measured by recording the maximum movement of the upper lid margin from maximal down-gaze to maximum up-gaze. It is important to prevent frontalis action when making this measurement; therefore fix the eyebrow, by pressing with one's thumb, when making the measurement. In a child that will not co-operate with measurements of the levator function, an estimate can be made from the depth of the skin crease; normal levator function is around 15 mm, and any figure above 10 mm is good.
4. Amblyopia, if it covers the pupil.
5. Failure of the lid to relax properly. On down-gaze, the lid in question will be higher than its fellow.
6. Occasionally there is associated weakness of the superior rectus muscle (double elevator palsy), which can be detected by a cover test. Any vertical squint should be corrected before correcting the lid. Overaction of the ipsilateral superior rectus muscle has also been described[1].
7. Presence of synkinesis (the Marcus Gunn phenomenon). This is movement of the jaw causing changes in the lid height, usually causing it to retract. Raising the lid to a more normal position makes these movements cosmetically more obvious, and conventional surgery will do nothing to abolish them.

ACQUIRED PTOSIS DUE TO APONEUROSIS INSUFFICIENCY

The features of acquired ptosis of aponeurosis insufficiency type are:

1. Ptosis, which is often mild and may be bilateral.
2. A raised, and often faint, skin crease
3. Levator function that is good to normal (i.e. greater than 10 mm)
4. The lid in question remaining lower on down-gaze
5. No association with synkinesis or oculomotility disorders
6. Frequent association with dermatochalasis
7. Frequent association with a deep upper lid sulcus due to the disinserted aponeurosis retracting and taking the orbital septum with it.

ANATOMY

Unfortunately, the nomenclature of the surgical spaces of the upper lid is not as clear as it should be, and accordingly precise definitions are given here for the terms used in this chapter (Figures 13.1, 13.2):

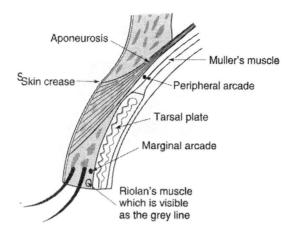

Figure 13.1 Anatomical cross-section of the upper lid.

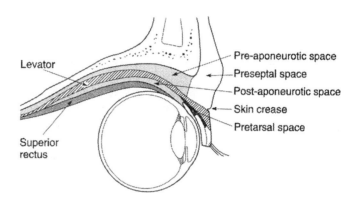

Figure 13.2 The four surgical spaces.

- *The skin crease.* The levator muscle inserts onto the upper one-third of the anterior surface of the tarsus and into the skin, and the skin crease marks the upper limit of this insertion. Generally the aim is to achieve symmetry with the opposing side, but in ptosis surgery the aim may be asymmetry. A low skin crease will help disguise a ptotic lid.
- *The preseptal space.* This is the space bounded by the orbicularis in front, the orbital septum behind and the levator below. The surface marking of the lower border is the skin crease. At and below the skin crease there is no well-defined space, because it is obliterated by fibres from the aponeurosis crossing it to insert into the skin.
- *The pre-aponeurotic space.* This is the surgical space behind the orbital septum and above the levator complex. It contains orbital fat. Some descriptions include the preseptal space as part of the pre-aponeurotic space.
- *The pretarsal space.* This is the surgical space between the aponeurosis/orbicularis oculi muscle and Muller's muscle/tarsus, and the upper border of the space is where Muller's muscle joins the levator aponeurosis. In it runs the peripheral arterial arcade, which is an important anatomical marker. The space can be entered particularly easily by the posterior approach.

- *The post-aponeurotic space.* This is the space between the levator aponeurosis and the superior rectus. The lower border is defined by the origin of Muller's muscle and is contiguous with the potential space between Muller's muscle and conjunctiva. Some descriptions include the pretarsal space as part of the post-aponeurotic space.

- *The pre-aponeurotic fat pad.* This is an exceptionally important surgical landmark as it has an invariant relationship with the aponeurosis, which lies just beneath it. The pre-aponeurotic fat pad is in direct continuation with the orbital fat. There is another fat pad just in front of the septum, which used to be called the pre-septal cushion of fat but is now known as 'SOOF' (sub-orbicularis oculi fat). The SOOF is a well-defined collection of fat that forms the upper border of the preseptal space and separates it from the 'dangerous area' of the scalp. It is adherent to the undersurface of the orbicularis muscle and the epicranial aponeurosis, and it extends from the brow and overlaps the orbital rim. It can extend down as far as the level of the upper lid sulcus.

- *The aponeurosis.* This is a glistening white structure that moves when the patient looks up and down. Superiorly the aponeurosis becomes the levator muscle, which looks like normal muscle. Whitnall's ligament is a clear band-like condensation of white connective tissue, and is found on the surface of the aponeurosis close to where it becomes the levator muscle. It runs from the trochlea to the lacrimal gland fascia and has been described as a pulley whose function is to redirect the action of the levator muscle, but it is probably truer to say that its function is not clear. It can be cut with impunity.

- *Muller's muscle.* This is a layer of smooth muscle located just beneath the aponeurosis. It can be reliably distinguished from orbicularis muscle by the orientation of its fibres, which are organized vertically (orbicularis oculi fibres are oriented transversely). Its origin is from the undersurface of the aponeurosis, and this can be helpful in finding a retracted aponeurosis. It inserts into the top of the tarsus, and directly beneath it is the conjunctiva.

- *The white line.* This should be clearly distinguished from the grey line, which is on the lid margin. The white line marks the point of fusion of Muller's muscle with the aponeurosis and, as its name suggests, it is relatively avascular. Cutting through Muller's muscle at this point allows entry to the second part of the post-aponeurotic space.

FINDING THE LANDMARKS

Despite the small structure of the upper lid, it is easy to become confused because bleeding orbicularis muscle is indistinguishable from bleeding Muller's muscle. There are a number of manoeuvres that can be helpful in correctly identifying tissues:

- The initial space to enter is the pretarsal space. The site of the incision at the skin crease marks the place where the preseptal space ends due to the fibres from the aponeurosis crossing it to insert into the skin. Aim for the upper part of the tarsus, and once on the upper third of the clean anterior surface of the tarsus you will unequivocally be in the pretarsal space.
- When in the pretarsal space, the tissue inserting directly onto the upper border of tarsus is Muller's muscle. Muller's muscle itself and its blood vessels run vertically. The presence of the peripheral arterial arcade on the surface of Muller's is a useful confirmatory landmark.
- The orbital septum is attached to the orbital rim and can be identified by pulling on it and palpating at the orbital rim[2]. The septum can be felt as an inelastic taut band. It is often translucent if there is no covering of orbicularis muscle, the orbital fat can be visualized behind it. Gentle pressure on the lower lid will cause the orbital fat to bulge forward, and this can be helpful in locating the septum before the fat can be directly visualized.
- When the septum is covered with orbicularis muscle, the edge of the aponeurosis can be found by looking at the muscle fibre orientation. The orbicularis fibres are orientated horizontally and Muller's muscle fibres are orientated vertically. Put the lower lid on traction to exposure the layers and grab the tissue where the muscle fibres change orientation (Figure 13.3). This is usually the edge of the aponeurosis. Dissecting down through the muscle above this line will usually result in finding the yellow orbital fat and the glistening white aponeurosis.

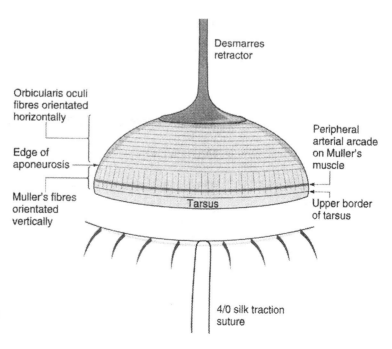

Figure 13.3 Finding the edge of the aponeurosis.

- The aponeurosis can also be identified by its mobility, which is why upper lid surgery is often easier under local anaesthesia. This mobility is often more easily felt (as a distinct tug) than seen when asking the patient to look up and down.
- The importance of finding the orbital fat is that it is located in the pre-aponeurotic space, and the layer directly beneath it is the aponeurosis. The aponeurosis is usually a shiny white colour.
- The pretarsal space is exaggerated by everting the lid over a Desmarres retractor (Figure 13.4). It is this trick that underpins the posterior approach. The same trick of lid eversion will also exaggerate the pre-conjunctival space, and this is useful for local anaesthetic injection and for separating Muller's muscle from conjunctiva.

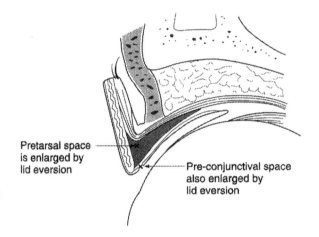

Pretarsal space is enlarged by lid eversion

Pre-conjunctival space also enlarged by lid eversion

Figure 13.4 Eversion of the lid exaggerates the pretarsal space (compare with Figure 13.2).

- The pretarsal space is seperated from the post-aponeurotic space by the white line. The white line is the point of fusion of Muller's with the aponeurosis. On cutting through Muller's at the white line, the relatively large post-aponeurotic space is entered.

THE FASANELLA–SERVAT PROCEDURE

INDICATION

This is indicated for those with good levator function and minimal ptosis of 1–2 mm because it reliably raises the lid by this amount. It does involve sacrificing normal tarsus and makes any subsequent upper lid surgery more difficult. Its major attraction is that it is a relatively simple operation to perform (and accordingly is often done inappropriately).

It is rarely, if ever, indicated for childhood ptosis due to levator dystrophy. It is occasionally useful for mild degrees of aponeurosis insufficiency, and it is often appropriate for the correction of ptosis due to Horner's syndrome.

PROCEDURE

Minimal equipment is required, and the operation takes about 15 minutes.

1. Place a traction suture at the upper lid margin at the high point on its curve, and evert the lid over a Desmarres retractor. Place two haemostats or arterial clips on the upper border of the tarsus (Figure 13.5a). This trick of eversion of the upper lid over a Desmarres retractor results in exaggeration of the pretarsal space. The tissues caught in the haemostats are the conjunctiva, upper portion of tarsus and the lower part of Muller's muscle.
2. Pass one end of a double-armed suture in and out just above the jaws of the haemostats, then release the haemostats.
3. Excise tissue by cutting along the crush marks.
4. Use the other end of the suture to approximate the two cut ends (Figure 13.5b).
5. Make a cut in the skin just beyond the lateral border of the lid, and bring both needles out through this. They can then be tied, cut and the ends buried under the orbicularis.

This operation does slightly lower the skin crease, but this is beneficial because the two conditions for which it is most commonly done (aponeurosis insufficiency and Horner's syndrome) are both characterized by an elevated skin crease.

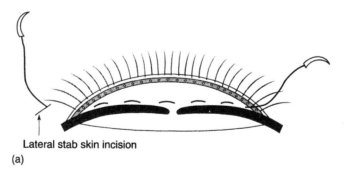

Lateral stab skin incision
(a)

Figure 13.5 The Fasanella–Servat operation. (a) Two haemostats are used to crush along the line of the planned incision. (b) Both ends of the suture emerge through the lateral skin incision and can then be tied and the knot buried.

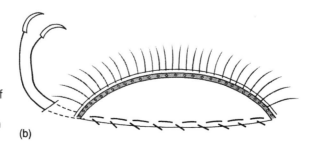

(b)

AFTERCARE AND COMPLICATIONS

Little is required by way of specific aftercare.

The single major complication is undercorrection (which implies inappropriate case selection).

APONEUROSIS SURGERY

INDICATION

The indication is surgery for ptosis of aponeurosis insufficiency type. The concept behind the operation is simple; if a muscle/tendon complex is weak, then it can be strengthened by shortening (as for strabismus).

CHOICE OF ANTERIOR OR POSTERIOR APPROACH

Surgery on the aponeurosis can be by an anterior or posterior approach. The advantage of the posterior approach is that there is no skin incision, but this is rarely a major issue because the skin crease incision heals remarkably well. The advantages of the anterior approach are that the conjunctival surface is untouched, which may be important (e.g. for contact lens wearers), and the procedure can be readily combined with blepharoplasty. This is particularly useful in the elderly, because aponeurosis disinsertion and dermatochalasis are both features of ageing.

PROCEDURE FOR ANTERIOR APPROACH

1. Mark the skin crease, and the point where the arch of the lid is highest (usually above the pupil when the eye is in the primary position of gaze). This is most easily done with the patient sitting up. Cover one eye, and ask the patient to stare directly at your eye (the patient's left eye should look at your right eye and *vice versa*) and then mark the point of the lid over the midpoint of the pupil. This mark is easily lost during surgery so, after infiltration of local anaesthetic, place the lid margin traction suture at this site to act as a permanent marker.
2. Make the skin incision, initially with a scalpel. With the help of an assistant, lift up the orbicularis of either side of the wound and buttonhole it to enter the pre-aponeurotic space, then enlarge the incision medially and laterally. As the orbicularis is divided into layers by the cutaneous insertions of the aponeurosis, it is very easy to make only a partial thickness hole, and tarsus should be clearly recognizable at the base of the hole before enlarging it. As muscle bleeds when cut, it is often best to diathermy prior to cutting.

3. Clean the anterior surface of the tarsus. Fibres from the aponeurosis insert into the bottom two-thirds, and these can be divided as required using the tips of spring scissors to clear enough space for suturing. To avoid damaging the lash follicles, do not get closer than 2 mm to the lid margin. The marginal arcade also runs in this area and runs the risk of being damaged, thereby causing unnecessary bleeding.

4. Find the aponeurosis. Looking up from the tarsus there is Muller's muscle, a band of connective tissue, and then orbicularis muscle. These layers can be exaggerated by putting the tissues under tension by pulling on the lid traction suture. The connective tissue layer (which is the aponeurosis) is at the point where the vertically oriented Muller's fibres meet the transversely oriented orbicularis fibres. In some cases of advanced aponeurosis deficiency the aponeurosis may have retracted back, but it can be located by identifying the Muller's muscle fibres and following them back to their attachment to the underside of the aponeurosis.

5. Open the orbital septum using spring scissors. It is overlaid by the orbicularis muscle, and pulling on the aponeurosis and cutting into this muscle usually reveals the pre-aponeurotic fat pad. To identify the septum, press gently on the lower lid and it will bulge forward along with the fat pad. Cut into the point of maximum bulging, and fully open the septum by making medial and lateral cuts with spring scissors.

6. Clean the superficial and deep surfaces of the aponeurosis. During this process, Whitnalls' ligament can be identified. At this stage, decide whether to preserve Muller's muscle – this choice only exists with the first operation, as scar tissue makes this very difficult if not impossible at subsequent surgery. Anecdotally, there are advantages in preserving Muller's muscle. It is innervated by the autonomic nervous system, and thus the tone in Muller's muscle varies with the state of alertness. For example, when tired the upper lids droop, and this is probably due to reduced tone in Muller's muscle. Preserving Muller's muscle therefore preserves these autonomic responses and helps maintain facial expressiveness.

7. If preserving Muller's muscle, it can be removed from the deep surface of the aponeurosis by either blunt or sharp dissection. Muller's muscle is about 15 mm long and then fuses with the undersurface of the aponeurosis, forming the white line. This point is relatively avascular. Cutting through Muller's muscle at this point enters the relatively large post-aponeurotic space. The correct orientation of the scissors' tips is 45° to the surface of the muscle.

Up until this point, the operation is the same whether it is for dystrophic levator or for aponeurosis deficiency. From now on the two procedures diverge, and will be described separately.

Aponeurosis repair
Unlike the levator resection, for aponeurosis repair the medial and lateral horns need not be identified. For mild degrees of ptosis it

may not even be necessary to clean the deep surface of the aponeurosis; it may be enough simply to reattach the aponeurosis to the tarsus without further dissection.

Raise the lid by using three sutures; one placed to form the centre of the lid arch and one each side. There are two problems: first, where to place the sutures in the aponeurosis, as this will determine the degree of shortening; and second, where to place them on the tarsus, as this will determine the lid contour.

The rules for determining shortening are different to those with congenital ptosis. Some guidelines are:

- Under local anaesthetic, aim to set the lid at the correct level on the table. Place the central suture and tie it on a bow; remove the operating lights so the patient can open the eye, and see if the lid has been set at the correct level[3]. This can be difficult due to paralysis of the levator muscle from the local anaesthetic. If there is paralysis of the levator muscle, then use the fellow eyelid and set the two lids at the same height on down-gaze.
- If the patient is under general anaesthesia, the gapping method can be used. The patient's eyelids should be closed when asleep; the surgery will open them, and this opening is the gap. The size of the gap should be 1 mm greater than the degree of ptosis being corrected – e.g. a 3-mm ptosis would require a 4–5-mm gap[4].
- Using the adjustable suture technique (described below), the lid can be adjusted to the correct height without the complicating effects of either local or general anaesthesia.

The second problem is that of lid contour. It is relatively easy to over-correct the lateral part of the lid and cause lateral flare; this is because the upper lid is more firmly attached laterally than medially and ageing exacerbates this. The result is that the lid tends to shift laterally; the midpoint of the tarsus also shifts laterally, and suturing to that point results in lateral or temporal flare. This is avoided by marking the peak of the arch prior to beginning surgery.

Once the levator has been shortened, the operation is completed with skin closure and skin crease reformation (see below).

Levator resection

Indication
Levator resection is the procedure of choice for congenital ptosis.

Procedure
After cleaning the deep surface of the aponeurosis, identify the medial and lateral horns by putting them under tension (i.e. pulling the aponeurosis medially when identifying the lateral attachment and laterally for the medial attachment). Once identified, cut the horns; the scissors should be angled in so as to avoid accidental injury to the lacrimal gland (related to the lateral horn) and the trochlea (related to the medial horn).

Next, decide how much to resect. This is arguably the most difficult part of the operation. As for aponeurosis deficiency, a number of rules have been proposed:

- Berke[5] proposed a method based on the position of the lid, and the endpoint is not the amount resected but where the lid lies relative to the superior limbus of the cornea on the table. This is rarely used.
- The gapping technique uses the degree of opening of the eye (the gap) on the table. The rule of thumb is that the gap should be equal to the degree of ptosis plus a 'fudge factor'; for congenital ptosis this 'fudge factor' is 3–4 mm (compared to 1–2 mm for acquired ptosis)[6].
- Benjamin Rycroft's principle states that 4 mm should be resected for every 1 mm of ptosis[6].
- It is most common to base the degree of resection on the levator function rather than the degree of ptosis, although there is a strong correlation between the two. A levator function of 8–10 mm requires 14–18 mm of resection; 6–7 mm requires 18–22 mm; and 4–5 mm requires 22–26 mm. If there is superior rectus weakness, then the resection should be increased by an extra 4 mm[7].

After shortening the levator complex and reattaching it to the tarsus, close the skin with reformation of the skin crease. This can be done either by using skin–apo–skin sutures, which attach the aponeurosis or tarsus to the site of skin crease reformation (Figure 13.6a) or by deep sutures from the aponeurosis into the orbicularis muscle (Figure 13.6b). Any suture material can be used if the stitches are to be removed at 1 week. In children, skin stitch removal may be difficult, and it may be easier to use a rapidly dissolving stitch (e.g. Vicryl rapide) or tissue adhesive.

Finally, insert a Frost suture (a 4/0 nylon suture placed through the inferior lid margin, used to pull the lower lid up and fixed to the forehead) to prevent lagophthalmos. A feature of congenital ptosis is dystrophic muscle, where there is failure of the lid both to rise and to relax. Accordingly, following surgery there is a real risk of lagophthalmos, particularly in the immediate postoperative period.

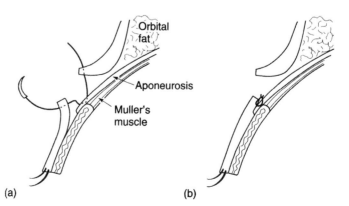

Figure 13.6 Two ways to ensure good skin crease formation: (a) skin–apo–skin; (b) deep closure.

(a)   (b)

COMBINING APONEUROSIS REPAIR WITH BLEPHAROPLASTY

Indication

Aponeurosis deficiency and dermatochalasis are both features of ageing and commonly coexist. Dermatochalasis is the result of laxity of the anterior lamella of the upper lid, and ptosis is due to laxity of the posterior lamella. Both can be corrected at the same time. It is a moot point in which order to do the procedures, but it seems, more logical to mark out and do the blepharoplasty first. This can be done in a totally standard manner, removing both skin and orbicularis.

Having removed orbicularis, expose and open the septum. If necessary, remove any orbital fat. This exposure should facilitate the aponeurosis repair, which can be done in the standard manner.

The advantage of doing the operation in this order is that it requires minimal deviation from the standard technique. However, the procedures can be done in the reverse order. The ptosis surgery represents no problems, and removing the muscle and skin may be easier because a superior muscle–skin flap has been raised. Both methods give good results.

Aftercare and complications

As the orbital septum has been opened, prescribe a short course of prophylactic antibiotics (e.g. augmentin 375 mg t.d.s. for 5 days) following the surgery.

The upper lid is prone to postoperative oedema; this is usually transient and of minor importance. Occasionally gross oedema results, with resulting stretching and distorting of the tissues. This oedema can be reduced by the use of routine ice packs applied for 5–15 minutes four to six times a day (a simple icepack is a packet of frozen peas).

Remove skin stitches at 5–7 days.

The complications are self-evident:

1. Undercorrection of the ptosis. This requires re-operation. If there is clear undercorrection that is immediately obvious, re-operation can be within the first week. Surgery is relatively easy at this stage. Otherwise, re-operation should be avoided between 1 week and 6 months after the initial surgery, due to increased vascularity of the tissues.
2. Overcorrection of the ptosis. A small degree of overcorrection is often desired when operating by the anterior approach, as the lid can be expected to fall by a small amount after the surgery. If the levator sutures are on the surface, their early removal can encourage the lid to drop. Lid massage can also help bring the lid down (ask the patient to grab the eyelashes and pull downwards while trying to gaze upwards, hold this for 60 s, and repeat the procedure three or four times a day).
3. Haemorrhage and infection. Any procedure that results in opening of the orbital septum carries a small risk of orbital haemorrhage and orbital infection.

PROCEDURE FOR POSTERIOR APPROACH

The technique is very similar to the anterior approach, the difference being the trick used to enter the post-aponeurotic space.

1. Mark the lid margin in the same way and place a traction suture.
2. Exaggerate the post-aponeurotic eversion over a medium-sized Desmarres retractor, and make an incision close to the top of the tarsal plate to enter the post-aponeurotic space. The tissue attached to the small strip of tarsus is Muller's muscle and conjunctiva (Figure 13.4). Dissect back along the anterior surface of Muller's muscle to its origin.
3. Find the aponeurosis, which is white and glistening and, in this approach, folded over to form a very visible white band. Cut through it close to the superior border of the tarsus. Pull it down and the orbital septum and the fat pad should be visible just above it. At this point remove the Desmarres retractor, reverse it and reinsert it. The orientation is now as for an anterior approach. Continue to open up the orbital septum. At this stage the pre-aponeurotic fat pad can be identified and is useful confirmation that the anatomy has been correctly interpreted.
4. Decide how much aponeurosis to resect, based on similar criteria to those for the anterior approach. For a resection (as opposed to a repair), the origin of Muller's muscle will need to be disinserted from the deep surface of the aponeurosis.
5. Suturing for closure is slightly more complex than for the anterior approach. Use double-ended sutures, making the first bite through the aponeurosis. Pass each needle through the end of the Muller–conjunctiva flap and then back through the tarsus to emerge on the skin at the site of reformation of the skin crease (Figure 13.7).

AFTERCARE AND COMPLICATIONS

These are essentially the same as for the anterior approach, the only difference being that there is tendency for the lid to rise with a posterior approach and drop with an anterior approach.

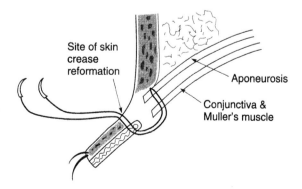

Figure 13.7 Suture technique for the posterior approach.

APONEUROSIS SURGERY ON ADJUSTABLE SUTURES

Given the problems of adjusting the lid to an ideal height, it is not surprising that adjustable suture techniques have been developed. Although not widely used, they are not difficult and are worthy of consideration – particularly if problems in judging lid height are anticipated.

Collin's method[8] uses 5/0 polygalactan (Vicryl®) sutures. Pass a double-ended suture through the aponeurosis and tie it to leave two equal lengths (Figure 13.8). Pass each needle through the upper part of the tarsus, and then one needle through the skin at the lower edge of the wound and the other needle through the skin at the upper edge. When tied, these sutures not only have the aponeurosis on what is effectively a 'hang back' suture, but also help to close the skin incision and reform the skin crease. Tie the sutures in a bow, which can be untied and adjusted 6–24 hours later. The sutures are slowly dissolvable, or can be removed at 4 weeks.

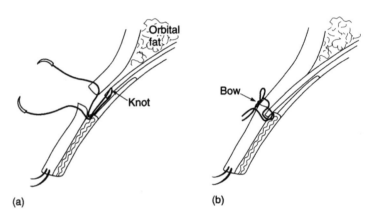

(a) (b)

Figure 13.8 The adjustable suture technique (Collin's method) for ptosis surgery.

REFERENCES

1. Steel, D. H. W. and Harrad, R. A. (1996). Unilateral congenital ptosis with ipsilateral superior rectus muscle overaction. *Am. J. Ophthalmol.*, **122**, 550–56.
2. Putterman, A. M. and Urist, M. J. (1974). Surgical anatomy of the orbital septum. *Ann. Ophthalmol.*, **6**, 290–94.
3. Hylkema, H. A. and Koornneef, L. (1989). Treatment of ptosis by levator resection with adjustable sutures via the anterior approach. *Br. J. Ophthalmol.*, **73**, 416–18.
4. Waller, R. P., McCord, C. D. Jr and Tanenbaum, M. (1987). Evaluation and management of the ptosis patient. In: *Oculoplastic Surgery*, 2nd edn (C. D. McCord Jr and M. Tanenbaum, eds), pp. 325–76. Raven Press.
5. Berke, R. N. (1959). Results of resection of the levator muscle through a skin incision in congenital ptosis. *Am. J. Ophthalmol.*, **61**, 177–201.
6. Mustarde, J. C. (1969). *Repair and Reconstruction in the Orbital Region*, 1st edn. E. & S. Livingstone Ltd.
7. Collin, J. R. O. (1989). *A Manual of Systematic Eyelid Surgery*, 2nd edn. Churchill Livingstone.
8. Collin, J. R. O. and O'Donnell, B. A. (1994). Adjustable sutures in eyelid surgery for ptosis and lid retraction. *Br. J. Ophthalmol.*, **78**, 167–74.

14

UPPER LID BLEPHAROPLASTY

INDICATIONS

Dermatochalasis (excess upper lid skin) is a normal phenomenon of ageing, and its removal is important to people who want to look younger. It is often associated with prolapse of the orbital fat, particularly medially, while the excess skin is usually more prominent laterally; thus blepharoplasty is often combined with orbital fat removal. There are three major indications for blepharoplasty:

1. Cosmetic ('rejuvenation'). This is the commonest indication, and it is one of the most frequently performed cosmetic operations.
2. Functional. When there is gross excess of upper lid skin, it can overhang the lid margin and cause a visual field defect.
3. Skin donor site. It is an ideal donor site for providing skin to close skin defects in another lid; this is particularly important for the upper lid, as the use of thick skin will result in an immobile lid. The choice of donor sites for closing such defects is, in order of preference, fellow upper lid skin, post-auricular skin, and supra-clavicular skin.

Ocular discomfort, which is common, is a relative contra-indication for blepharoplasty.

ASSESSMENT

1. Look for ocular discomfort. As a general rule, the more open the lids the greater the ocular discomfort, and the narrower the palpebral aperture the greater the ocular comfort. Blepharoplasty may impair lid closure, and therefore pre-existing ocular discomfort is a relative contra-indication.
2. Check lid closure and for Bell's phenomenon. Blepharoplasty is relatively contra-indicated if there is a risk of postoperative ocular exposure.
3. For cosmetic blepharoplasty, enquire about patient expectations (preferably with a mirror). Blepharoplasty will not remove fine

lines and wrinkles such as crow's feet at the lateral canthus, although there are other techniques that may help with these.

4. Check for brow ptosis. If this is present, the correct procedure is correction of the brow ptosis. Blepharoplasty will only make subsequent correction of the brow ptosis difficult.
5. Check for lacrimal gland prolapse. It is a major disaster if a prolapsed lacrimal gland is mistaken for prolapsing orbital fat and excised. Ask the patient to look down and inwards while elevating the brow; lacrimal gland prolapse will be seen as lump appearing in the outer part of the upper lid.
6. Measure the upper lid skin crease on down-gaze of both eyes. This is important, as the skin crease will be reset with the surgery. A key part of the cosmetic result of the operation is symmetry of the skin crease.
7. Check upper lid position. There is often a degree of upper lid ptosis of the aponeurotic insufficiency type. Aponeurosis repair can be readily combined with blepharoplasty.
8. Check visual fields if there is the requirement to demonstrate a functional component.
9. Check visual acuity and oculomotility, as loss of vision and restriction of oculomotility are very rare but well described complications of the surgery.

PROCEDURE

1. Mark the skin crease, which will form the lower border of the excision. It is important not to go too medially as an epicanthic fold may result, and the medial limit of the incision is a vertical line running through the upper lid punctum. The skin crease is usually 8 mm from the lid border in women and 10 mm in men, and this is the distance from the lid margin. The crease follows a gentle curve and approaches the lid margin both medially and laterally, but should not get any closer than 5 mm. The incision from the lateral canthus to the orbital rim can either be a horizontal line or slope upwards at 45°; the latter may result in slightly less skin removal, but helps ensure that the two edges of the wound are of equal length for subsequent closure. The incisions should never go beyond the lateral orbital rim (Figure 14.1).

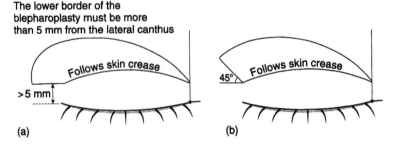

Figure 14.1 Marking out the blepharoplasty. The majority of the excess skin is usually lateral. The lateral limit must not go beyond the orbital rim or the medial limit beyond the punctum.

2. The upper border determines the amount of skin to be excised. The excess skin normally forms a fold, and a fold of 3 mm corresponds to 6 mm of excess skin. The exact amount can be determined by asking the patient to look down and gently pinching the skin with a pair of forceps. There are two methods of dealing with excess medial skin (Figures 14.2, 14.3).

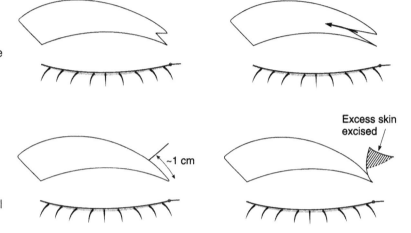

Figure 14.2 The W-excision to deal with excess medial skin. The tip of the W is advanced temporarily with the closure.

Figure 14.3 An alternative method to remove excess medial skin.

3. Having marked out the incision, inject local anaesthetic.
4. Excise the skin. First cut the edges of the excision with a no. 10 scalpel. The skin or skin muscle can then be removed either by undermining and cutting with spring scissors, or by lifting the skin up by a corner and removing it using the scalpel. In the latter approach the muscle is relatively firmly attached to skin, and the plane of the excision is usually between the muscle and the septum. The result is a skin–muscle blepharoplasty. If only skin is wanted, then the former approach is probably better.
5. Removal of the prolapsing orbital fat is a frequent adjunct to the cosmetic procedure, but is not necessary for functional blepharoplasty or when simply harvesting skin for a graft. The simplest method is just to remove the medial fat, but it can be removed from the medial, central and lateral fat compartments. The most direct way is to open up the orbital septum fully and remove fat from all three compartments directly. For cases of thyroid eye disease this is probably the best technique as, due to previous orbital inflammation, the fat does not flow freely. For cosmetic blepharoplasty it is not necessary to open the orbital septum fully. Make a stab incision with sharp pointed scissors and spread, then let the excess fat prolapse out (Figure 14.4a). This can be encouraged by gentle pressure on the lower lid (Figure 14.4b). It is important not to pull on the fat, as this may cause deep orbital bleeding. Clamp the prolapsed fat with an artery forcep, cut it off and apply diathermy to the stump before releasing the artery clip and letting the stump flow back behind the septum. This process can be done for all three compartments.

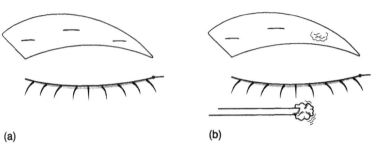

Figure 14.4 Removal of orbital fat. (a) Sites of stab incisions for removal of fat. Medial and temporal fat pads are yellow; nasal fat is white. (b) Gentle pressure on the lower lid causes fat to prolapse.

6. Reform the skin crease. The skin crease is formed by the insertion of the aponeurosis and is not affected by this procedure; however, it is sensible to put a couple of stitches in to ensure a good crease.
7. Close the skin. The site heals well, and a number of suture materials can be used, either continuous or interrupted, or even tissue adhesives. As always, the skin sutures should be removed at day 5.

AFTERCARE

It has been suggested that the patient be left unpadded afterwards and the vision tested hourly for the first few hours so as to be able to detect deep orbital bleeding that may lead to optic nerve compression. However, an alternative school of thought is that leaving the patient unpadded theoretically increases the risks of a bleed, and therefore a pressure dressing should be maintained for as long as possible. Regardless, the development of severe pain after the operation is an absolute indication to examine the eye and check the vision to exclude this extremely rare but devastating complication.

The upper lid is a site where oedema readily collects, and regular ice packs can help to minimize this.

Skin stitches should be removed at 7 days. If the orbital septum has been opened, then consideration should be given to prescribing a short course of systemic broad-spectrum antibiotics (e.g. augmentin). Ocular lubricants should also be prescribed in the early postoperative phase, particularly last thing at night, as transient lagophthalmos is common.

The aftercare for blepharoplasty closely resembles that for ptosis surgery.

COMPLICATIONS

VISUAL LOSS

This is a rare but well described complication of the procedure[1], and the estimated frequency is 0.04 per cent. There are at least 75 cases reported in the literature, all of which were characterized by opening of the orbital septum and removing fat. The exact mechanism is not clear, but it is suggested that it is due to bleeding causing compression of the central retinal artery.

LAGOPHTHALMOS

A more common complication is the inability to close the eyelids after surgery. It usually occurs only transiently, and is most marked in the first postoperative week. Mild cases can be treated with ocular lubricants, but the only solution for severe cases is to replace the excised skin. For this reason, in cases of cosmetic blepharoplasty it is recommended that the excised skin should be wrapped in a damp swab and stored in a sterile container for 3 days at 4°C. Under these conditions the skin usually remains viable, and it can be replaced if necessary.

LID MALPOSITION

This is more of a problem with lower lid blepharoplasties. Ptosis (and diplopia) can occur, presumably as a result of poor dissection with damage to deep structures. Ptosis will occur with damage to the levator complex, and the commonest cause of diplopia is damage to the superior oblique tendon, particularly around the trochlea.

REFERENCE

1. Lowry, J. C. and Bartley, G. B. (1994). Complications of blepharoplasty. *Surv. Ophthalmol.*, **38**, 327–50.

15

RETROBULBAR ETHANOL INJECTION

INDICATION

Chapters 16 and 17 describe ways of removing the eye, and the commonest indication for this is a chronically painful and blind eye. However, if the blind and painful eye is cosmetically acceptable and there are no concerns over possible subsequent sympathetic endophthalmitis or an intraocular tumour, a simpler procedure is to inject pure ethanol into the retrobulbar space to kill the nerves to and from the eye.

This technique is irreversible and kills all the nerves including the optic nerve, so if the patient has any sight at all (e.g. perception of light) this will be lost. It can also cause a ptosis by destroying the innervation to the levator, but this is rare (occurring in 5 per cent or less). An advantage of absolute ethanol is that its action is extremely localized and there is no risk of distant toxic effects due to diffusion, since its toxicity is a function of concentration and once diluted from 100 to 70 per cent it will not kill tissue. There have been no reports of brainstem complications following this procedure.

PROCEDURE

This is as for any retrobulbar injection.

1. The patient should be lying down and in a place where full resuscitation facilities are available.
2. Use a retrobulbar needle and insert it with the aim of placing the tip of the needle in the retrobulbar space (see Chapter 8).
3. Initially, inject 2 ml of 2% lignocaine and leave the needle *in situ*, then wait 5 minutes to make sure that no ptosis has occurred. Pure ethanol injection is potentially very painful and lignocaine provides anaesthesia as well.

4. If after 5 minutes all is well, inject 0.5 ml of absolute ethanol down the same needle.

If the first injection does not work, a second one can be given after a few days.

16

EVISCERATION

INDICATIONS

The commonest indication for evisceration is a blind and painful eye following ocular infection. There is concern that enucleation may exposure the patient to the risk of meningitis, as cutting the optic nerve effectively results in entering the CSF space; the risk is clearly greater if there has been perforation of the globe.

The cosmetic result with evisceration is often claimed to be better than enucleation and orbital implant, but it is not clear how real this advantage really is.

A disadvantage of evisceration for trauma is that, unlike enucleation, it does not completely abolish the risk of sympathetic endophthalmitis.

It should be noted that evisceration is never an appropriate technique for managing intraocular tumours.

PROCEDURE

1. First, ensure that surgery is being performed on the correct eye (check the consent form and notes; mark the eye preoperatively; check the eye on the table)!
2. Perform a 360° peritomy, followed by blunt dissection in the four quadrants using straight, blunt-tipped scissors. Push these into the area between the two recti muscles under Tenon's and the conjunctiva and spread them; this effectively mobilizes the conjunctiva and Tenon's.
3. Make a cut in the sclera 2 mm behind the limbus and enter the suprachoroidal space. The purpose of the operation is to remove the uveal tract with the retina, lens and vitreous from the eye. The uveal tract is only anchored to the sclera at two significant sites, the scleral spur and the optic nerve, and while there are other attachments in the form of the emissary vessels, these are weak. Push a blade of a pair of spring scissors into the suprachoroidal space and cut round as close as possible to the scleral spur. The

result will be corneo-scleral disc attached to what will be the surgical specimen at the scleral spur.

4. Pass an evisceration spoon backwards and around in the supra-choroidal space, breaking the attachments of the emissary vessels (Figure 16.1). Break the final attachment at the optic nerve by scraping firmly with the spoon against the sclera and the uvea and its contents can be removed as one specimen, lifting it out by the corneo-scleral disc.

5. Alternatively, simply cut off the cornea and scrape the contents of the eye out with the evisceration spoon. A disadvantage of this method is that the specimen is much harder (or impossible) to interpret histologically.

6. Next, decide whether to place an orbital implant. The cosmetic results are so much better with such an implant that there must be a good reason not to (such as active infection).

7. The implantation technique is straightforward. First, open up the posterior sclera to allow a bigger implant to be placed – an 18-mm ball implant can generally be used. Place the implant in or behind the sclera and then close the tissue in layers over it, starting with the sclera, then Tenon's and finally conjunctiva. Use Vicryl® 4/0–5/0 for deep closure and 5/0–6/0 for conjunctiva. Finally, place a conformer shell, aiming for the largest size that will fit while making sure that the eyelids can close.

AFTERCARE

A pressure dressing will minimize swelling and bruising, and should be left in place for as long as is tolerable (2–5 days). A prophylactic 5-day course of a broad-spectrum antibiotic is appropriate.

The first fitting of an artificial eye can be carried out 4 weeks after surgery. The first eye fitted is usually a temporary pre-made shell, and

Figure 16.1 (a) First cut around as close as possible to the scleral spur to generate a corneo-scleral disc, then (b) use an evisceration spoon to dissect in the suprachoroidal space. The emissary vessels are delicate and easily divided, and the only area of significant resistance is the attachment to the optic nerve.

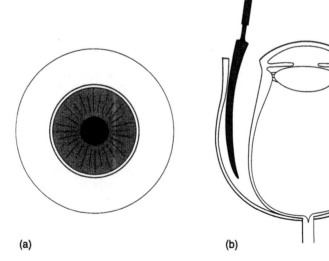

(a)   (b)

a custom-built hand-painted eye can usually be fitted at around 3 months after surgery.

With second-generation implant materials, which are porous, there is the option of drilling the implant with a view to fitting a peg to enhance oculomotility.

17

ENUCLEATION

INDICATIONS

The major indications for enucleation are intraocular malignancy (usually uveal melanoma), a blind and painful eye, and following trauma when there is a perceived high risk of sympathetic ophthalmitis. In all cases, the psychological impact of enucleation can be lessened by good cosmetic rehabilitation.

There are very few situations when it is not appropriate to use an implant. For example, it has been argued that an implant should not be used in cases of ocular melanoma as it may mask local recurrence, but this concern is unfounded. Local recurrence is both uncommon and can be predicted, as it only occurs following incomplete excision (i.e. transected extrascleral extension on histology[1]) and can be prevented by orbital radiotherapy.

PROCEDURE

Implantation of a Medpor® ball with attachment of the four recti muscles is described here.

1. As with evisceration, first check that surgery is being performed on the correct eye! The eye may not always look abnormal on gross examination (as with intraocular tumours), so it is worth dilating the eye and checking the fundoscopy on the table.
2. Mark the superior fornix with a double-ended suture, such as a 4/0 silk, by passing the needles through the superior fornix to emerge through the skin. Not only does this mark the fornix, but it also acts to protect the upper lid levator complex from accidental damage during the procedure. The inferior fornix can be marked, if desired, in a similar manner.
3. Insert a lid speculum, which must be more rigid than a wire speculum (e.g. a Clark's speculum) because the lids become very floppy once the globe has been removed.
4. Perform a 360° peritomy, which should be 1.5 mm back from the limbus so as to disinsert both Tenon's and conjunctiva. Next, use scissors to blunt dissect in all four quadrants (as described in the previous chapter).

5. Disinsert the recti muscles. Strip fascia off each muscle in turn, starting with the nearest and following the spiral of Tillaux (medial, inferior, lateral and superior: MILS), and secure each muscle with a double-ended 5/0 absorbable suture. The technique is identical to that used for strabismus surgery. Use two squint hooks to lift the muscle clear of the globe, taking care not to perforate the sclera; this is exceptionally important if enucleating for retinoblastoma, as perforation will commit the patient to adjunctive treatment (usually orbital radiotherapy). Stripping the fascia back a long way is important at the end for recreating the fornices.

6. Cut the muscles off using spring scissors following diathermy. Next attach 4/0 silk traction sutures to the stumps; these will be used to lift the globe out.

7. Identify and cut the superior and inferior oblique tendons. They insert under the superior and lateral recti respectively, and are readily found once the recti have been disinserted.

8. Cut the optic nerve, using either scissors or the Foster snare (Figure 17.1a); the latter is cleaner. To ensure a good length of

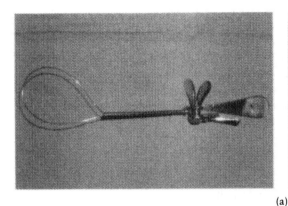 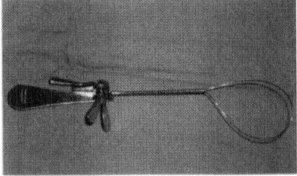

(a)

(b)

Figure 17.1   (a) Foster snare; (b) Foster snare with straight artery clip attached.

optic nerve, which is important if enucleation is being performed due to an intraocular malignancy, put a straight artery clip on the tip of the snare's loop (Figure 17.1b) and then use this to push the loop down the medial orbital wall as far as it will go. Ensure that the lids are not caught and that the four recti muscles and their sutures are outside the snare. Lift the globe by gentle traction on the traction sutures in the recti muscle insertions, and slowly tighten the snare to take up the slack. It is prudent to have the lateral canthus protected by a squint hook to prevent accidental damage to the lids. Then disengage the artery clip and complete the process – this requires four hands; two for the snare, one to lift the globe, and one to disengage the artery clip from the tip of the snare. The globe should just lift out when the nerve is cut. An advantage of the snare is that often little bleeding occurs. The alternative (or if the snare breaks) is to use enucleation scissors, which are passed behind the eye to the orbital apex and all tissue is cut. Enucleation scissors can cause considerable bleeding from the cut end of the retinal artery, but this can be controlled by pressure on the socket packed with gauze.

9. Prepare the implant. A 20-mm diameter ball can usually be fitted. If it is an acrylic or hydroxyapatite ball, it will need wrapping in sclera, Vicryl® mesh or Mersilene® mesh to allow the muscles to be sutured to it. Sclera has the best handling properties, but its use is being phased out because of the problem of prion disease. Medpor® implants do not need to be covered; they also have the advantages of being porous, less inflammatory than hydroxyapatite and completely synthetic.

10. Insert the implant. The insertion technique depends upon the implant used. A sclera-covered ball has a smooth surface and is simply pushed into the intraconal space. Implants covered with Mersilene® mesh and Medpor® implants have a rough surface, and any attempt to place them directly in the orbit will result in subsequent extrusion because they catch on the orbital tissue and do not slide past it. The secret of success is to place the implant deep in the orbit and ensure a good covering; the trick is to use a finger from a disposable glove to form a temporary covering to the implant (Figure 17.2). This has a smooth, slippery surface, allowing deep placement of the implant, and the glove finger can then be pulled out using an instrument placed down the inside of it, leaving the implant behind.

11. Suture the recti muscles to the front of the implant by passing the sutures forward and tying. It is important to have an instrument pushing the implant back while suturing, as there is a tendency to pull it out while trying to pass the needles.

12. Close the Tenon's with a purse-string suture using 4/0 absorbable suture (e.g. Vicryl®), and close the conjunctiva with a fine (6/0) suture.

13. Put a conformer shell in. They come in a number of sizes labelled A to F, and generally a D or an E shell can be fitted. The shells are egg-shaped, and the wider end goes laterally. The purpose of the

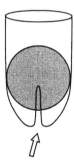

Figure 17.2 Use of disposable glove for implantation. The implant is placed in the thumb of the glove, and a relieving cut is made in the tip so the ball can be pushed through the glove without removing it.

shell is to maintain the fornices. This is not usually a problem for uncomplicated cases, when it can be omitted.

VARIATIONS ON THE BASIC PROCEDURE

There are a large number of described variations on the basic procedure.

- Some advocate suturing the inferior oblique muscle to the implant as this may prevent subsequent inferior fornix shallowing[2]. The rationale is that the inferior oblique is closely associated with the anterior capsulopalpebral fascia, and therefore by doing this the normal anatomy can be restored[3]. This, so far, has the status of conjecture, with no hard evidence to support it.
- A refinement on the suturing technique is to recreate the fornices. When the muscles are stitched onto the implant, the suture is tied but the needles are left on. The needles are then passed back through Tenon's and conjunctiva and tied after the Tenon's and conjunctiva have been closed. The idea is to reduce postoperative swelling and to help recreate the fornices.
- Removing the four recti muscles is really no different from any squint muscle recession procedure. These muscles are often 'lost' during the procedure but, unlike in squint surgery, can easily be found following the removal of the globe. The muscles retract into the extraconal space and form dimples or pockets in Tenon's.

AFTERCARE AND COMPLICATIONS

Aftercare is very similar to that for many lid surgical procedures. A pressure dressing left on for a few days will minimize postoperative swelling, and this can be further helped by the use of ice packs. A short course of systemic antibiotics is advisable.

There is no particular need for the conformer shell to be removed for daily cleaning, and initially the patient usually prefers for the socket to be left alone. A temporary artificial eye can be fitted at 4 weeks, and a permanent one at 3 months.

Implant extrusion is the major short-term complication. Extrusion rates as high as 29 per cent have been reported with Mersilene®-mesh covered implants[4], but the problem is probably generic to all implants with porous surfaces because they grip tissue and there is failure to get deep implantation. Extrusion rates are almost certainly technique related. Rates as low as 3 per cent have been reported with hydroxyapatite in good hands[5].

Post-enucleation socket syndrome is the major long-term complication. The clinical features are enophthalmos of the artificial eye, deep upper lid sulcus (reflecting loss of orbital volume), shallowing of the inferior fornix, and lower lid laxity. It is thought that a major contributory factor to the lower lid laxity is mechanical stretching from a large prosthesis secondary to a loss of orbital volume.

REFERENCES

1. Starr, H. J. and Zimmerman, L. E. (1962). Extrascleral extension and orbital recurrence of malignant melanomas of the choroid and ciliary body. *Int. Ophthal. Clin.*, **2**, 369–85.
2. Sloan, B. H. and McNab, A. A. (1997). Complications of hydroyapatite implants (letter). *Ophthalmology*, **104**, 1982–3.
3. Goldberg, R. A., Lufkin, R., Farahani, K. *et al.* (1994). Physiology of the lower eyelid retractors: tight linkage of the anterior capsulopalpebral fascia demonstrated using dynamic ultrafine surface coil MRI. *Ophthal. Plast. Reconstr. Surg.*, **10**, 87–91.
4. Yalaz, M., Demircan, N., Yagmur, M. and Haciyakupoglu, G. (1997). Mersilene® mesh: long-term results in oculoplastic surgery. *Orbit*, **16**, 217–23.
5. Oestreicher, J. H., Liu, E. and Berkowitz, M. (1997). Complications of hydroxyapatite orbital implants. A review of 100 consecutive cases and a comparison of Dexon® mesh (polyglycolic acid) with scleral wrapping. *Ophthalmology*, **104**, 324–9.

18

ORBITAL IMPLANTS

INDICATIONS

There are two major types of orbital implants; an intraconal orbital implant, which is indicated for the anophthalmic socket, and an orbital floor implant, either to act as a barrier (as in orbital floor fractures) or to augment orbital volume. This chapter concentrates solely on the first of these indications.

There are three reasons why an intraconal orbital implant is desirable:

1. It improves the cosmetic result. The single biggest factor for a poor cosmetic result is a deep upper lid sulcus, which is a feature of volume loss from the orbit.
2. It improves oculomotility by allowing the muscles to be in a more physiological position.
3. It allows a reduction in size of the subsequent prosthesis. This is easier for the lower lid to support, and can be more mobile.

There are two relative contraindications. The first is in situations where lining may be a problem – for example, in those who have previous ocular surgery, where it may be impossible to remove the eye without removing a considerable amount of conjunctiva. In this situation, consideration should be given to using dermis fat. The second is following trauma where Tyers and Collins reported a relatively high extrusion rate[1] for 'baseball' implants, and this may also be due to loss of lining. Secondary implants may also have an increased risk of migration[2].

PROPERTIES OF IMPLANT MATERIALS

Implant materials should ideally have the following properties:

1. They should be non-toxic and resist infection. The risk of prion infection makes the use of sclera less desirable, and this is a factor against the use of acrylic balls and hydroxyapatite implants.
2. They should handle well and it should be possible to attach sutures to them. Only high density polyethylene (Medpor®) meets these criteria.

3. They should retain volume. All implants (with the exception of dermis fat) are excellent in this respect.
4. There should be potential for including a mechanical coupling between the implant and the prosthesis. The porous implants are candidates.
5. They should be inexpensive. The cheapest is the acrylic ball, and the most expensive is hydroxyapatite.

COVERING MATERIALS

These provide a substrate for suture attachment in those implants that are too hard to allow direct suture.

Sclera[3] is an excellent covering material, as its smooth surface allows for easy implantation. However, it is not sterilized and there is a theoretical risk of contamination and there is a particular concern over prion disease. Although no cases of transmission by this route have yet been reported and the risk must be considered remote, there are four case reports of patients developing Creutzfeld-Jacob disease having had corneal grafts from donors who have died from this same disease[4].

Mersilene® mesh[5] can be likened to a porous coat and thus provides a rough surface. This makes deep implantation difficult, and there is the need for a temporary smooth covering (see Figure 17.2). High extrusion rates have been reported from some centres and reflect the increased technical difficulty[6]. Vicryl® mesh[7,8] and Dacron mesh[9] are also available.

IMPLANT MATERIALS

Implant materials can be classified as vital (i.e. dermis fat) or non-vital, and the latter substances can be subclassified into first- and second-generation materials. First-generation materials included glass, plastic and gold, all of which are inert and well tolerated.

SECOND-GENERATION IMPLANT MATERIALS

Second-generation implant materials are characterized by being porous, which allows in-growth of host tissue into the implant. The major advantage is that once vascularized there is a reduced risk of late extrusion (because the implant can sustain a thin covering) and of late migration (because the implant is much more firmly anchored). It will also allow subsequent drilling because the hole will re-epithelialize, although it takes 6 months for the implant to become vascularized (this can be checked by either an MRI scan or by a technetium bone scan).

The most important criterion for tissue in-growth is pore size, which should be a minimum of 40 μm and ideally 150 μm. The pore size for hydroxyapatite is $400\,\mu$m, and it is $100-200\,\mu$m for the high density porous polyethylene implants used for orbital floor implants and facial remodelling.

Hydroxyapatite

This was the most commonly used material (56 per cent) in the USA in 1995, and it was most frequently wrapped in sclera (59 per cent)[10]. However, it is too hard to attach sutures to directly and therefore needs to be covered. It has also been reported to cause more post-operative pain[11-13] than other implants materials.

High density porous polyethylene (Medpor®)

The polyethylenes are straight-chain aliphatic hydrocarbon chains created under high pressure and temperature. The length of the chains depends upon the conditions under which the polymerization occurs. Short chains act as lubricants, while long chains form solids. High density porous polyethylene (HDPP) was licensed for use as a medical grade implantable material by the FDA in America in 1985, but it was first used for facial reconstruction in 1947[14].

Although experience with HDPP is more limited than with hydroxyapatite, it appears to give similar results[15].

Drilling and fixing a peg for cosmesis

The only clear advantage of the porous implants is that they allow the fitting of a mechanical coupling device for oculomotility. This causes a significant improvement in the prosthetic motility, but it is not clear how this translates to improvements in patient quality of life.

Infection and porous materials

All foreign materials are vulnerable to chronic infection, and the presence of inert material somehow enhances micro-organism survival. The incidence of infection with porous materials is low, but two cases of *S. epidermidis* have been described with hydroxyapatite[16] and a case of *Actinomyces* with HDPP[17]. Several big series have reported no infections[9,13,18].

BIOLOGICAL MATERIALS – DERMIS FAT

Dermis fat has several advantages:

1. There is no risk of extrusion.
2. Infections can be treated as for any soft tissue infection, without the need of removal of the implant.
3. Fat can also provide an increased lining as well as volume augmentation.
4. It provides good oculomotility, which at least equals that seen with spherical implants[19].

These advantages make a dermofat graft the technique of choice where there is concomitant shortage of linking of the socket. It does have disadvantages in that there is variable resorption, making volume replacement achieved unpredictable, and there can be complications at the donor site.

CHOICE OF SHAPE AND SIZE

SHAPE

The eye is crudely spherical, and this is therefore the obvious shape for an implant. The key difference is that the surface of the eye is exposed, while it is necessary to ensure that all implants are covered; hence volume implanted must be less than that of the removed eye. Final volume enhancement is with the ocular prosthesis.

The first orbital implants were hollow glass spheres[20], which were implanted into Tenon's capsule and the extraocular muscles imbricated in front of them. The problem with this was that the implant tended to migrate outside the muscle cone[21]. As a result two sets of solutions were hit upon, both relying on the extraocular muscles being attached to the implant. The first method was to provide channels through which the muscles could be threaded, such as the Castrovejo, Allen and Roper-Hall implants (Figure 18.1). The other technique was to wrap the implant in a material to which the muscles could be directly sutured. The scleral-wrapped acrylic ball implant was described in 1976 by Frueh and Felker[22], who proposed its use as a secondary implant; it has since become apparent that they work equally well as a primary implant[23].

There are two problems with the Castrovejo/Roper-Hall/Allen implants, both due to them being effectively hemispheres. They are of relatively low volume and, if they rotate, give 'edge effects' (i.e. from the rim), giving an uneven surface. This makes fitting of a prosthesis more difficult and causes thinning of the covering.

Despite the large amount of work on implant material, it appears that shape is more important. The Bristol group reviewed their patients and, although numbers were small, they could show no benefit of hydroxyapatite versus acrylic balls. However, spherical implants appeared to do better than Castrovejo implants, and all did better than non-implanted sockets[24]. Other shapes, such as the conical implant, are being developed which may be an improvement on the ball implant[25].

SIZE

The volume of a normal eye is approximately 8 ml. Ball implants come in a range of sizes in 2 mm steps, and a small increase in size makes a big difference to the increase in volume – an 18-mm diameter implant is about 3 cm^3 in volume, whilst a 20-mm implant is about 4 cm^3. This is only half the removed volume, and the extra volume is generally provided by the prosthesis. If more volume is required, the standard

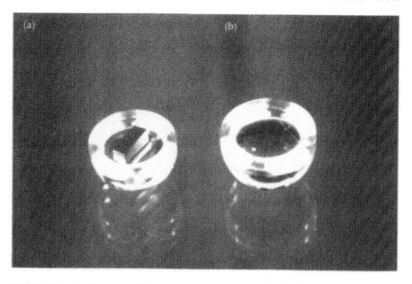

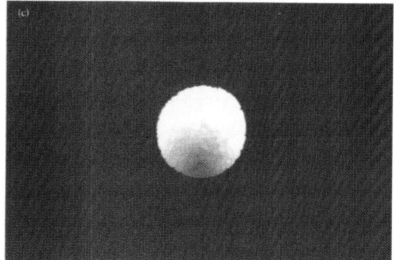

Figure 18.1 Two examples of hemispherical implants. (a) The Roper–Aleen implant with a magnet incorporated to enhance motility and (b) The Allen implant. (c) A ball implant made from high density polyethylene (Medpor®).

approach is to perform an orbital floor implant. Too large an implant should, however, be avoided, as room must be left to fit a prosthesis.

WHICH IMPLANT IS BEST?

This cannot be answered definitively[26], given the lack of any controlled trials comparing shape, technique or material. That said, a HDPP 20-mm ball implant for enucleations and an 18-mm ball for eviscerations is the author's current practice.

REFERENCES

1. Tyers, A. G. and Collin, J. R. O. (1985). Baseball orbital implants: a review of 39 patients. *Br. J. Ophthalmol.*, **69**, 438–442.

2. Leatherbarrow, B., Kwartz, J., Sunderland, S. *et al.* (1994). The 'baseball' orbital implant: a prospective study. *Eye*, **8**, 569–76.
3. Soll, D. B. (1974). Donor sclera in enucleation surgery. *Arch.Ophthalmol.*, **92**, 494–5.
4. Lang, C. J., Heckmann, J. G. and Neundorfer, B. (1998). Creutzfeldt-Jakob disease via dural and corneal transplants. (Review.) *J. Neurol. Sci.*, **160(2)**, 128–39.
5. Hughes, J. D., Downes, R. N. and Kemp, E. (1992). The Mersilene® covered intraorbital implant. *Eye*, **6**, 484–6.
6. Yalaz, M., Demircan, N., Yagmur, M. and Haciyakupoglu, G. (1997). Mersilene mesh: long-term results in oculoplastic surgery. *Orbit*, **16**, 217–23.
7. Jordan, D. R., Ells, A., Brownstein, S. *et al.* (1995). Vicryl®-mesh wrap for the implantation of hydroxyapatite orbital implants: an animal model. *Can. J. Ophthalmol.*, **30**, 241–6.
8. Jordan, D. R., Allen, L. H., Ells, A. *et al.* (1995). The use of vicryl mesh (polyglactin 910) for implantation of hydroxyapatite orbital implants. *Ophthal. Plast. Reconstr. Surg.*, **11**, 95–9.
9. Oestreicher, J. H., Liu, E. and Berkowitz, M. (1997). Complications of hydroxyapatite orbital implants. A review of 100 consecutive cases and a comparison of Dexon® mesh (polyglycolic acid) with scleral wrapping. (Review.) *Ophthalmology*, **104**, 324–9.
10. Hornblass, A., Biesman, B. S. and Eviatar, J. A. (1995). Current techniques of enucleation: a survey of 5439 intraorbital implants and a review of the literature. *Ophthal. Plast. Reconstr. Surg.*, **11**, 77–88.
11. Waterman, H., Leatherbarrow, B., Slater, R. *et al.* (1998). The hydroxyapatite orbital implant: post-operative pain. *Eye*, **12**, 996–1000.
12. Waterman, H., Slater, R., Leatherbarrow, B. *et al.* (1998). Post-operative nausea and vomiting following orbital hydroxyapatite implant surgery. *Eur. J. Anaesthesiol.*, **15**, 590–94.
13. McNab, A. (1995). Hydroxyapatite orbital implants. Experience with 100 cases. *Aust. NZ J. Ophthalmol.*, **23**, 117–23.
14. Rubin, L. R. (1983). Polyethylene as a bone and cartilage substitute: a 32-year retrospective. In: *Biomaterials in Reconstructive Surgery*, 1st edn (L. R. Rubin, ed.), pp. 484–93. CV Mosby.
15. Karesh, J. W. and Dresner, S. C. (1994). High-density porous polyethylene (Medpor®) as a successful anophthalmic socket implant. *Ophthalmology*, **101**, 1688–96.
16. Jordan, D. R., Brownstein, S. and Jolly, S. S. (1996). Abscessed hydroxyapatite orbital implants: a record of two cases. *Ophthalmology*, **103**, 1784–7.
17. Karcioglu, Z. A. (1997). Actinomyces infection in porous polyethylene orbital implant. *Graef. Arch. Clin. Exp. Ophthalmol.*, **235**, 448–51.
18. Shields, C. L., Shields, J. A., De Potter, P. *et al.* (1993). Lack of complications of the hydroxyapatite orbital implant in 250 consecutive cases. *Trans. Am. Acad. Ophth. Otolaryngol.*, **91**, 177–95.
19. Bosniak, S. L., Nesi, F., Smith, B. C. *et al.* (1989). A comparison of motility: autogenous dermis-fat vs. synthetic spherical implants. *Ophthal. Surg.*, **20**, 889–91.
20. Mules, P. H. (1885). Evisceration of the globe with artifical vitreous. *Trans. Ophthal. Soc. UK*, **5**, 200–206.
21. Allen, L. (1983). The argument against imbricating the rectus muscles over spherical orbital implants after enucleation. *Ophthalmology*, **90**, 1116–20.
22. Frueh, B. R. and Felker, G. V. (1976). Baseball implant: a method of secondary insertion of an intraorbital implant. *Arch. Ophthalmol.*, **94**, 429–30.
23. Smit, T. J., Koorneef, L., Mourits, M. *et al.* (1990). Primary versus secondary intraorbital implants. *Ophthal. Plast. Reconstr. Surg.*, **6**, 115–18.
24. Ghabrial, R., Potts, M. J., Harrad, R. A. *et al.* (1997). Assessment of the anophthalmic socket with dynamic cine-MRI. *Orbit*, **16**, 207–16.
25. Rubin, P. A. D., Popham, J., Rumelt, S. *et al.* (1998). Enhancement of the cosmetic and functional outcome of enucleation with the conical implant. *Ophthalmology*, **105**, 919–25.
26. Downes, R. (1996). Orbital implants: food for thought. *Eye*, **10**, 1–3.

19

LACRIMAL SURGERY

SYRINGING AND PROBING

INDICATION

This is the treatment for congenital nasolacrimal duct obstruction, and should be limited to second-line treatment following the first-line treatment of observation. Up to 20 per cent of infants are born with nasolacrimal obstruction; 96 per cent of them will have resolved spontaneously by the end of the first year[1], and another two-thirds by their second birthday[2]. Probing at 1 year will shorten the time to resolution, but there is no significant difference at 2 years for those probed and not-probed[1]. Spontaneous resolution has also been observed in the third year of life.

Probing into the lacrimal sac is helpful diagnostically for acquired nasolacrimal obstruction, but passing the probe down the nasolacrimal duct is of little, if any, therapeutic value in contrast to congenital obstruction.

INSTRUMENTS

Three special instruments are required for this and all lacrimal procedures; a lacrimal cannula, a punctal dilator and lacrimal probes.

PROCEDURE

The key issue when performing syringing and probing is to be gentle. Traumatic probing may cause scarring of the lacrimal system and do more harm than good.

1. First locate the punctum. This is situated one-sixth away from the medial end of the lid, and it is the anatomical mark that divides the lid into ciliary and lacrimal portions. It is situated in line with the grey line and is usually easily identified in children although it can be difficult in adults. The normal puncta is directed backwards and is only visible if the lid is slightly everted. It is also surrounded

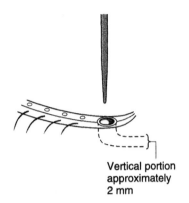

Figure 19.1 The initial part of the inferior canaliculus is vertical to the ampulla.

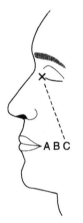

Figure 19.2 The surface anatomical markings for the nasolacrimal duct. In the lateral view, the direction of the probe is from the corner of the eye towards the first upper molar tooth. It is in a slightly posterior direction. A, angle of mouth at the canine teeth; B, modiolus (the knot of muscle of the interdigitating orbicularis oris) located at the second premolar tooth; C, first molar tooth.

by a ring of fibrous tissue, which is avascular and thus appears white. If there is a problem with one canaliculus, try the other one.

2. Dilate the punctum to allow passage of a probe. A Nettleship dilator is the most commonly used, and it should be noted that the initial course of the canaliculus is vertical to the ampulla (Figure 19.1); it then becomes horizontal. Any kinks in the passage can be straightened by pulling the lid laterally.

3. Following dilatation, insert a probe and advance it until it is in the lacrimal sac, where its passage will be halted by the bone lining the lacrimal fossa (hard stop). If it cannot advance that far (soft stop), then abort the procedure.

4. Next, pass the probe down the nasolacrimal duct by rotating it 90°. The duct travels in a slightly postero-lateral direction, so aim in the direction of the ipsilateral first upper molar tooth (Figure 19.2). Gently advance and withdraw the probe, and keep changing its position until there is no resistance; advance again until reaching a hard stop. The probe has entered the duct if it can be released and remain vertical. The presumed aetiology of congenital nasolacrimal obstruction is membranous obstruction, which the probe breaks. However, it is very unusual to feel such an obstruction.

After probing, prescribe a short course of topical antibiotics (e.g. chloramphenicol q.d.s. for 1 week).

PUNCTAL SURGERY – THREE-SNIP PROCEDURE

INDICATION

Punctal surgery is indicated for a stenosed punctum with easily patent syringing. The classical causes of punctal scarring are herpes simplex and blepharitis.

PROCEDURE

The procedure is exactly as the name suggests – three snips (Figure 19.3).

1. Snip 1 – use St Martin's forceps to grasp the punctum, and make a vertical cut with Vanna's scissors between the punctum and conjunctival mucosa.

2. Snip 2 – cut along the lid margin as posteriorly as possible (i.e. close to the mucosal surface), but do not extend the cut into the common canaliculus.

3. Snip 3 – peel back the posterior flap and make a second cut on the mucosal side.

It will heal and end up with a smaller orifice with time.

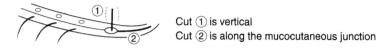

Cut ① is vertical
Cut ② is along the mucocutaneous junction

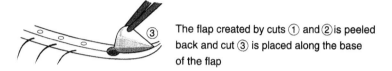

The flap created by cuts ① and ② is peeled
back and cut ③ is placed along the base
of the flap

Figure 19.3 The three-snip operation.

DACROCYSTORHINOSTOMY

The purpose of dacrocystorhinostomy is to create an anastomosis between the mucosa of the lacrimal sac and the nasal mucosa, which requires the removal of the intervening bone. The new opening into the nose occurs just in front of the middle turbinate, which occasionally needs removing. Toti is usually credited with devising the operation and gave a description of it in 1904[3], but it was Dupuy-Dutemps and Bourguet, in 1920–1921, who suggested that the lacrimal and nasal mucosa should be formally anastomized to create an epithelial-lined fistula. The operation has undergone only minor modifications since, and the published success rates are in excess of 90 per cent.

INDICATIONS

The major indications are:

1. Watering of the eye in association with a blocked nasolacrimal duct.
2. A persistent lacrimal mucocoele causing symptoms. This must be distinguished from a chronic canaliculitis, which is usually due to *Actinomyces israeli* (see Chapter 29).
3. Recurrent attacks of dacrocystitis.

The pathology in all these cases is a blockage of the nasolacrimal duct. In most cases the cause of the blockage is unknown, but it is commoner in the elderly and in women rather than men.

The operation is technically easier if there is a mucocoele, as that implies a large lacrimal sac.

THE BLEEDING PROBLEM

Dacrocystorhinostomies are notorious for problems with bleeding. Despite such a small incision the total blood loss can, on occasion, even threaten the haemodynamic stability of the patient. Bleeding also

obscures all the anatomical landmarks, making the operation technically formidable, and the following steps should be taken to minimize
this problem:

1. Ask the patient to avoid aspirin and related drugs for a week
   before the operation. Try to avoid operating on patients taking
   anticoagulants or with a known bleeding diathesis.
2. Ask for a degree of hypotension from the anaesthetist.
3. In addition to the general anaesthetic, inject the site of the skin
   incision, the superior and inferior canalicular area and the infra-
   trochlear region with a vasoconstrictor (e.g. lignocaine 2% with
   1 : 200 000 adrenaline).
4. Pack the nose with a vasoconstrictor such as cocaine (e.g. Moffet's
   solution).
5. At surgery, avoid cutting the orbicularis muscle and go through
   this layer by blunt dissection.
6. Remember, all bleeding can be stopped with pressure. Use traction
   sutures routinely.
7. There is a constant but unnamed branch of the infraorbital artery
   that runs in the suture of Notha (or the sutura longitudionalis
   imperfeta of Weber). It gives off a number of minute twigs that
   enter the 'suture' and supply the nasal mucosa. This structure
   should be routinely diathermied.

PROCEDURE

Preparation and anaesthesia

Minimize bleeding as described above. This is one of the remaining
clinical uses of cocaine, which is a powerful local anaesthetic and
vasoconstrictor. Moffet's solution is cocaine hydrochloride 6% with
adrenaline 0.05% in 2 ml, to which 2 ml of sodium bicarbonate 2% is
added just prior to use. Apply this after the patient is asleep and has a
throat pack in. The area that needs packing is the area just in front of
the middle turbinate, as this will be the internal site of the osteotomy
(Figure 19.4). Pack it with ribbon gauze soaked in Moffet's solution,

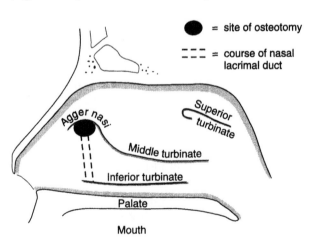

● = site of osteotomy

▬ ▬ ▬ = course of nasal
lacrimal duct

Agger nasi

Superior turbinate

Middle turbinate

Inferior turbinate

Palate

Mouth

Figure 19.4 Internal view of the
lateral wall of the nasal cavity.

or deposit the solution straight down the nostril with the patient lying horizontally with a slight chin up position. It will then form a pool over the sphenoidal bone and in particular the sphenopalatine foramen, through which the sphenopalatine artery (the main blood supply to the nose) passes. A combination of the two methods may be used.

A less effective alternative is to soak two or three cotton buds with 1 : 1000 adrenaline and place these up the nose, again trying to place them just in front of the middle turbinate.

Inject lignocaine 2% with 1 : 200 000 adrenaline under the site of the skin incision, below the inferior canaliculus and above the superior canaliculus, and use an infra-trochlear block to further help to minimize bleeding. The major blood supply to the anterior ethmoidal air cells is from the anterior ethmoidal artery, and the infra-trochlear block will vasoconstrict this vessel.

Making the incision

There are a number of minor variations on the exact location of the skin incision because there are two conflicting desires. The first is to avoid the angular vein, which classically runs across the medial canthal tendon 8 mm from the medial canthus, on the flat side of the nose. The second is deliberately to site the incision on the flat of the nose, as a scar that runs across a hollow has a tendency to bowstring as it contracts, resulting in an epicanthic fold; this is probably the more important consideration.

Make an incision about 2 cm long, starting just above the medial canthal tendon and running straight down along the flat of the nose.

Locating the medial canthal tendon

Dissect down to the bone. The key landmark is the orbital rim (Figure 19.5), and dissection can be quickly completed with blunt-tipped scissors, which can be burrowed down to the orbital rim and then spread, first along the rim and then at right angles. Perform this dissection above and below the medial canthal tendon. Identify the tendon itself, by blunt dissection, as a white structure, and cut the tendon along with the periosteum just in front of the anterior lacrimal crest using a no. 15 Bard Parker or the cutting edge of a Roulet rougine.

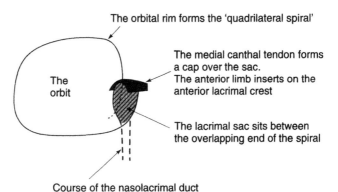

The orbital rim forms the 'quadrilateral spiral'

The orbit

The medial canthal tendon forms a cap over the sac.
The anterior limb inserts on the anterior lacrimal crest

The lacrimal sac sits between the overlapping end of the spiral

Course of the nasolacrimal duct

Figure 19.5 Anatomy of the medial canthal tendon.

Strip the periosteum off the side of the nose, working medially, then place four traction sutures (e.g. 4/0 silk) to make the wound into a square opening (placement can be helped by the principle of 'half and half again' – see Figure 19.6). The two medial sutures can take in periosteum. If bleeding is heavy at an earlier stage, use the sutures earlier and more generously (e.g. four for the skin, four for the orbicularis and then two or more for the periosteum). All bleeding can be stopped with pressure, and traction sutures are especially useful if the source cannot be identified.

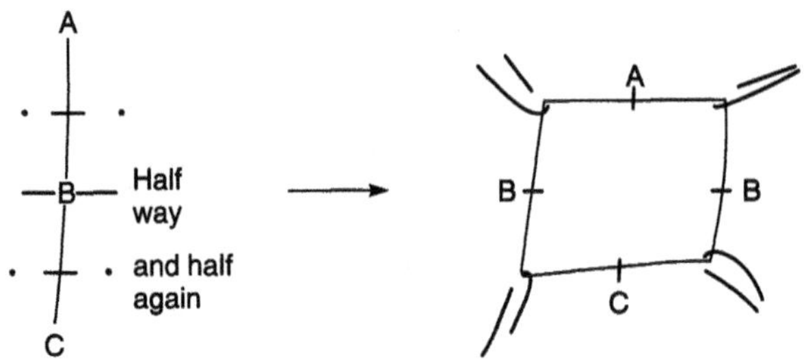

Figure 19.6. The principle of half and half again for the placement of traction sutures.

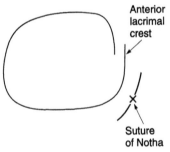

Figure 19.7 Position of the suture of Notha.

At this stage there will invariably be bleeding from the 'suture of Notha' (Figure 19.7), and this should be diathermied as soon as it is identified. This suture has also occasionally been mistaken for the lacrimal suture, although it lies medial and anterior to the anterior lacrimal crest, whereas the lacrimal suture always lies within the lacrimal fossa (i.e. behind the anterior lacrimal crest). Notha means 'bastard' or 'illegitimate', and was so-named by anatomists because it is not a proper suture. It was well named.

Locating the lacrimo-maxillary suture and the anterior ethmoidal air cells

The periosteum can easily be stripped going back into the lacrimal fossa. Its only firm point of attachment is the lacrimo-maxillary suture; tear this attachment and strip the periosteum back beyond this to expose the whole floor of the lacrimal fossa. The usual way to commence the osteotomy is to dislocate the lacrimo-maxillary suture using an instrument such as a Traquair's periosteal elevator. It is much easier to enter the lacrimo-maxillary suture by pressing on the lacrimal bone part of it. Do this as high up the suture as possible in order to increase the chance of entering an air cell and therefore reduce the likelihood of tearing the nasal mucosa[4].

The lower half of the lacrimal fossa directly borders the nasal cavity, but the upper half is usually separated by anterior ethmoidal air cells. The bone covering these air cells is the lamina papyracea (literally paper-thin) and can be entered easily by pressure with any blunt instrument[5], and an easier way to commence the osteotomy is to look for an anterior ethmoidal air cell. In over 90 per cent of cases the anterior air cells border the posterior part of the lacrimal fossa; however, there is considerable anatomical variation of the air cells, which can make life difficult (Figure 19.8).

Figure 19.8 Anatomy of the anterior ethmoidal air cells. (a) The superior part of the lacrimal sac is bordered by anterior ethmoidal air cells, which form the agger nasi (see Figure 19.4). The lower part borders the nasal cavity directly. (b) The dotted lines mark the anterior extension of the ethmoid air cells in relation to the upper half of the lacrimal fossa, with the percentage marked above.

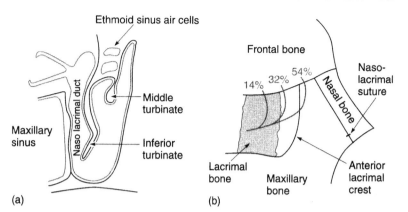

Figure 19.9 Making the osteotomy: removing the bone. Starting from the lacrimal-maxillary suture, go forward (1), then down along thin bone (2) and back (3), leaving the thick bone of the anterior lacrimal crest until last.

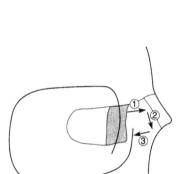

Making the osteotomy

Remember to remove the nasal pack before beginning the osteotomy. The osteotomy needs to be about 2 × 2 cm, and the hardest part is where the bone is thickest, which is the frontal process of the maxilla where it forms the anterior lacrimal crest. Figure 19.9 shows the suggested order for removing the bone.

The osteotomy often starts from within an ethmoidal air cell. The easiest approach is to remove the thin bone first using up- and then down-cutting bone punches, and so undermine the thick bone; taking care not to damage the nasal mucosa by ensuring that the mucosa is separated from the bone using a Traquair periosteal elevator between each bite. A second problem is the possibility of causing a saddle nose by removing the bone that forms the bridge of the nose. The osteotomy may reach, but should not cross, the naso-maxillary suture (Figure 19.9). The osteotomy should extend posteriorly to close to the posterior lacrimal crest and include the floor of the fossa.

Deboning the medial wall of the nasolacrimal duct

Three bones form the nasolacrimal canal – the maxilla, lacrimal and inferior nasal concha. The anterior part of the nasal surface of the maxilla has a groove called the sulcus lacrimalis. The descending process of the lacrimal bone forms the medial wall, and it articulates with the inferior concha, which overlies the opening of the duct in the deepest part of the inferior meatus. The lacrimal bone can be safely removed in its entirety.

Deboning the nasal mucosa

The osteotomy usually starts in an anterior ethmoidal air cell, and although the deep tissue may look like mucosa, it usually contains bone. Debone this area by feel (it gives a gritty or grating sensation), using toothed forceps, or the posterior nasal flap will not be mobile and fall back into a good position.

Size of the osteotomy

There is a belief that success rates are related to the size of the osteotomy but, although a 2 × 2 cm osteotomy has been suggested, there is little evidence to support this. Osseous closure is a rare cause of DCR failure[5], and there is little relation between the size of the osteotomy and the size of the final drainage passage, which is often ten times smaller than the bony osteotomy[6]. In endolaser DCR, the size of the osteotomy is only 2×2 mm and the flaps are not sutured, but still the success rate is in excess of 60 per cent.

Creating the nasal flaps

It is sensible to make the nasal flaps before the lacrimal sac flaps, as this opens up the nose and increases the working space. Before cutting the nasal flaps, make sure that the mucosa has been adequately deboned. Create the flaps by inserting a Stallard or a handle for a Bard-Parker up the nose to press against and making a cut with a no. 11 blade, then complete with spring scissors if necessary; the ratio of the anterior flap to posterior flap should be $2:1$. The anterior flap can then be retracted using a 6/0 Vicryl® suture; leave the needle on and secure the two ends of the suture with a bull-dog, and this same suture can then be used later for anastomosing the anterior flaps.

Opening the lacrimal sac

The sac is defined by passing a lacrimal probe through either the upper or the lower canaliculus. The sac can be made more prominent by inflating it with viscoelastic or hypromellose or marking it with a dye, but it is usually found easily enough without such manoeuvres. The lacrimal fascia is in continuity with the medial canthal tendon, and lifting the cut lateral end or inserting a lacrimal probe should result in tenting the lacrimal fascia and sac; this should help in avoiding accidental damage to the common canaliculus when making the stab incision with a no. 11 or no. 12 blade (Figure 19.10).

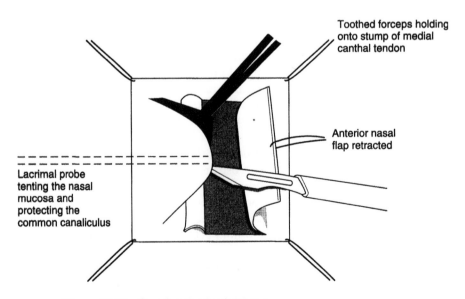

Toothed forceps holding onto stump of medial canthal tendon

Anterior nasal flap retracted

Lacrimal probe tenting the nasal mucosa and protecting the common canaliculus

Figure 19.10 Entering the lacrimal sac.

Pass the end of a squint hook into the sac through the stab incision and use this to tent the sac open while extending the incision initially downwards using spring scissors (Figure 19.11). It is surprisingly easy not to open the lacrimal sac, which has a very well defined fascia and a thin and loosely adherent mucosa, such that a lacrimal probe can pass through the mucosa and tent the lacrimal fascia. This can be opened and mistaken for the sac, so pass an instrument down the nasolacrimal duct to ensure that the sac is opened. Failure to open the sac is probably the commonest cause for DCR failure, and leads to the presence of a 'sac remnant' when a DCG is performed on a patient who has had unsuccessful DCR surgery. Once the sac is defined, open it with, ideally, a single cut. Then angle the scissors upwards and extend the cut to the roof (or fundus) of the sac and again make two relieving cuts to create the flaps.

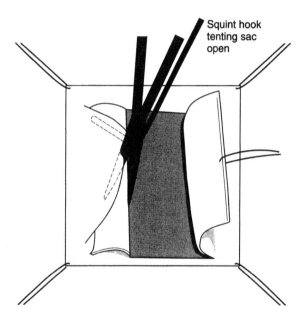

Squint hook tenting sac open

Figure 19.11 The squint hook tents the sac open and lets the blade from a pair of spring scissors slip in and open it.

Extend the vertical opening of the lacrimal sac to include the nasolacrimal duct; failure to do so results in a blind pouch of the nasolacrimal duct remaining, which can cause the sump syndrome.

Having cut down, make two relieving cuts in order to turn the slit into flaps and then angle the scissors upwards and extend the cut to the roof of the sac and again make two relieving cuts to create the flaps.

Making the anastomosis

The posterior nasal and lacrimal flaps should spontaneously lie back and appose each other. The posterior nasal flap may not fall back because it is still supported by bone, either residual lamina papyracea or the middle turbinate which, in 15 per cent of cases, encroaches across the osteotomy. The middle turbinate is attached to the cribriform plate, so it is most safely removed by 'nibbling' – do not simply grab and pull!

Suture the posterior flaps using a fine absorbable suture (three stitches are standard). Some surgeons do not suture the posterior flaps, and occasionally it is impossible if there is heavy bleeding that obscures the view. It is suspected that failure to suture the posterior flaps compromises the success rate of the operation, but it should be noted again that with endolaser DCR the opening that is created is much smaller and there is no effort to perform mucosa-to-mucosa anastomosis, but the success rate still approaches 70 per cent[7,8]. When suturing down a deep hole, it is easiest to use a half-circle or five-eighths needle.

Suture the anterior flaps together. Access is not difficult; use three to five 6/0 Vicryl® sutures. If the anterior nasal flap has been damaged or destroyed during the surgery, then suture the anterior lacrimal flap to the nasal periosteum.

Closure

Deep closure is usually limited to one stitch to reform the medial canthal tendon (or suture the lateral stump to the nasal periosteum). The orbicularis muscle does not require suturing, and the skin is closed in the standard manner.

MODIFICATIONS AND OPERATIVE DIFFICULTIES

Bleeding is the single most common problem encountered during surgery (as discussed above).

The use of silicone tubes is often considered to be the universal panacea for difficult DCR surgery. The standard indications are usually listed as: active infection in the sac (as may occur in a chronic mucocoele); the presence of common canalicular disease or a membrane covering the opening of the common canaliculus; intra-operative haemorrhage; and endolaser DCR. All these situations are risk factors for surgical failure, and a stent is used to maintain patency of the lacrimal system during the healing process. There is no consensus on how long they should remain[9], and it is not even clear whether they help the operation success rate[10]; there is even a suggestion that routine use in uncomplicated surgery may jeopardize it by promoting granulation tissue and subsequent closure of the nasal ostium[9].

Nasal mucosa is easily damaged and it may be impossible to construct neat flaps. The standard solution is the use of bridging sutures from the lacrimal flaps to the remnants of the nasal mucosa.

The lacrimal sac may be damaged. It is not uncommon, when learning to perform this operation, to find that when passing the lacrimal probe it immediately appears in the operation site. This means that the lacrimal sac has already been inadvertently opened. The major problem is that the opening is usually small and failure to open it properly will result in a high risk of failure. A squint hook is ideal for searching for the opening and, when found, the hook can be passed into the sac and used to tent it; it will not pass between fascia and lacrimal sac mucosa. This makes it relatively easy to slip a blade of the spring scissors into the sac and then fully open it.

LACRIMAL FISTULA

There are two sorts of lacrimal fistulas; congenital and acquired. Acquired fistulas occur secondarily to dacrocystitis. The correct treatment is as for any acquired fistula – ignore it and re-establish the correct flow pathway (i.e. a DCR) and the fistula will spontaneously close.

By contrast, congenital fistulas are epithelialized tracks and there is no blockage in the normal drainage pathway. The correct approach is to dissect out and remove the tract.

COMPLICATIONS

The major complications are:

1. Soft tissue infection. The incidence can be markedly reduced by prophylactic antibiotics[11].
2. Nose bleed. A small amount of blood from the nose is normal in the immediate postoperative period.
3. Delayed or secondary haemorrhage. About 1 per cent of patients suffer a severe haemorrhage at around day five after the surgery; at this stage the patient is usually at home and this is therefore a particularly frightening complication for the patient. It requires urgent admission, possible blood transfusion and help from the ENT surgeons to pack the nose. This is usually thought to occur as a result of wound infection, and thus it seems sensible to maintain prophylactic antibiotics for the first postoperative week and not simply rely on an intra-operative bolus dose. A second risk factor for postoperative infection is the formation of a crust at the internal osteotomy, and this can be prevented by nasal douching.
3. Recurrent epiphora – that is, the surgery has failed to help the patient. The published success rates are in excess of 90 per cent, but this is an area where a successful outcome is poorly defined. Notwithstanding that, it is a highly successful operation for those patients who have epiphora secondary to nasolacrimal obstruction.
4. The sump syndrome. This is a rare complication, where the epiphora has been successfully treated but the remnant of the nasolacrimal duct forms a cup in which stagnant fluid can collect and become infected[12]. It requires re-operation, classically by open surgery with the aim of fully opening up the wall of the nasolacrimal duct.

POSTOPERATIVE CARE

Postoperative care varies considerably between surgeons, but a typical standard regime is:

1. Prophylactic broad-spectrum antibiotics for 7 days
2. Nasal douching twice a day for 2 weeks
3. Guttae Betnasol-N q.d.s. for 4 weeks, to reduce the inflammatory phase of healing with the idea of improving fistula patency rates
4. Skin stitches out at 5–7 days
5. Silicone tubing out (if used) at 12 weeks (times vary from 6 weeks to 6 months, with no evidence to favour one time point over another).

REFERENCES

1. MacEwen, C. J. and Young, J. D. H. (1991). Epiphora during the first year of life. *Eye*, **5**, 596–600.
2. Young, J. D. H., MacEwen, C. J. and Ogston, S. A. (1996). Congenital nasolacrimal duct obstruction in the second year of life: a multicentre trial of management. *Eye*, **10**, 485–91.
3. Toti, A. (1904). Nuovo metodo conservatore di cura radicale delle suppurazione del sacco lacrimale (cadriocistorhinostomia). *Clin. Moderna (Firenze)*, **10**, 385.
4. Blaylock, W. K., Moore, C. A. and Linberg, J. V. (1990). Anterior ethmoid anatomy facilitates dacrocystorhinostomy. *Arch. Ophthalmol.*, **108**, 1774–7.
5. McLachlan, D. L., Shannon, G. M. and Flanagan, J. C. (1980). Results of dacrocystorhinostomy: analysis of the reoperations. *Ophthalmic Surg.*, **11**, 427–30.
6. Linberg, J. V., Anderson, R. L., Bumsted, R. M. and Barreras, R. (1982). Study of intranasal ostium external dacrocystorhinostomy. *Arch. Ophthalmol.*, **100**, 1758–62.
7. Boush, G. A., Lemke, B. N. and Fortzbach, R. K. (1994). Results of endonasal laser-assisted dacrocystorhinostomy. *Ophthalmology*, **101**, 955–9.
8. Kong, Y. T., Kim, T. I. and Kong, B. W. (1994). A report of 131 cases of endoscopic laser lacrimal surgery. *Ophthalmology*, **101**, 1793–1800.
9. Allen, K. and Berlin, A. J. (1989). Dacrocystorhinostomy failure: association with nasolacrimal silicone intubation. *Ophthalmic Surg.*, **20**, 486–9.
10. Walland, M. J. and Rose, G. E. (1994). The effect of silicone intubation on failure and infection rates after dacrocystorhinostomy. *Ophthalmic Surg.*, **25**, 597–600.
11. Walland, M. J. and Rose, G. E. (1994). Soft tissue infections after open lacrimal surgery. *Ophthalmology*, **101**, 608–11.
12. Jordan, D. R. and McDonald, H. (1993). Failed dacrocystorhinostomy: the sump syndrome. *Ophthalmic Surg.*, **24**, 692–3.

20

EXCISING LID TUMOURS

The majority of lesions removed from the eyelids are benign, such as cysts, chalazia, skin tags, papillomas etc. However, some lesions are more serious, including the various types of skin cancers.

CLASSIFICATION

Tumours may be benign or malignant, the latter being either primary or secondary. Precise classification depends upon the cell type of origin, but the key point is that the surgical technique should be tailored to the nature of the lesion. Clinical diagnosis can be wrong, and it is good practice to submit specimens for histological examination, especially those lesions that have recurred at the same site.

MARSUPIALIZATION

The majority of cysts arise from blocked ducted secretory glands (such as cysts of Moll). Although these cannot be unblocked directly, a new passage may be made. This works particularly well for serous glands but much less well for mucinous glands.

The simplest technique is to make a hole into the cyst with a hypodermic needle. This carries a success rate of approximately 50 per cent. A more definitive procedure is to make a bigger hole which is unlikely to close spontaneously and this is often termed marsupialization (from the latin marsupium, meaning pouch). True marsupialization involves resecting the anterior wall of a cyst and formally anastomosing the cut ends of the wall to the skin, but on the lid the procedure usually done is de-roofing.

CURETTAGE

Benign epidermal lesions, such as basal papillomas, skin tags, molluscum contagiosum, actinic keratosis etc., can be readily removed by curettage. This is a simple technique that can be used in outpatients. It effectively removes the lesion, leaving a partial-thickness skin defect which will usually heal without scarring. It is quick because there is no need for any type of closure.

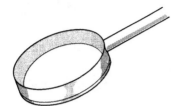

Figure 20.1   Supersharp curette.

The neatest way to do it is to score around the lesion with the point of a no. 11 scalpel blade and then remove it using a disposable super-sharp curette (Figure 20.1), which come in a number of sizes.

INCISION AND CURETTAGE

This technique is used for removal of meibomian cysts or chalazions. The key point in draining chalazia is to do it from the inside of the lid.

Inject subcutaneous and subconjunctival lignocaine 2% with adre-naline. The major problem is bleeding, which is most easily controlled by a clamp; this also facilitates everting the lid (Figure 20.2).

Lance the chalazion with a no. 11 blade and then extend this to a vertical cut, avoiding the lid margin. The chalazion is often visible as a subtle grey-yellow discoloration of the tarsus, and this should be the site of the stab incision. The contents will often ooze out, and the process is completed by insertion of a curette and scraping. Sebaceous cell carcinoma can mimic a chalazion, so the curettings from a recurrent chalazion at the same spot should be sent for histo-logical examination.

Firm pressure following removal of the clamp will minimize bruising (this can be applied by the patient using the heel of the hand and pressing for at least 6 minutes). It is standard to prescribe a short course of a topical antibiotic.

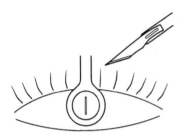

Figure 20.2   Incision and curettage for a chalazion. The lid is everted with a chalazion clamp and a vertical stab incision is made.

PRINCIPLES OF BIOPSY

There are several biopsy techniques (Figure 20.3), and the purpose of the biopsy must be clear in the surgeon's mind before performing it. In many cases where full excision would require extensive reconstruction and an error in diagnosis would have profound implications, the diag-nosis is clear clinically and the biopsy is confirmatory (e.g. basal cell carcinoma of the lid). In this situation an incisional biopsy is relatively contraindicated if the plan is to perform subsequent excision using histological control of the margins. As with any operation there is an inflammatory infiltrate afterwards, and inflammatory cells can look very similar to tumour cells in frozen and Moh's sections. An incisional biopsy can therefore compromise a Moh's procedure, and in this situation a shave biopsy from the tumour surface is the preferred technique. Most reconstruction techniques involving flaps or grafts do not lend themselves to repeating, and it is therefore imperative to ensure that excision is complete before reconstructing.

However, if the diagnosis is really not clear an incisional biopsy is preferable, and a number of points will make the pathologist's job easier:

1. Most importantly, give sufficient clinical information to the pathologist.

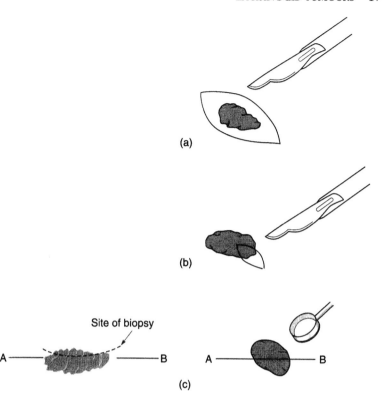

Figure 20.3 Three types of biopsy: (a) excisional; (b) incisional; (c) shave or surface biopsy.

2. The biopsy should involve the margin and include normal tissue. Simply biopsying the centre of a necrotic lesion would be uninformative.
3. Careful handling of the specimen helps avoid crush artefact; similarly, try to avoid direct infiltration of anaesthetic solution into the biopsy site.
4. Prompt fixation is important, but there are situations where unfixed material may be helpful. For example, routine processing of tissue into paraffin results in removal of lipid. For sebaceous cell carcinoma the demonstration of fat is an important diagnostic feature, and accordingly the specimen requires special processing. In this situation a fresh specimen (fixed specimens do not adhere well to glass slides without embedding) for frozen sections is helpful. The problem with fresh material is that it requires immediate handling (to avoid tissue autolysis), so the laboratory needs to be informed in advance and prompt transport for the specimen arranged.

EXCISION OF BASAL CELL CARCINOMA

It is a moot point whether basal cell carcinomas (BCCs) should be considered truly malignant as they do not metastasize, but they can certainly be invasive. Squamous cell carcinoma (SCC) of the skin is also of limited metastatic potential and can initially be managed along similar lines to BCCs. All other malignant neoplasms of the lid (e.g. melanoma and sebaceous cell carcinomas) are highly malignant and should be referred to an appropriate team.

The aim of treatment is to remove the BCC completely while preserving as much normal tissue as possible. Usually only one good reconstruction can be made using flaps, and margin control of excision is imperative if it will not be possible to close the posterior lamella defect by direct closure.

The standard margin for a BCC is 4 mm, and 98 per cent are adequately excised by such a margin[1] because the average subclinical extension of nodular BCC is 2.1 mm. By contrast, the subclinical extension of morpheaform tumours has been estimated at 7.2 mm[1], and they accordingly require margin control.

If the tumour is confined to skin and far enough away from the lid margin that none of the tarsus needs to be sacrificed, then it is reasonable to consider skin graft to close the defect without the expense and trouble of margin control. The limiting factor for good reconstruction is the posterior lamella. Full-thickness defects of one-third to half (with lateral cantholysis) of the lid can be closed directly, but if more than half of the posterior lamella of the lower lid has to be sacrificed, then reconstruction becomes problematic. The best replacement for tarsal plate is tarsal plate, which is in very short supply. Most BCCs affect the lower lid, and it is possible split the upper tarsal plate horizontally and bring it down on a pedicle (Hughes and Hewes tarso-conjunctival flaps). Such cases should be referred at the outset to an appropriate team.

SIMPLE EXCISION

It is best to plan full-thickness skin excisions as an ellipse with pointed ends so as to facilitate closure (Figure 20.3). The orientation of the long axis depends upon the line of the scar (one consideration is to hide this in a pre-existing structure such as a skin fold) and the fact that, following closure, the short axis is under tension but the long axis is not. Therefore the long axis is usually orientated to point at the lid margin so as to prevent secondary ectropion.

DIRECT CLOSURE

This is in effect performing a full-thickness wedge resection as for a lid-shortening procedure. With time the lid tissue stretches, although there is no accompanying increase in the number of skin appendages such as lashes.

LATERAL CANTHOLYSIS

A defect of about one-third of the lid can be closed directly, and an extra 2–4 mm can be gained by cutting the lateral canthal tendon.

First, find the lateral canthal tendon. Make a small lateral cut with scissors through the lateral canthus, and the lateral canthal tendon can be identified by putting the lower lid on tension and feeling a tense band. It can be isolated by putting the tips of scissors parallel to it and then spreading them, and doing this on both the conjunctival and the orbicularis surfaces of the tendon. Blunt dissect downwards under the skin and under the conjunctiva on either side of what is the lateral canthal ligament. Away from the lateral angle the conjunctiva and the lateral canthal tendon separate, leaving a clear potential space (normally occupied by a small pocket of orbital fat) in which blunt dissection is possible.

Cut the tendon. There is always bleeding at this stage, as the peripheral arterial arcade is invariably cut. Next, extend the cut with the scissors along the outer two-fifths of the orbital rim. Cut the lateral orbital septum as well as the tendon in order to mobilize the lid. Much of this procedure has to be done by feel and is not under direct vision; it is facilitated by pulling the lid medially and putting the attachments of the lid under tension.

SKIN GRAFTS

These are indicated for larger full-thickness skin or anterior lamella defects of the eyelids where direct closure is not possible and secondary intention healing is considered inappropriate.

There is a clear hierarchy in choice of donor sites, and the principle behind this is that the skin thickness should match. Upper lid skin is preferred, followed by post-auricular skin and finally supraclavicular skin. This is less important for lower lids, but is essential for the upper lid preseptal region (Figure 20.4), which is exceptionally mobile. Thick skin at this location will compromise lid opening and closing.

To perform a graft, first harvest skin. Grafts tend to shrink, and the graft should be oversized by about 10 per cent to allow for this. Next, prepare the donor site. For any defect the tissue dies back about $200\,\mu$m over 24 hours, and therefore it is necessary to debride this surface layer in old wounds.

After lack of a recipient blood supply, the single most important adverse factor is movement, which will shear nascent capillaries. The graft site must be immobilized, and the single most effective way of doing this is with bolsters – flavine-soaked cotton wool is a popular choice (Figure 20.5). When suturing the graft in place the tails of the stitches should be left long so that they can be sewn over the bolster. The bolster ensures good apposition of graft to bed, prevents haematoma formation and prevents the graft moving with respect to its bed. It should remain in place for 1 week. An alternative, currently being explored by the author, is botulinum toxin injection at least 3 days before the surgery to immobilize the graft site.

The dressing should be kept on for 1 week, after which the stitches can be removed. A healthy graft is a normal skin colour and a failed graft goes black and necrotic, but in the early postoperative period

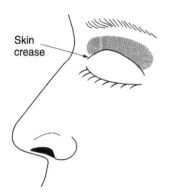

Figure 20.4 The shaded area is where skin flexibility is essential.

Skin crease

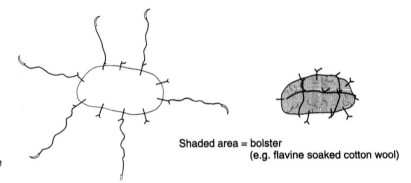

Shaded area = bolster
(e.g. flavine soaked cotton wool)

Figure 20.5.   The use of flavine wool as a bolster.

(1–2 weeks) a graft may look as if it has failed and yet still take successfully, so do not be tempted to debride it at this stage.

REFERENCE

1. Salasche, S. J. and Amonette, R. (1981). Morpheaform basal-cell epitheliomas: a study of subclinical extensions in a series of 51 cases *J. Dermatol. Surg. Oncol.*, **7**, 387–94.

21

EXTRAOCULAR MUSCLE SURGERY

The aetiology of most cases of eso- and exotropia is simply a mystery. Nevertheless, the principles behind squint surgery are extremely simple. The muscles can be thought of as guy ropes controlling a tent pole (the line of gaze), and the position of the pole can be adjusted by slackening or tightening the ropes as desired. The purpose of surgery is to try and align the poles (lines of gaze) so that they both point in the same direction. The major problem with this type of surgery is that, even following successful realignment, there is no guarantee that they will stay aligned, because the motor drive to the muscles may alter. The other principles are: first, in squints due to restrictive myopathies (such as thyroid eye disease) only recessions should be performed; and secondly, blind eyes tend to diverge with time.

While the purpose of surgery is to realign the eyes, for exotropia this is best achieved by deliberately aiming for a small overcorrection of 4–20 prism dioptres[1,2].

ANATOMY

There are several important points of anatomy:

- The relationships of the layer's of Tenon's capsule and the conjunctiva at the limbus. Tenon's fuses with the globe about 1.5 mm from the limbus, whereas conjunctiva fuses at the limbus. The correct plane to enter is the sub-Tenon's plane, and this is done by lifting conjunctiva and Tenon's 2 mm from the limbus (Figure 21.1).
- The course of the extraocular muscles can be subdivided into extracapsular or intracapsular, and most extraocular muscle surgery is on the intracapsular portion (Figure 21.2).
- Most descriptions of intermuscular septa refer to structures outside Tenon's capsule in the muscle cone, which is a continuation of the capsule from the site where the muscle penetrates it back along the muscle to fuse with its sheath. However, there are also intermuscular septa in Tenon's space, and these are variously described as falciform folds of Guerin[3], adminicula of Merkel[3] or the intracapsular ligaments of Lockwood[4]. Whatever the name, they can easily be seen and felt. For example, they form the resistance to passage of

Figure 21.1 Diagram of the limbal anatomy showing the correct place to enter the sub-Tenon's plane. (1) Tenon's fuses with the episcleral tissue 1.5 mm from the limbus; (2) the conjunctiva fuses at the limbus; (3) 2 mm from the limbus both Tenon's and conjunctiva can be lifted together using forceps.

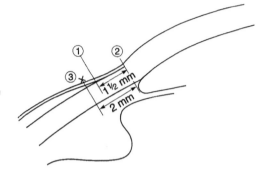

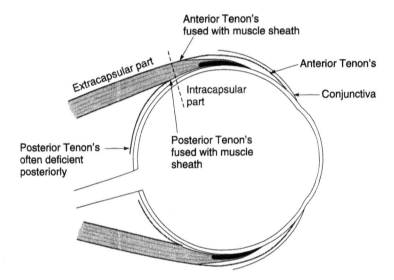

Figure 21.2 The course of the recti muscles.

a cannula when trying to perform a sub-Tenon's block, and prevent retraction of the extraocular muscles when their tendons are cut. During extraocular muscle surgery this tissue is stripped off the muscle and, if let go (or 'lost'), the muscle will recoil outside Tenon's capsule and leave a dimple in the capsule to mark its exit.

• The blood supply to the anterior segment of the eye is via the anterior ciliary arteries. These vessels run along the surface of the extraocular muscles and for this reason not more than two recti muscles should be operated on at the same time in an adult (three in a child). Although vessel-sparing techniques have been described[5,6] the results are too unpredictable to be relied upon.

HORIZONTAL RECTUS RECESSION

In any recess–resect operation, always start with the recession. This creates space.

The only difference between the medial and lateral rectus is that the lateral rectus inserts a little further from the limbus than the medial rectus. The distance of the insertions from the limbus are 5.5 mm for the medial rectus, 6.5 mm for the inferior, 7.0 mm for the lateral and

8.0 mm for the superior rectus (this orderly sequence is called the spiral of Tillaux, see Figure 22.3.

Preoperative drops (adrenaline 0.01% or phenylephrine 2.5%) can be used just before starting surgery. They are vasoconstrictors as well as dilating drops, and help reduce the bleeding.

Insert 5/0 traction sutures (on microspatulate needles) to help manipulate the globe. With bilateral muscle surgery, the obvious places for the traction sutures are at 6 and 12 o'clock, at the limbus through the conjunctiva and episclera, so that they can be used to pull the globe in either direction.

The conjunctival incisions can be made over the tendon insertion, but they heal better if the incisions are made near the limbus. Tenon's fuses with the globe about 1.5 mm from the limbus, whereas conjunctiva fuses at the limbus. The ideal plane to enter is the sub-Tenon's plane, and this is done by lifting conjunctiva and Tenon's 2 mm from the limbus and making a cut using Westcott scissors. One or two relieving incisions will be required later, and therefore it is reasonable to align the initial cut along the line of one of the future relieving incisions. A blade of the spring scissors can then be entered into the sub-Tenon's space and pushed forward to the point where Tenon's fuses with the episcleral tissue close to the limbus; with the curve of the blade oriented to follow the limbus, the peritomy can be made.

Next make the relieving incisions straight back parallel to the muscle borders. One cut results in a L-shaped incision; this is easier to close neatly, and if the relieving cut is superior, then it will be largely covered by the upper lid. Two relieving cuts give better access, but if the conjunctiva has been somewhat 'mauled' it can be hard to put back neatly.

The next step is to make a passage to allow passage of the squint hook. At the muscle insertions there are reflections of Tenon's into the sub-Tenon's space (the intermuscular septa); however, they can easily be broken by lifting the Tenon's capsule and passing blunt-tipped scissors beneath it and spreading. This should be done both above and below the muscle to prevent the squint hook getting entangled in these intermuscular septa. Having done this, lift Tenon's to reveal a dark empty space into which a squint hook can be passed. It is easy to hook only part of the muscle or to split it by the passage of the squint hook, and this is particularly likely to occur if the muscle is hooked in the wrong plane; it should be hooked in the same plane that it is lying (Figure 21.3). Therefore always hook each muscle at least twice, first from one side and then from the other side to make sure that the whole muscle is hooked. The lateral rectus insertion overlies the inferior oblique insertion, so make sure that the final hooking of the lateral rectus is from above to avoid accidentally hooking the inferior oblique.

The intracapsular portion of the muscle is covered by a sheath, which is continuous with the intermuscular septa. These can be dissected off with forceps and scissors, but the neatest way is to strip them off. Lifting up the Tenon's will reveal falciform folds of fine fascial material, which are the remnants of the intermuscular septa; grab this with a pair of forceps adjacent to one end of the muscle insertion and

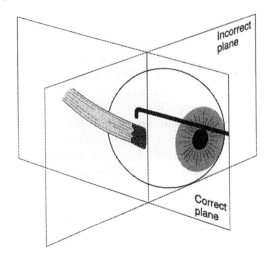

Figure 21.3 Hook the recti muscle. The squint hook should be in the same plane as the muscle.

then strip backwards along the muscle border on both sides (Figure 21.4).

The next step is to place stitches in the muscle, using an absorbable suture (e.g. 5/0–6/0 Vicryl®) on a spatulate needle. Take two bites with each suture, full thickness and partial thickness, and lock the two throws by passing the needle through the loop of suture material created when taking the second bite. Each suture incorporates the lateral third of the muscle, and it is important that the stitches are not too close to the insertion so that there is room to cut the muscle off without risk of cutting the stitches.

Next apply diathermy to the muscle along the cutting line and then cut the muscle off with spring scissors, taking care not to cut sclera. Rediathermy the stump, as the anterior ciliary arteries permit two-way flow.

Squint surgery is notoriously unpredictable. Table 21.1 gives the amounts of horizontal muscle surgery suggested by the American

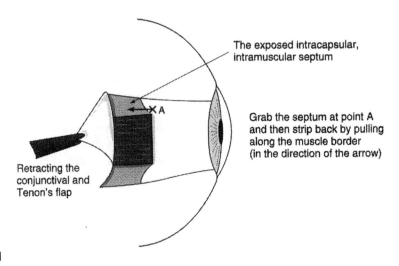

The exposed intracapsular, intramuscular septum

Grab the septum at point A and then strip back by pulling along the muscle border (in the direction of the arrow)

Retracting the conjunctival and Tenon's flap

Figure 21.4 Stripping the fascial attachment of the muscle.

Table 21.1 Amount of horizontal muscle surgery to perform for horizontal strabismus of different sizes. The figures are suggested amounts only[12], and do not take into consideration such factors as A or V patterns, previous surgery or the individual surgeon

	Symmetrical	
Esotropia (D)	Recess medial rectus (mm)	Resect lateral rectus (mm)
15	3	4
20	3.5	5
25	4	6
30	4.5	7
35	5	8
40	5.5	8
50	6	9
	Monocular recess and resect	
Esotropia (D)	Recess medial rectus (mm)	Resect lateral rectus (mm)
15	3	4
20	3.5	5
25	4	6
30	4.5	7
35	5	8
40	5.5	8
50	6	9
	Symmetrical	
Exotropia (D)	Recess lateral rectus (mm)	Resect medial rectus (mm)
15	4	3
20	5	4
25	6	5
30	7	6
	Monocular recess and resect	
Exotropia (D)	Recess lateral rectus (mm)	Resect medial rectus (mm)
15	4	3
20	5	4
25	6	5
30	7	6
	Exotropia with poor vision	
Angle (D)	Recess lateral rectus (mm)	Resect medial rectus (mm)
40	8	6
50	9	7
60	10	8
70	10	9
80	10	10

The maximum that a medial rectus can be recessed or resected is approximately 6 mm, and for a lateral rectus 8 mm, without causing a restriction on oculomotility[13].

Academy of Ophthalmology. It should be noted that squint surgery is only an approximate art, despite measurements given to the nearest half millimetre.

The muscle can be sutured back in two ways. First, it can be stitched directly to the sclera at the appropriate place by taking a partial-thickness bite of sclera, and the sutures can be aimed outwards (which will spread the muscle – Figure 21.5a) or inwards. The

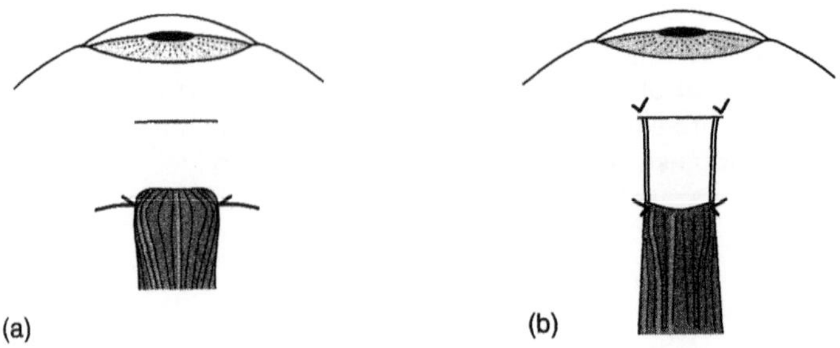

Figure 21.5 Two ways of reattaching the muscle. (a) The muscle is directly sutured to the sclera; (b) it is reattached by hangbacks.

advantage of doing this is that it is then relatively easy to move the muscle insertions up or down if desired for the correction of A or V patterns. A disadvantage is that for large recessions access can be difficult, and sometimes the sclera is extremely thin. The second method is to use hangback sutures (Figure 21.5b), which are technically much less demanding. The suture is stitched through the insertion and the muscle is left on a loop of thread. Both techniques work well.

Next close the conjunctiva, taking care not to accidentally include Tenon's capsule into the closure. The conjunctiva is slightly pink, but Tenon's is avascular (helpful in its identification) and will appear a bright white against the pink background. A tip to ensure that Tenon's has not been included is to use balanced salt solution; Tenon's will hydrate if balanced salt solution is injected into it but conjunctiva will not.

Occasionally with large recessions or reoperations it is worthwhile recessing the conjunctiva. It is fine to leave bare sclera, as it rapidly reconjunctivalizes.

Finally, give subconjuctival bupivacaine for postoperative pain relief.

HORIZONTAL RECTUS RESECTION

All the steps up to exposure and hooking the muscle are the same as for recession, but the technique diverges after the muscle has been successfully hooked. Once this has been done, pass second Chavasse squint hook (Figure 21.6), which is designed to spread the muscle.

Pre-place sutures at the distance back along the muscle belly that will correspond to the amount of the muscle to be resected. Then cut the muscle in front of the suture and remove its stump before suturing the muscle back to the insertion. Note that the effectiveness of the resection depends on how far back the sutures were placed, and not on how much is cut off.

Close the conjunctiva as for a recession.

CORRECTION OF A AND V PATTERNS

The terms A and V patterns are purely descriptive, and estimates of the incidence in the strabismic population range from 13–88 per cent[3]. An A pattern is when the eyes are more esotropic/phoric on up-gaze and

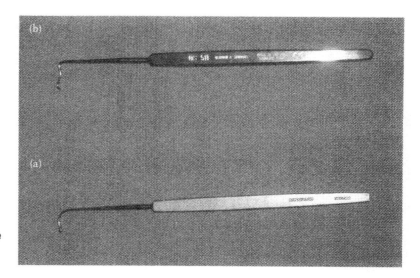

Figure 21.6 (a) The standard squint hook and (b) the Chavasse squint hook.

exotropic/phoric on down-gaze, and a V pattern is the reverse. A difference of 15 D between down- and up-gaze is diagnostic of a V pattern, and 10 D of an A pattern[7].

Just because an A or V pattern exists does not mean that it is either functionally or cosmetically significant, nor that it must necessarily be corrected. If it is to be corrected, the next step is to decide whether there is inferior oblique overaction causing the V pattern or superior oblique overaction for the A pattern. If there is a V pattern with inferior oblique overaction, then the horizontal muscle surgery can be combined with an inferior oblique weakening procedure. As always with inferior oblique weakening procedures they seem to be self-adjusting, with the same operation having a large effect when there is a large V pattern and a small effect when there is a small V pattern. An A pattern with superior oblique muscle overaction is probably best treated by surgery on the superior oblique tendon (see Figure 21.7 for posterior oblique tenotomy for correction of A patterns in association with superior oblique overaction.

When there is no clear oblique muscle overaction, then the A or V pattern can be corrected along with the horizontal deviation at the time of horizontal muscle surgery. This is done by shifting the muscle

Figure 21.7 The Fells technique for posterior oblique tenotomy (a) The incision is parallel to the limbus and centered on the lateral border of the superior rectus muscle with the globe rotated down and in. The aim is to remove a posterior triangle of the S.O. insertion as shown in (b). (b) Find and remove a triangle of superior oblique tendon, taking care to avoid any vortex veins.

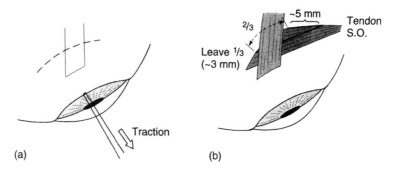

insertions (Figure 21.8). If a horizontal rectus muscle is shifted upwards it will have a greater effect on up-gaze and *vice versa* for down-gaze. Accordingly, for an A pattern shift the medial rectus insertion up and the lateral rectus insertion down by a half to one insertion width in addition to the recess–resect appropriate for the angle in the primary position. For a V pattern, move the lateral rectus upwards and the medial rectus down, again by half to one insertion width.

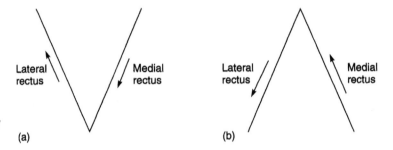

Figure 21.8 Direction required to move insertions to correct (a) V pattern and (b) A pattern.

The amount of surgery to correct the horizontal deviation is determined and performed independently of any additional procedures to correct an associated A or V pattern.

ADJUSTABLE SUTURE TECHNIQUES

Squint surgery is unpredictable, and the option to be able to fine-tune the operation with the patient awake therefore seems a very attractive option. However, it is not clear how useful this is for routine use, as there is a poor correlation between the results at 1 day and 1 month[3]. The technique is most useful if there is potential for binocular single vision but only a small fusion range, as can occur in some horizontal strabismus and most vertical deviations in an adult.

The two basic techniques for adjustable surgery are the Fells technique and the Jampolsky technique, and they differ in how the suture is passed through the sclera, but they have much in common. The operation is very similar to the standard operation (except that two conjunctival relieving incisions are necessary) and is the same up to the point of putting the suture material in the muscle, and a double-ended suture is required for both. The same material and needle type is used as for non-adjustable surgery, but this time take a bite in the middle third of the muscle, then repeat it and tie. Then with each needle, take a full-thickness and a partial-thickness bite of the edge of the muscle and lock the suture (i.e. pass it through the loop of suture material) before cutting the muscle off as for conventional surgery. For the Fells technique, pass the needles through the ends of the insertions and then loop them back and pass them through the insertion for a second time but on this occasion at the centre (Figure 21.9a). Tie the sutures as a bow and leave them with the needles cut off but the ends long for readjustment. For the Jampolsky technique, pass each needle through

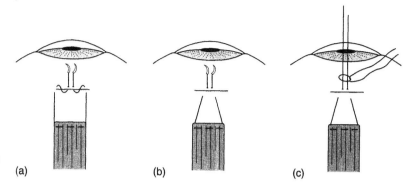

Figure 21.9 The adjustable suture techniques: (a) The Fells technique; (b) and (c) the Jampolsky techniques. In (c) there is a tie tied tightly around the two sutures with a surgical knot to increase the resistance to movement of the adjustables.

(a) (b) (c)

a tunnel of sclera so they re-emerge close together (Figure 21.8b, c). Place a tie around the two sutures to make the situation more secure.

Suture the conjunctiva, but this time to the level of the insertion. The bare sclera regains a conjunctival covering very quickly by secondary intention.

Carry out adjustment as soon as is practical after the surgery.

General points

1. A strong suture (e.g. 4/0 nylon) can be placed in front of the muscle insertion to act as a handle to facilitate subsequent adjustment, but this is not necessary.
2. The techniques can be done on either the recessed or the resected muscle or both, but on bilateral horizontal muscle surgery the majority choose to do it on just the recessed muscle.

It does not matter which technique is used. The Jampolsky technique is easier to adjust, particularly in allowing the muscle to be recessed further, but it is the less 'secure' of the two techniques, with a greater chance of the muscle 'slipping'. With the Fells technique there is tendency for the suture to 'lock', and it can be difficult to adjust; however, it is usually secure enough that it can, if necessary be left without tying off. With the Jampolsky technique, the suture must always be tied off.

INFERIOR OBLIQUE SURGERY

Inferior oblique surgery can be readily combined with horizontal muscle surgery.

The general principle in squint surgery is that a standard operation has a large effect for a large deviation and a small effect for a small one. The ultimate expression is in myotomy for inferior oblique recession, when the same procedure is indicated for small, moderate or large overaction. There are two procedures described; the first is myotomy and the second is recession, and the procedures give equivalent results.

MYOTOMY

Make the incision in the inferotemporal quadrant, running from the inferior insertion of the lateral rectus to the lateral border of the inferior rectus. This can be estimated as being a circumferential incision 5 mm from and parallel to the limbus.

Locate the muscle: The inferior oblique runs just posterior to this incision, and it can be found in one of two ways. The first is simply to hook it with a squint hook. The muscle crosses Tenon's capsule to enter the intracapsular space as it crosses the inferior rectus and then it runs just deep to it and is connected to it via the intramuscular septa. There is a marked intermuscular septum that comes off the posterior border of the muscle, and the tip of the squint hook will catch up in this and need angling out of the incision. Retract Tenon's and poke the end of the squint hook through this intermuscular septum. Alternatively, pull the Tenon's and intermuscular septum forward 'hand over hand', using two pairs of forceps, and this should pull the muscle into view so it can then be hooked under direct vision.

A problem with either technique is that it is possible to split the muscle with the squint hook and not be aware of it. Therefore pass a second squint hook adjacent to the first and separate them slightly, and look in the gap to make sure that there is no part of the muscle left behind because this will greatly reduce the effect of the operation. It is also worth checking that it is the inferior oblique that has been found and not the wrong muscle. The inferior oblique looks different from all the other muscles (it is cylindrical rather than strap-like), it lacks a tendon, and pulling on it causes the globe to elevate and extort. However, the consequence of performing a myectomy on the lateral or inferior rectus is unequivocally disastrous, and if there is any doubt it is worth formally identifying the inferior and lateral rectus, by hooking with a squint hook, before proceeding to the next step.

Perform the myotomy. All muscle bleeds when cut. Along the course of the inferior oblique there are one or two surface blood vessels, and these should be directly diathermied. The standard technique is to crush the muscle with an artery clip, cut it just lateral to the artery clip and then cauterize the stump with diathermy before releasing the artery clip.

Close the incision with fine absorbable material (e.g. 6/0 Vicryl®) and, as always, take care to make sure that Tenon's is not incorporated into the closure.

INFERIOR OBLIQUE RECESSION

Performing a recession allows the surgery to be graded but, given the muscle's oblique course, it is difficult to directly measure the amount. Accordingly, it is usual to express the recession in terms of the co-ordinates where the end of the muscle is reattached to the globe. The co-ordinates are:

- For a large or '10 mm' recession, 3 mm posterior and 2 mm lateral to the lateral edge of the inferior rectus insertion
- For a moderate or '8 mm' recession, 6 mm anterior and 6 mm inferior to the inferior corner of the lateral rectus insertion.

The procedure is very similar to the myotomy, with the incision, location and disinsertion being the same. The difference is that the muscle is then reattached with an absorbable suture on a spatulate needle using the above co-ordinates prior to conjunctival closure.

AFTERCARE

Aftercare is similar for all the procedures, and a topical antibiotic and a topical steroid are appropriate for a couple of weeks after the surgery (e.g. Predsol-N q.d.s. for 2–4 weeks after the surgery).

COMPLICATIONS

Squint surgery is remarkably safe. Although complications are rare the list of reported problems is considerable, and the following is not exhaustive.

1. *Double vision.* Only a minority of patients with strabismus have potential for binocular single vision, and those often have a very limited fusion range. However, if adult patients with strabismus are questioned directly, the large majority report intermittent experience of double vision, which they do not describe as a problem. This is very different from acquired double vision (e.g. following a sixth nerve palsy or a blow-out fracture), which is very disturbing. Most patients want strabismus surgery for cosmetic rather than functional reasons. The eyes are an important part of facial expression, and a wandering gaze can be taken as being rude. Severe strabismus is probably best considered a disfigurement rather than a cosmetic defect. It is sensible to warn all patients who undergo strabismus surgery for cosmetic reasons of the possibility of postoperative double vision, and to document this warning.
2. *Under- and overcorrection.* The commonest complication is under- or overcorrection. The amount of surgery performed is on the basis of normograms but, as in all biological systems, there is a degree of unpredictability. This is best corrected by further surgery once the angle of deviation has been shown to be constant over a suitable period of time (3–6 months). It should be noted that a small amount of overcorrection is usually the aim for exo-deviations.
3. *Haemorrhage.* A degree of haemorrhage or bruising is to be expected, and is usually minor.
4. *Perforation.* Scleral perforation can occur in three ways; blunt trauma, cutting with scissors, or needle track. The commonest is

by needle track, and one series found evidence of this in 9 per cent of cases[8]. Complications as a result of accidental perforation are extremely rare, but retinal detachment and endophthalmitis have been reported[8,9,10]. The sclera can be cut when disinserting the muscle, and excessive traction on the muscle can also cause the sclera to tear or rupture if it is very thin. The management is common sense; repair the defect, dilate the pupil, and look for and treat (or arrange treatment for) any associated retinal damage.

5. *Infection*. Stitch abscesses, endophthalmitis and orbital cellulitis are all rare but reported complications. In one very large series, 87 cases of endophthalmitis were reported out of 300 000 cases, and while the role of accidental scleral perforation is not clear in this, it is likely to be a risk factor[11].

6. *Stitch reactions and granulomas*. These used to reported quite frequently with some of the older suture materials. Acute allergic reactions to the suture material present at 1–7 days, causing chemosis and conjunctival hyperaemia, while delayed reactions and stitch granulomas present at 2–8 weeks. The treatment is topical steroids. These reactions are much rarer with modern synthetic dissolvable materials such as polyglactin 910 (Vicryl®).

7. *Anterior-segment ischaemia*. The blood supply to the anterior segment comes from the anterior ciliary arteries, which run on the recti muscle and are therefore cut with the standard technique. The clinical features are corneal oedema, anterior chamber flare, iris atrophy, cataract and hypotony.

8. *The lost muscle*. This is when there is failure to reattach the muscle at surgery, and is a rare but serious complication that causes a severe oculomotility defect. The management of this is early surgical exploration to try and find the lost muscle – which is notoriously difficult. Reported suggestions that may help include:

- Having two assistants to help retract, as access is a problem
- Trying to identify the intermuscular septum and follow this back; however, this may well have been stripped and therefore this method will fail.

The author's experience is confined to looking for 'lost muscles' in the context of enucleation surgery, when the muscle clearly retracts outside Tenon's capsule, leaving a dimple when viewing it from the inside. In this situation, the muscle can be readily found by lifting and spreading Tenon's with two pairs of forceps, looking for this dimple and then grabbing the tissue at its base with a pair of forceps; the muscle is found there.

REFERENCES

1. Raab, E. L. and Parks, M. M. (1969). Recession of the lateral recti: early and late postoperative alignment. *Arch. Ophthalmol.*, 82, 203–8.
2. Scott, W. E., Keech, R. and Marsh, A. J. (1981). Postoperative results and stability of exodeviations. *Arch. Ophthalmol.*, 99, 1814–18.
3. Van Noorden, G. K. (1980). *Binocular Vision and Ocular Motility*, 2nd edn. C. V. Mosby.

4. Duke-Elder, A. and Wybar, K. C. (1961). *System of Ophthalmology, Volume II. The Anatomy of the Visual System*, 1st edn. C. V. Mosby.
5. Freedman, H. L., Waltmann, D. D. and Patterson, J. H. (1992). Preservation of anterior ciliary vessels during strabismus surgery: a non-microscopic technique. *J. Ped. Ophthalmol. Strab.*, **29**, 38–43.
6. McKeown, C. A., Lambert, H. M. and Shore, J. W. (1989). Preservation of the anterior ciliary vessels during extraocular muscle surgery. *Ophthalmology*, **96**, 498–506.
7. Stuart, J. A. and Burian, H. M. (1962). Changes in horizontal heterophoria with elevation and depression of gaze. *Am. J. Ophthalmol.*, **53**, 274.
8. Gottlieb, F. and Castro, J. L. (1970). Perforation of the globe during strabismus surgery. *Arch. Ophthalmol.*, **84**, 151–7.
9. Basmadjian, G., LaBelle, P. and Dumas, J. (1975). Retinal detachment after strabismus surgery. *Am. J. Ophthalmol.*, **79**, 305–9.
10. Havener, W. H. and Kimball, O. P. (1960). Scleral perforation during strabismus surgery. *Am. J. Ophthalmol.*, **50**, 807.
11. Knoblach, R. and Lorenz, A. (1962). Über ernste komplikationem nach Schieloperationem. *Klin. Monatsbl. Augenheilkd.*, **141**, 348.
12. American Academy of Ophthalmology (1994). *Pediatric Ophthalmology and Strabismus*. American Academy of Ophthalmology.
13. Mein, J. and Trimble, R. (1991). *Diagnosis and Management of Ocular Motility Disorders*, 2nd edn. Blackwell Scientific Publications.

22

PENETRATING KERATOPLASTY

Stephen Tuft MChir MD FRCOphth

It is a common misconception that a penetrating keratoplasty is a technical exercise. Although the technique is relatively easy to master, this is only one of several important aspects in the management of the patient. Careful patient selection and meticulous attention to detail during postoperative review can avoid many of the complications. Success cannot be defined solely in terms of graft clarity, and corneal astigmatism is still a major postoperative problem. Visual rehabilitation usually requires the prescription of glasses or contact lenses, but further refractive surgery is necessary in some eyes. Many patients therefore take as long as 2 years to achieve full visual potential.

Although Zirm performed the first successful human penetrating keratoplasty in 1905[1], the procedure was rarely performed before the 1950s. The development of suitable needles, monofilament sutures, the operating microscope, tissue preservation and effective topical steroid preparations led to the more widespread use and an improved outcome from surgery. The development of intermediate corneal storage at 4°C and long-term storage by organ culture has meant that the majority of cases can be performed electively, with time for safety checks to be performed on the donor material, and tissue matching if required.

There are two broad types of keratoplasty; full and partial thickness. The most commonly performed is the full-thickness transplantation or penetrating keratoplasty (PK) of the central zone of the cornea. The transplanted corneal endothelium is the major target for allograft rejection, and endothelial cell loss after rejection is the commonest cause for corneal graft failure after a PK. A partial-thickness or lamellar keratoplasty (LK) involves transplantation of the corneal stroma and, as the endothelium is not transplanted, rejection is very uncommon. An LK can be of any depth, but a dissection to the level of Descemet's membrane prior to transplantation of the donor material has become known as a deep lamellar keratoplasty.

A tectonic graft describes an operation to seal a perforation or support a thinned cornea, and this may either be a PK or an LK. The mechanical effect is the primary objective, and the visual benefits are secondary. Indeed, the grafted tissue may only involve peripheral corneal tissue and not cross the visual axis.

INDICATIONS

The majority of PKs are performed to improve the vision from the eye. This is achieved by removal of irregular surface astigmatism that is not correctable by simpler management options such as spectacles or a contact lens, as is often the case with advanced keratoconus. A PK may also be needed to remove an axial corneal scar or stromal haze secondary to injury or inflammation.

The second most frequent indication for a PK is relief from discomfort arising from bullous corneal oedema secondary to endothelial cell loss in the aphakic or pseudophakic eye. There may often be an improvement of vision after surgery for corneal oedema, although cystoid macular oedema is common in eyes that have experienced previous traumatic surgery. A PK is not appropriate if the eye is blind, when a conjunctival flap is the preferred option.

A PK to eliminate infection is rarely indicated, as the outcome is usually better after the infection and the associated inflammation has been controlled. However, early surgery may be necessary if there is a corneal perforation, but even then the procedure should be delayed until therapeutic tissue levels of antibiotic have been achieved by systemic and intensive topical treatment. Similarly, a PK is not usually an early treatment option for amoebic infections, where elimination of the organism prior to surgery reduces the risk of recurrence of the disease and subsequent rejection. A therapeutic PK is necessary in most cases of fungal keratitis due to filamentary organisms, as these respond poorly to medical therapy.

A tectonic PK can be used to support the globe or seal a perforation. The most common indication is for inflammatory melting that develops as a complication in patients with rheumatoid arthritis who have dry eyes. However, a LK is the preferred option if there has been active corneal melting.

PATIENT SELECTION

To be able to provide patients with an informed discussion about the risks of surgery the surgeon must be aware of the common complications, such as allograft rejection, postoperative astigmatism and recurrence of disease. The common risk factors for allograft rejection are corneal neovascularization, previous graft surgery, glaucoma, and active inflammation. If there is a severely dry eye or active ocular surface disease, as is often the case in advanced Stevens–Johnson syndrome or ocular cicatricial pemphigoid, graft failure is almost inevitable unless supplementary treatment is performed to protect the ocular surface. Surgery in this group of patients should only be undertaken after careful consideration and discussion with the patient. Because of the risk of rejection and failure and the refractive problems associated with graft surgery, patients with unilateral disease should be carefully appraised of their likely outcome, not only in terms of graft survival but also in terms of visual potential, prior to undertaking surgery. Patients are unlikely to be satisfied with the results of surgery, no matter how good the outcome, if the final corrected acuity is worse than the uncorrected visual acuity in the contralateral eye[2]. Conversely, no matter how poor the outcome, the patient is likely to be pleased if it becomes their better eye.

DONOR MATERIAL

Donor corneal material may be stored fresh for up to 48 hours in a moist pot to prevent drying. It can also be kept for 5–7 days at 4°C in corneal storage medium, or for as long as 30 days in organ culture. The age of the donor is not a contra-indication to use, as long as the endothelium is healthy with a cell density in excess of 2300 cells/mm^2. However, the presence of an arcus can be a cosmetic problem in young patients with a dark iris, and donor material from infants less than 1 year of age is subject to late ectasia. In the United Kingdom, consent should be sought from relatives prior to the retrieval of material.

Blood from prospective donors should be screened for HIV antigen and hepatitis B and C antigen prior to use, and the GP should be contacted to determine if there has been a history of neurological disease or brain surgery. Tissue matching takes several days, and can only be performed on tissue from patients who have been ventilated for a period prior to death, or on material that is stored in organ culture.

PATIENT PREPARATION

The best chance for surgical success is for the ocular pressure to be normal and the ocular surface healthy. Accordingly, any pre-existing ocular hypertension/glaucoma should be controlled. Any ocular infection and inflammation or severe ocular surface disease (e.g. allergic conjunctivitis, dry eye, trichiasis) and exposure should be treated and controlled.

Constrict the pupil with two drops of pilocarpine 2% if the eye is phakic, but the pupil must be dilated if simultaneous cataract extraction and lens implantation is planned.

If a PK combined with a cataract extraction or lens exchange is planned, calculate the intraocular lens power. The axial length can be measured as normal with ultrasound, but if the corneal surface is irregular the keratometry can either be taken from the contralateral eye or estimated using a 'typical' keratometry reading of 7.8 mm. Two drops of cyclopentolate 1% is often all that is needed to dilate the pupil for open-sky surgery, and the iris can then be constricted at the end of the procedure to keep a lax iris out of the wound during suturing.

PROCEDURE

The majority of corneal graft procedures in the United Kingdom are performed under general anaesthesia, although surgery under local anaesthesia is possible in most cases.

Prepare the eye in the standard manner for intraocular surgery.

1. Align the eye: The centre of the cornea should be vertical to avoid parallax errors during trephination of the cornea, and a traction suture (7/0 silk) placed at the limbus or through a rectus insertion may occasionally be required to stabilize the eye and to help alignment.

2. A scleral support (e.g. Flieringa) ring may be used to support the globe during surgery. The aim of the support ring is to prevent collapse of the globe, which can prolapse the ocular contents or distort the donor rim. Secure the ring with at least four scleral sutures placed just anterior to the rectus insertions, and leave the superior and inferior sutures long and secure them to the drapes to provide anterior traction to the globe (Figure 22.1). A support ring is not usually necessary for phakic eyes or for combined corneal graft surgery and extracapsular cataract extraction. If in doubt use a ring, as it is very difficult to insert when the eye is soft after surgery has started. The use of a ring is strongly recommended for a PK after intracapsular surgery, on paediatric eyes, and when performing large diameter PKs (> 10 mm) that cross the limbus.

3. Insert a paracentesis at the limbus of the host cornea, prior to trephination. This allows the aqueous to be replaced with viscoelastic to prevent sudden shallowing of the anterior chamber, which can risk damage to the iris or lens from the trephine blade. A paracentesis also provides access for reformation of the anterior

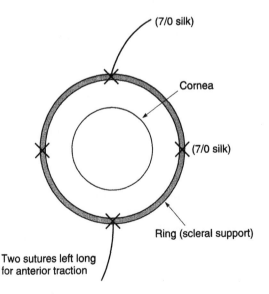

Figure 22.1 Use of a scleral support ring (Flieringa ring). It is secured with four sutures (e.g. 7/0 silk) with the two sutures at six and twelve o'clock left long for anterior traction.

(7/0 silk)

Cornea

(7/0 silk)

Ring (scleral support)

Two sutures left long for anterior traction

chamber during the procedure and removal of viscoelastic at the end of surgery.

4. Mark the centre of the cornea as an aid to centration of the trephine. Centring the trephine on the cornea can be difficult, but should be done carefully – it is important to centre on the cornea and not on the pupil of the eye. An effective technique is to estimate the centre visually, mark the cornea, and then check that this mark is equidistant from the superior and inferior limbus using callipers. Some surgeons use a radial keratotomy marker to mark the cornea at 8 or 12 peripheral points, which aids suture placement, and this is especially helpful in aphakic eyes, when the cut rim of the cornea can collapse and becomes distorted.

5. Cut the donor material. Most surgeons do this after the diameter of the host trephination has been decided, but before actual trephination. This is essential when there is no reserve donor material to use, in case the donor cornea is inadvertently damaged. The simplest way to cut the donor material is with a circular Superblade punch from the endothelial surface, with the cornea supported in a moulded silicone block. Use a trephine punch 0.25 mm larger than the diameter of the host trephine, with the trephine held vertically and placed equidistant from the limbus. After punching the cornea, take care to ensure that the endothelial surface of the donor button is protected from drying with storage medium or a viscoelastic.

6. Cut the cornea of the host. This can be done in several different ways. First, check centration. The cornea can be cut freehand after the epithelium has been marked with a trephine; this is the technique of choice if there is a perforation and the eye is soft or if an irregular shape is required. If the eye is firm, the cornea can be cut with either a hand-held Superblade trephine or a semi-automated suction trephine. The diameter of the trephination is a compromise determined by the size necessary to encompass the pathology and the risk of rejection. Grafts of less than 6 mm are often not optically effective, and grafts of greater than 8 mm have an increased risk of rejection. The majority of grafts consist of a 7.75-mm donor button placed into a 7.50-mm host trephination.

7. In the phakic eye the aim of trephination is to just enter the anterior chamber rather than to cut a complete disc, as this risks damage to the iris and to the lens. Once the anterior chamber has been entered, cut the rest of the disc with either a diamond blade or corneal scissors. Suction trephines usually have a crosshair to aid centration during cutting, but as most of the cornea is obscured during the cutting process large errors of centration can occur if care is not taken. Parallax error from using crosshairs can occur, and it is good practice to confirm centration by viewing the cornea from the side and top. Avoid the temptation to press on the globe during trephination, as this increases undercutting of the host cornea by the blade of the trephine as the cornea passes into the barrel of the trephine blade (Figure 22.2). Gently lift the suction trephine during cutting to reduce undercutting. Bleeding

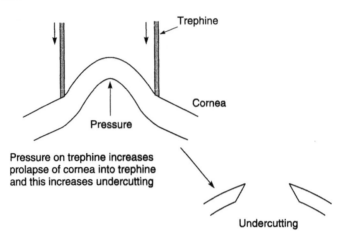

Pressure on trephine increases
prolapse of cornea into trephine
and this increases undercutting

Figure 22.2 Mechanism for undercutting with a trephine.

from corneal new vessels during cutting of the disc can obscure the view later; control this by irrigating the field with saline containing 1 : 10 000 adrenaline, or an assistant can 'blow' the blood from the wound with a viscoelastic or saline.

8. Combined cataract extraction and graft surgery is normally performed as an open-sky technique after the corneal button has been completely removed. Perform a continuous curvilinear capsulorhexis, as this helps to maintain intraocular lens centration later. There is a strong tendency for a capsulorhexis to tear peripherally due to anterior lens pressure, and if the view is adequate it is a good idea to perform this manoeuvre via a paracentesis before the cornea has been trephined. The nucleus of the lens can be removed by hydroexpression following hydrodissection of the cortex, or by open-sky phakoemulsification. After aspiration of the cortical lens remnants, place the intraocular lens implant within the capsular bag. A previous implant does not need to be removed if it is not mobile, however, remove vitreous within the anterior chamber. An angle supported (Multiflex) intraocular lens is suitable for implantation in the aphakic eye, or a posterior chamber lens can be used if there is adequate capsular support. Sutured lenses are more difficult and time consuming to insert, and have no apparent clinical advantage. Perform an iridectomy if there has been previous intraocular inflammation; this is not indicated in phakic eyes, such as in keratoconus.

9. Suture the graft. There are several different techniques of graft suture, and there is little evidence to show that the method of suturing affects the final astigmatism. In general, interrupted sutures are used if there has been corneal melting or ocular surface disease such that there is a possibility that one or more of the bites of the suture could become loose and need to be replaced. A single or double running suture is suitable for almost all other cases, and it is quicker to insert.

10. Use four cardinal sutures of 10/0 nylon to hold the donor button in approximation before performing final suturing (an alternative is to use overlay crossover sutures of 7/0 or 8/0 silk, but these have

to be inserted prior to trephination when the eye is still firm). The first two cardinal sutures of 10/0 nylon are the most difficult to insert as the graft is still mobile, and it is easiest to insert sutures beneath the fixating forceps to prevent the tissue rolling between the needle and the forceps. The cardinal sutures should be replaced until there is approximately the same amount of tissue in the four quadrants (Figure 22.3a), and the tension lines generated by these sutures should form a square (Figure 22.3b). When using a continuous suture, place the first bite within the corneal stroma adjacent to a cardinal suture and use 16–24 bites to complete the closure, with the knot tied within the corneal wound. Radial sutures are the easiest to insert (Figure 22.4), although anti-torque sutures can be used. The oblique throws between the bites of a radially placed continuous suture exert a circumferential torque force when the suture is tightened, and this force tends to rotate and distort the graft. If the suture bites and the connecting throws are placed at the same angle to the wound, the resultant force is radial and there is no rotational torque force. For interrupted sutures, insert the additional sutures radially and equidistant between the cardinal sutures until eight sutures are inserted, and then repeat the process.

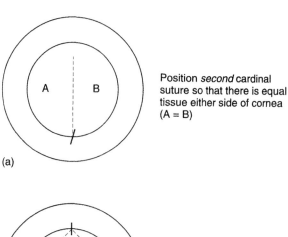

Position *second* cardinal suture so that there is equal tissue either side of cornea (A = B)

(a)

Figure 22.3 Insertion of the four cardinal sutures. (a) Position the second cardinal suture so that there is equal tissue either side of the cornea (A = B). (b) After the third and fourth cardinal sutures have been positioned, the tension lines on the surface of the cornea should form a square.

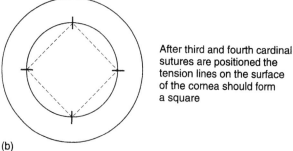

After third and fourth cardinal sutures are positioned the tension lines on the surface of the cornea should form a square

(b)

11. Place the sutures as deep as possible in the cornea to prevent posterior wound gape, which can lead to wound instability and astigmatism after suture removal (Figure 22.5). However, it is more important to approximate the epithelial surfaces than the

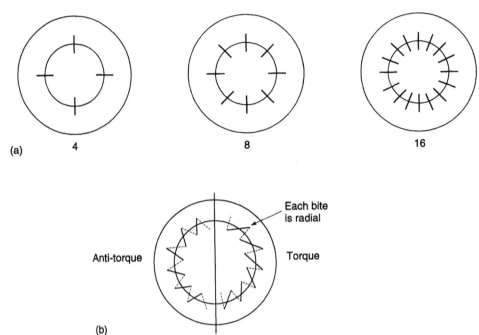

(a)   4   8   16

Figure 22.4 (a) Interrupted sutures. Start with the four cardinal sutures, then add four more bisecting the fist four, and repeat the process. (b) Continuous sutures showing the difference between torque and anti-torque sutures.

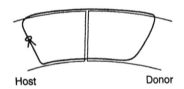

Figure 22.5 Suture placement. The suture is placed deeply and the knot rotated to bury it in host tissue and facilitate removal.

endothelial surfaces if there is a difference between the thickness of the donor and host material. Place each suture bite first into the donor to emerge just anterior to the Descemet's membrane. Then place the tip of the needle as deeply as possible in the surface of the host cornea, again just anterior to the Descemet's membrane, and advance the suture. A useful sign to confirm an adequate depth in a clear cornea is a 'bow-wave' originating from the tip of the needle (Figure 22.6). Bring the tip of the needle out just short of the limbal vascular arcade using counterpressure. When inserting a continuous suture, take care not to damage the needle half way through suturing; some surgeons prefer to use a double-ended

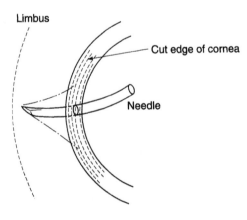

Figure 22.6 Corneal graft suturing technique. A bow-wave tension line in the cornea arises from Descemet's membrane and indicates that the needle is at the appropriate depth.

suture so that the suturing can be completed in the other direction if one needle is damaged.

12. Remove the cardinal sutures after the continuous suture has been inserted, and tighten the sutures to close the margins of the wound. Add a bit of extra tension until there is slight whitening of the cornea at the wound margin. In general it is preferable to leave the sutures too tight than too loose, but an over-tight suture can lead to delay in epithelialization, dellen formation, or a persistent epithelial defect. After tightening and tying off the suture, restore the pressure within the eye by injecting saline through the paracentesis and adjust the distribution of tension between the sutures by viewing the reflex of a keratoscope on the central cornea. Remove excess fluid from the corneal surface to minimize the meniscus effect before viewing this reflex. Adjust the tension in a continuous suture by feeding the suture circumferentially toward the steep meridian (Figure 22.7); replace interrupted sutures that are too tight. After tying the knot and trimming it carefully, bury the ends of a continuous suture within the wound. Rotate the knots of interrupted sutures to leave the knot on the side of the host tissue, as this makes later removal safer.

13. Remove viscoelastic from the eye at the end of surgery and check the wound to ensure there is no leak and no iris incarcerated within the wound. Insert additional sutures if necessary. Give a subconjunctival injection of antibiotic and steroid (e.g. betamethasone 4 mg/ml and cefuroxime 125 mg/ml). Because of the risk of a postoperative spike in pressure that can lead to iris ischaemia in eyes with keratoconus (the Urrets–Zavalia syndrome), some surgeons give Diamox 250 mg stat at the end of surgery, which is repeated q.i.d. for 24 hours.

Apart from cataract extraction and lens implantation, other combined techniques are rarely performed at the same time as graft surgery because of the high risk of complication and failure. For this reason, glaucoma procedures such as trabeculectomy are usually performed as a separate procedure. Cyclodiode therapy for uncontrolled glaucoma can be performed after wound closure, but intensive topical steroid treatment is needed to control postoperative inflammation.

MODIFICATIONS

A lamellar keratoplasty is an alternative to a PK if the corneal endothelium of the host appears to be normal. It is therefore used to treat superficial scars, some corneal stromal dystrophies, and keratoconus if there has not been a previous episode of acute corneal hydrops. Mark the diameter of the graft on the cornea as for a PK, but dissect the cornea carefully until as much as possible of the stroma has been removed over the Descemet's membrane.

Prepare donor material for a superficial lamellar graft from a whole globe by lamellar dissection after marking the cornea with a trephine

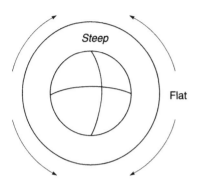

Figure 22.7 Correction of astigmatism by manipulating a continuous suture. The running suture is fed toward the steep meridian.

the same size as the host, or 0.25 mm larger. A deep LK can be completed using a full-thickness donor button prepared as for a PK. Some surgeons wipe the endothelial cells off a full-thickness donor button or mechanically remove the Descemet's membrane to reduce the risk of a second anterior chamber forming between the donor and the recipient Descemet's membrane. The LK is then secured as for a PK.

If the corneal opacities are limited to the very anterior layers, such as the superficial opacities of Reis Buckler's dystrophy, remove them by excimer laser photoablation.

Tectonic grafting is often indicated and performed on a soft eye after there has been a perforation. If the corneal disease is the result of a systemic process such as rheumatoid arthritis, immunosuppress the patient initially with systemic steroid to reduce the risk of recurrence of the melting disease in the graft. Perform lamellar surgery if possible to reduce the risk of wound leak at the edge of the graft from continued corneal melting. Extend the dissection beyond the edges of the thinned cornea into cornea of normal thickness. Mark the area to be excised and deepen the incision freehand using a guarded micrometer diamond blade. Cut a template to show the size and shape of the graft from a piece of sterile drape laid over the wound, and then lay this onto a whole donor globe. Cut the margins of the donor LK and complete the lamellar dissection. Complete the excision of the diseased host cornea as a lamellar dissection. It is preferable to use interrupted sutures to secure the graft if there has been melting prior to surgery.

COMPLICATIONS

Small wound leaks or suture track leaks are common after graft surgery. As the majority of leaks seal spontaneously, no intervention is necessary if the anterior chamber is deep; however, if the anterior chamber is shallow the pressure should be checked to ensure that the cause is not aqueous misdirection. If the pressure is low a bandage contact lens can be inserted, but an anterior chamber that remains shallow after 24 hours usually requires additional corneal sutures.

If donor material has been stored for more than 2–3 days, it is common for the donor epithelium to be lost entirely by the first postoperative examination. Delay in re-epithelialization can occur if there is drying or active ocular surface disease. If there is a complete epithelial defect immediately postoperatively, the use of non-preserved drops should be considered and the eye should be kept well lubricated until epithelialization is complete. A bandage contact lens or a botulinum toxin tarsorrhaphy are occasionally needed to protect the regenerating epithelium. Filaments forming at the margin of the wound or over sutures can be uncomfortable and lead to early suture loosening, and can be managed by adding acetylcysteine drops 10% q.i.d.

Transmission of infection has been reported in approximately 0.02 per cent of cases following PK. Bacterial infection is the most common, and the case must be managed as a potential endophthalmitis.

Primary graft failure due to damage to the donor endothelium is rare. Delayed clearing of the graft is especially common in diabetic patients and, as late clearing can occur, primary graft failure should not be diagnosed until at least 2–3 weeks after surgery.

In even the lowest risk groups (e.g. keratoconus), allograft rejection occurs in about 30 per cent of cases. Fortunately, the majority of rejection episodes can be reversed using intensive topical steroid drops alone. There is no clear benefit from adjunctive treatment of rejection with subconjunctival or systemic steroids. The overall risk of graft failure is determined by several factors, many of which can be identified preoperatively[3].

Recurrence of disease can occur following corneal grafting. There is no proof that keratoconus can recur in a PK, but stromal dystrophies can recur. For this reason there has been a move toward lamellar surgery for these conditions, as the surgery can be repeated if necessary. Infections can recur in a graft, most notably herpes simplex disease and fungal keratitis.

AFTERCARE

Postoperatively, it is usual to prescribe a topical antibiotic (chloramphenicol 0.5%) q.i.d. for 1 week, or until the cornea has re-epithelialized. Topical steroid is used at a frequency of one drop every 2 hours for the first week, reducing to q.i.d. for the next month. The subsequent reduction in topical steroid treatment depends upon the clinical indication for surgery and the associated risk of graft rejection. For low risk grafts it is usual to reduce the treatment by one drop per day per month, but to continue low dose treatment with FML daily for 12–18 months.

If the graft was performed for herpes simplex keratitis, oral antiviral treatment (e.g. Aciclovir 400 mg b.d.) should be given in the immediate postoperative period. This is less toxic than topical treatment. It is not known for how long this should be continued, but the majority of clinicians will continue treatment for 6–12 months. Because of the expense, it is recommended that a diagnosis of herpes keratitis is confirmed by checking the host button for herpes antigen, and that treatment is stopped if there is no immunological support for the diagnosis.

The large majority of patients do not require systemic immunosuppression after surgery, and this should only be considered for high-risk grafts, and probably only then if it is an only eye. Oral steroid is effective at controlling acute inflammation, while cyclosporin (4 mg/kg) is suitable for long-term maintenance therapy. Blood pressure, renal function and trough levels of cyclosporin need to be closely monitored. The risk of potentiating malignancies and the increased risk of lymphoma need to be discussed with the patient before the starting cyclosporin. Because inflammation that may require systemic immunosuppression may develop after surgery, consideration of this risk must be made before undertaking high-risk surgery for unilateral disease.

Patient reviews are usually conducted 1 week after surgery, at 1 month, and then at 3-monthly intervals until the sutures are removed. At each visit the intraocular pressure is checked, and the graft inspected to make sure the sutures are buried and that there is no neovascularization or rejection. The patient needs to be aware of the risk of direct injury to the eye. Effective adjustment of a continuous suture or selective removal of interrupted sutures can be performed from the early postoperative period, and it is thus advisable to obtain a refraction or keratometry within the first month of surgery. However, there is no convincing evidence that selective suture adjustment reduces astigmatism after all sutures have been removed.

Loose sutures should be removed, as they are a potential source of infection and a stimulus for corneal neovascularization and subsequent graft rejection. Interrupted sutures can be removed individually, but a continuous suture that has become loose early may need to be replaced in part or completely.

It is recommended that all corneal sutures be removed electively. Sutures eventually degenerate and break, and they can act as a source of infection or a stimulus for neovascularization and rejection. Sutures are normally removed 12–15 months after surgery, but they can be left for 3–4 years if there is low corneal astigmatism. Unfortunately, there can be large unpredictable changes in astigmatism after suture removal. Sutures can be safely removed at the slit lamp using 1% amethocaine anaesthesia, although some surgeons prefer to do this under an operating microscope. No matter how long the sutures have been in position, there is a small risk that the wound may slip after suture removal, although wound dehiscence is infrequent. Patients must be warned that the suture may have to be replaced if there is leakage through the wound at the time of suture removal. After suture removal, topical antibiotic should be used for at least 3 days, and topical steroid should be used for approximately 1 month to reduce the risk of a rejection episode.

Visual rehabilitation after corneal graft surgery may require glasses or a contact lens. A prescription may be given before final suture removal, although the patient should be warned that this will need to be changed after suture removal as the refraction changes. A contact lens may be fitted from approximately 6 months after surgery and prior to suture removal, although only a gas-permeable material is recommended to reduce the risk of neovascularization.

Finally, all patients should be warned of two long-term risks. First, although the risk of rejection of the graft reduces over time after the surgery, it never disappears entirely. Patients should be reminded of the symptoms of late rejection and the importance of immediate consultation, particularly if they are discharged from the clinic. Secondly, the strength of the graft–host junction is never as strong as a normal cornea, and there is always a risk of graft dehiscence following even relatively mild blunt trauma, which should therefore be avoided.

REFERENCES

1. Zirm, E. (1906). Eine erfolgreiche totale keratplatik. *Graefes Arch. Ophthalmol.*, **64**, *580–93*.
2. Williams, K. A., Roder, D., Esterman, A. *et al.* (1992). Long-term outcome after corneal transplantation. Visual assessment and patient perception of success. *Ophthalmology*, **99**, 403–14.
3. Williams, K. A., Muehlberg, S. M., Bartlett, C. M. *et al.* (eds) (2000). *The Australian Corneal Graft Registry. 1999 Report.* Snap Printing.

REFERENCES

23

GLAUCOMA SURGERY

Alexander J. E. Foss DM FRCOphth and
Peter Shah FRCOphth

There is much about the management of glaucoma that simply is not clear, and key question as to the indications and timing of surgery are subjects of controversy. This chapter describes the commonly performed procedures of peripheral iridectomy and trabeculectomy.

PERIPHERAL IRIDECTOMY

INDICATION

Iridectomy is indicated where relative pupil block is thought to be a contributory mechanism in the process of angle closure.

PROCEDURE

1. Anaesthetize the eye as for any ocular procedure.
2. Consider a paracentesis to help anterior chamber reformation at the end of the procedure.
3. Use either a limbal or a clear corneal approach, but the latter is probably preferable, leaving the conjunctiva intact in case a subsequent drainage procedure is required. Make a reverse sloping corneal section of 2–3 clock hours; the commonest surgical error is to make this incision too small.
4. Grasp the iris with a pair of fine-toothed forceps and perform the iridectomy with a pair of fine scissors (e.g. Vanna's or DeWecker's). Ensure that it is full thickness, by checking that the pigment layer is present on the posterior surface of the excision specimen.
5. Reposition the iris and reform the anterior chamber reformed, if required.
6. Close the section.

AFTERCARE AND COMPLICATIONS

As with any intraocular procedure, the standard postoperative care is prevention and/or treatment of any postoperative iritis with topical steroids ± cycloplegia as well as antibiotic cover. A typical regime is maxidex q.d.s., chloramphenicol q.d.s. and cyclopentolate 1% o.d. for 4 weeks.

The most common complication is an incomplete peripheral iridectomy. Raised intraocular pressure may also persist following a peripheral iridectomy as, although it alleviates relative pupil block, there may be other mechanisms at play (e.g. aqueous misdirection or irreversible angle closure). There is also a problem with the steroid responder in that one cause of raised ocular pressure – relative pupil block – is replaced by another, which may be very hard to recognize. Newer potent steroids such as rimexolone are thought to have less tendency to elevate the IOP, and non-steroidal anti-inflammatory drops are an alternative.

Other complications include cataract formation, anterior synechiae, hyphaema (usually clears spontaneously), wound leak (requires resuturing) and endophthalmitis.

TRABECULECTOMY

This operation can have an extremely high success rate, but success is by no means guaranteed. The postoperative care is every bit as crucial as the operative technique, and the surgical procedure should be regarded as the first step in a 2–3-month period of active bleb management. In general, most cases who have this operation in this country are elderly Caucasians, and this demographic group has high success rate and a relatively low complication rate. There are a large number of variations in technique described, and two techniques are described here. The first has been developed for high-risk cases (such as re-do surgery and developmental glaucomas) and, while time-consuming, is designed to avoid the problem of immediate postoperative hypotony, and to maximize the chances of achieving good bleb morphology and long-term pressure control. It is suspected that most long-term complications are related to poor bleb morphology (bleb leaks, late-onset endophthalmitis, failure to control pressure) and hypotony (the risk of subsequent cataract formation and maculopathy). The second technique is the 'standard' trabeculectomy, which has the advantages of simplicity and, in the favourable subgroups, an excellent success rate. It is less suitable for high-risk cases or with mitomycin C use.

HISTORY

While Richard Bannister observed the association between glaucoma and raised ocular pressure in 1622, it was not generally accepted until the nineteenth century. In 1830 MacKenzie tried to lower the ocular pressure by sclerotomy or paracentesis, but the benefit was short-lived. A number of procedures such as trephination and thermosclerostomy were developed with a view to draining aqueous, but all were complicated by hypotony and often by very thin blebs, which are a feature of any full scleral thickness fistula procedure, with a high risk of subsequent endophthalmitis.

In 1961, Sugar introduced a new approach based on the excising a portion of trabecular meshwork in the hope that aqueous would flow into the cut ends of Schlem's canal. Cairns (1968) and Watson (1970) reported achieving good success rates with trabeculectomy[1,2], which became popular because the complication rates were lower than with the standard operation of the time and not because success rates were higher[3]. As understanding improved it became clear that the operation worked by creating a fistula, and that success rates were unaffected but complications fewer if the excised internal block was in clear cornea and did not include the trabecular meshwork[4].

The recognition that most failures of pressure control were due to subconjunctival scar tissue, with the Tenon's fibroblast the major effector cell in this process, led to the introduction of cytotoxic agents. At this time the standard trabeculectomy typically resulted in a brief period of postoperative hypotony, lasting for 1–2 weeks, which terminated with the formation of subconjunctival scar tissue. With the use of such wound-modifying agents this period of hypotony can be greatly prolonged, thus increasing the risk of serious complications, and one solution to this problem is to temper the degree of wound healing inhibition to the anticipated degree of healing response. A second solution has been the development of surgical techniques, still actively evolving, which aim to achieve the same pressure control while avoiding the period of hypotony by setting the resistance to aqueous outflow at the level of the scleral flap. This makes the use of wound-modifying agents much safer. This modified trabeculectomy we have termed 'the modern trabeculectomy', and the driving force behind it is the reduction of complication rates[5]; however, it probably does have superior control rates. A feature of hypotony is breakdown of the blood–aqueous barrier, and such aqueous will almost certainly stimulate healing and therefore be a risk factor for late failure.

INDICATION

The purpose of the operation is to lower the intraocular pressure, but there is no consensus on the exact indications for trabeculectomy. It has been estimated that over half of all patients with chronic simple glaucoma will subsequently require surgery (although since these studies three new classes of medication have appeared on the scene; the topical carbonic anhydrase inhibitors, the alpha 2-agonists and the prostaglandin analogues)[6,7] and that previous topical medication lowers the subsequent success rate of surgery[8]. While some surgeons advocate an aggressive surgical approach, claiming a 98 per cent success rate[8], others highlight the risks of surgery and argue for caution[9].

Accordingly, there is no consensus on the exact place of surgery other than to lower the intraocular pressure in patients who have either progressive or advanced optic atrophy with cupping.

Trabeculectomy should be approached with caution in eyes with angle-closure glaucoma; such eyes are at high risk of developing malignant glaucoma, and serious consideration should be given to the possibility of lens extraction before[10] or with glaucoma filtration surgery.

BLEB MORPHOLOGY

Long-term problems are mainly bleb-related, and a driving force behind recent developments is the aim of reproducibly producing the perfect bleb. The ideal characteristics are:

1. A normal vasculature – excessive vasculature is associated with an excessive wound healing response, while an avascular bleb is usually thin and prone to leaks.
2. A microcystic but otherwise normal mucosa – fine epithelial microcysts are a feature of a normally draining bleb.
3. Not macrocystic – macrocysts are a feature of two complications; they form over 'blow holes' (i.e. full-thickness sclerostomies) and are of high risk of forming leaks and subsequent late-onset endophthalmitis, and are also a feature of the encapsulated bleb.
4. Diffuse – this means a low level of elevation over a large area.
5. Posterior draining – i.e. with no corneal overhang, which is a feature of anterior draining blebs.

In the normal eye and in chronic simple glaucoma, resistance to aqueous outflow is at the trabecular meshwork. With a trabeculectomy, the resistance to outflow is determined by the scleral flap and the episcleral tissue. In the initial postoperative period there is low episcleral resistance, which forms with the healing response, and the only resistance is the scleral flap. The long-term results are determined at the level of Tenon's and conjunctiva (the episcleral resistance). A major cause of failure is the development of a 'ring of steel', a barrier of episcleral tissue around the bleb and thickening of Tenon's and conjunctiva, causing encapsulation and preventing posterior drainage. A high, thin macrocystic bleb clearly has aqueous entering the bleb, but it has difficulty leaving it; these blebs are the most at risk of late leaks and infection, in addition to giving poor pressure control. The strength of the healing response can be assessed by the vascularity, as a vascular response is a feature of a vigorous wound healing response.

HYPOTONY

The consequences of a period of hypotony are:

1. Breakdown of the blood–aqueous barrier – this can be seen clinically as the development of flare; it is likely that with loss of the

blood–aqueous barrier the altered aqueous humour is a major factor in stimulating Tenon's fibroblasts, and accordingly is a potential risk factor for late failure

2. Cataract progression – hypotony may cause cataract progression, and subsequent cataract surgery is a major risk factor for subsequent trabeculectomy failure

3. Anterior chamber shallowing and peripheral anterior synechiae formation – a flat or very shallow peripheral anterior chamber will result in peripheral anterior synechiae formation

4. Immediate and delayed suprachoroidal haemorrhage – hypotony results in fluid collecting in the suprachoroidal space, and vessels crossing this space are at risk of bleeding.

5. Hypotonous maculopathy – this is characterized by persistent choroidal and retinal folds, which occur as a result of 'scleral collapse' and are a particular risk in myopic eyes in young patients[11,12].

Resistance at the level of Tenon's and conjunctiva takes at least 10 days to start developing, and up until then the resistance is determined by the scleral flap. Therefore the way to avoid a period of hypotony is by meticulous creation and suturing of the scleral flap.

PROCEDURE

The technique described here is as refined by the glaucoma unit at Moorfields Eye Hospital, and addresses the two major problems of preventing 'ring of steel' formation and an immediate postoperative period of hypotony.

Site of trabeculectomy and the corneal traction suture

A standard trabeculectomy is sited superiorly under the upper lid; while the operation can in principle be placed at any location, the incidence of endophthalmitis is higher elsewhere[13,14]. Given that the superior location is the ideal site, a corneal traction suture (e.g. 7/0 silk on a microspatulate needle) is required to rotate the globe downwards (see Figure 23.2). A superior rectus traction suture is not ideal as injury to the conjunctiva may stimulate an increased healing response, cause bleeding and buttonhole the conjunctiva, so a corneal traction suture is used. However, it is important not to perforate, because of hypotony.

Conjunctival flap

There is still considerable controversy over whether the conjunctival flap should be fornix- or limbal-based (Figure 23.1). The latter are associated with adverse bleb morphology and tend to encapsulate, so fornix-based flaps are preferable. They have the added advantage of being easier to perform. With fornix-based flaps anterior leaks are common, particularly with the use of antimetabolites; however, this can be solved with good suturing technique.

Raise the flap by lifting both Tenon's and conjunctiva at the limbus and then make a small buttonhole with a pair of spring scissors; pass

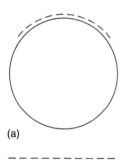

(a)

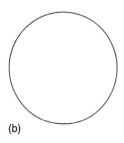

(b)

Figure 23.1   (a) The site of a fornix-based flap and (b) a limbus-based flap. The nomenclature is confusing, with the actual incision made at the limbus for a fornix-based flap and *vice versa*.

one blade of the spring scissors into the buttonhole, press it against the limbus and cut. The peritomy needs to be about 6 mm long, and no relieving incisions should be made. The purpose of the operation is to allow aqueous to drain posteriorly, and to encourage this it is worthwhile blunt dissecting under the flap (by passing and spreading blunt-tipped scissors either side of the superior rectus muscle).

Scleral flap and preplaced sutures

Next choose the site of the trabeculectomy; the key point is to avoid any perforation of blood or aqueous vessels in the flap because this can effectively turn the guarded procedure into an unguarded one. Make the site avascular with bipolar diathermy, taking care to apply it as lightly as possible consistent with closing the blood vessels. It must be done well, as diathermy done after cutting the scleral flap causes flap shrinkage.

Cut a partial-thickness flap, typically 2–3 mm posteriorly by 4.0 mm wide (Figure 23.2). The flap has two features that encourage the aqueous to drain posteriorly (Figure 23.3); the dimensions of the flaps (which should have a posterior edge about twice the length of the sides), and radial incisions that go about 80 per cent of the way towards the limbus but not quite the whole way (in young people, under the age of 30 years, this should be shorter at 60 per cent or less). Next raise the scleral flap with a crescent or pocket knife and extend it into clear cornea.

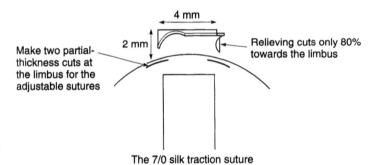

Figure 23.2 Construction of the scleral flap.

The next stage is to pre-place the adjustable/releasable sutures. It is much easier to suture into a firm eye than a hypotonous eye, and the sutures also allow rapid closure of the eye if there are problems. These sutures were originally designed as being releasable. The suture technique has changed, as has the concept behind their use, and they are better termed 'adjustables'. The original idea is that they could easily be removed by leaving an accessible loop on the cornea, which could be grasped, and the knot designed so that it would unravel by pulling. A releasable suture is an all-or-nothing event and does not give the desired level of control; it also offers little, if anything, over interrupted sutures and argon laser suturolysis. Rather than removing these sutures, if the loop is buried they can be adjusted by applying pressure behind the scleral flap, which will cause them to loosen. This allows

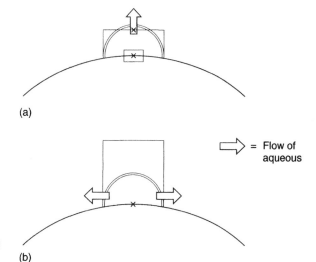

(a)

= Flow of
aqueous

(b)

Figure 23.3 Rationale behind scleral flap design. (a) The rectangular, correctly designed flap; the arrow marks the shortest path to the internal sclerotomy. (b) A poorly designed, square scleral flap will encourage anterior drainage.

for a graded response, which is particularly important when antimetabolites are used. As they are buried, they may remain in place indefinitely (i.e they will not loosen spontaneously or become exposed), and this is particularly important when mitomycin C is used because hypotony may result following routine suture removal even after several weeks or months. Use a 10/0 nylon suture on a microspatulate needle (Figure 23.4).

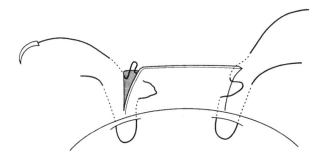

Figure 23.4 Pre-placement of the two releasable/adjustable sutures. The loops of suture on the cornea will be buried in the limbal incisions.

Paracentesis

Make a paracentesis with a MVR blade. It is essential to avoid accidental damage to the lens, and this is best done by using an oblique course. The paracentesis allows the anterior chamber to be reformed at will using balanced salt solution using a cannula. For high-risk cases (e.g. Sturge–Weber syndrome, highly myopic eyes) an infusion line can be used (Lewicky infusion line) through the paracentesis so that there is no period of hypotony.

The trapdoor

Release any pressure on the traction suture or the anterior chamber will be flattened on entering it. Above a critical size the size of the trapdoor does not matter, and laser sclerostomies giving a fistula of

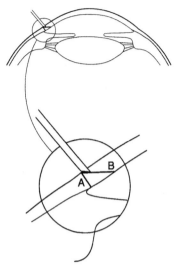

Figure 23.5 Direction of incision into the anterior chamber showing the difference between cataract and glaucoma surgery. A, trapdoor incision; B, cataract surgery incision.

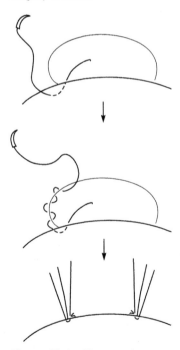

Figure 23.6 The suturing technique for the corners of the conjunctival flap. (a) First, anchor suture with a sclero-corneal bite; (b) then essentially do a purse string; (c) when tied, the conjunctiva will form a pleat.

0.2 mm diameter are quite large enough to cause hypotony and effectively give no resistance to the passage of flow[15]. The internal ostium provides no significant resistance to outflow.

Make a slit incision into the anterior chamber, using a sharp blade and entering down towards the iris (this is different to the angle used in small incision cataract surgery, where the aim is to enter in a plane parallel to the iris plane with the intention for the incision to be self-sealing) (Figure 23.5); the incision must be 50 per cent longer than the width of the scleral/Descemet's punch used (0.75 mm across for the Kelly punch, down to 0.5 mm for the newer punches). The punch is used in a very similar manner to a down-cutting bone punch for DCR surgery, and the aim is to take one good full-thickness bite.

Peripheral iridectomy
Failure to perform an iridectomy may result in the iris plugging the internal opening. Grasp the iris with a pair of plain or microgrooved tipped forceps through the trapdoor and then cut it with a pair of scissors.

Adjustable sutures
Close the scleral flap by tying the two adjustable sutures with three throws and a loop, then place one or two more adjustable sutures and tie them in an identical manner. Adjust the tension and inflate the anterior chamber. If it cannot be inflated, then the sutures are either too loose and should be tightened, or too few and more need to be added, or both.

Suturing the conjunctiva
Suture the conjunctiva with the same material, 10/0 nylon on a microspatulate needle. The needle blunts quite easily, so be prepared to use a second suture.

At each end, use small buried purse-string sutures anchored to the sclera (Figures 23.6, 23.7). In the centre, use one or two buried mattress stitches with the conjunctival bites slightly closer together than the scleral bites to help ensure a watertight fit[16].

The standard trabeculectomy
A standard trabeculectomy is described here in order to illustrate the spectrum of surgical technique. It differs in most aspects from the surgical principles espoused above, and yet still has a very high success rate in low-risk cases. It is significantly easier and quicker to perform than the above technique.

1. Insert a superior rectus traction suture.
2. Use a limbal-based flap raised 8 mm from the limbus.
3. Make a scleral flap as before – the exact size can vary from 4 × 4 mm to 2 × 2 mm (microtrabeculectomy[17,18]). The smaller flap size gives rise to fewer complications (such as induced astigmatism) than the large, with no reduction in pressure control rates. A paracentesis may or may not be performed.

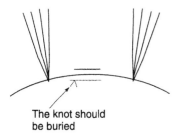

Figure 23.7 Central box suture. Note that the corneal bite is wider than the conjunctival bite.

The knot should be buried

4. Make the trapdoor.
5. Close the scleral flap with two interrupted 10/0 nylon sutures.
6. Close the conjunctiva with a locking 8/0 or 10/0 Vicryl® on a round-bodied needle (to prevent leakage from the needle tracks).

A number of interesting techniques have been described, all with the aim of trying to prevent postoperative hypotony. Methods include tying the scleral flap sutures tightly and then releasing them by argon laser suture lysis[19], the use of a compression shell[20], and the use of 10/0 Vicryl® tied tightly for the scleral flap[21]. The 10/0 Vicryl® will dissolve over 10 days and loosen at the time that the episcleral resistance starts to form. Another interesting approach is for an air bubble to be injected via the paracentesis, blocking the internal ostium of the drainage site, but it lasts only a couple of days, which is shorter than the usual period of postoperative hypotony. However, this approach may be worth exploring using other gases that persist for a longer period, such as sulphahexafluoride.

These approaches all work with high success rates for low-risk cases. Problems arise in high-risk cases requiring powerful adjunctive therapy such as mitomycin C (MMC). With MMC, the episcleral response is greatly delayed or absent and in this situation, if the scleral flap is not correctly sutured, then the result will be prolonged hypotony.

MODIFICATION WITH WOUND-HEALING AGENTS

Wound modification agents act on either the first (inflammatory) stage or the second (cellular) stage. Corticosteroids are effective wound-healing inhibitors and act predominantly on the inflammatory stage of wound healing, which occurs during the first 1–2 months.

In principle, any cytotoxic agent or radiotherapy will inhibit cellular proliferation and thereby the cellular phase of wound healing. Of all the available agents, the two that have been extensively used are 5-fluorouracil (5-FU) and mitomycin C (MMC). These agents probably act on the inflammatory phase as well as the cellular phase. They seem to have different clinical effects to each other, and they are not equivalent.

Corticosteroids
A clear beneficial effect of topical steroids has been shown in a study of rabbits[22]; the single clinical study shows a benefit of topical steroids but no added benefit of oral steroids[23]. Intensive topical steroids do not as yet appear to add benefit for high-risk cases[24]. A typical regime would be dexamethasone 0.1% four to eight times per day for the first month, then tapering off over the next 1–2 months.

5-fluorouracil
The initial use of 5-FU was by subconjunctival injection separate from the operative site performed twice daily for 1 week and then daily for a second week[24], but this time-consuming regime has now been replaced

by application of 5-FU at the time of surgery. It can be supplemented by injections during the postoperative period if required.

In applying antimetabolites, two distinct sites need to be considered; under the scleral flap with the idea of preventing of the scleral flap failing, and under the Tenon's surrounding the future bleb with a view to preventing encystment. It is particularly important not to treat the edge of the conjunctival/Tenon's flap.

A cellulose sponge is soaked in a solution of 50 mg/ml of 5-FU and then cut into small fragments because the sponge swells on getting wet. The edge of the flap is best protected (e.g. with a muscle clamp) and lifted clear and the pieces of sponge are placed deep underneath it. At the same time, an assistant dabs off any excess fluid and keeps the edge of the conjunctiva/Tenon's flap dry. The swabs should be counted in and out.

The treatment usually takes 3–5 minutes. The effect is partly time-dependent, and for reasons of comparability it is desirable that this should be standardized; 3 minutes appears to be becoming the standard. At the end of this time the swabs are removed and the area is copiously irrigated with at least 30 ml of balanced salt solution. The run-off is potentially toxic and should be collected (with paper towels) for special disposal.

Mitomycin C

MMC is an alkylating agent and a powerful antiproliferative agent. The effect can be titrated by the dose, and the range used is from 0.1–0.5 mg/ml. The effect is exponential, and 0.1–0.2 mg/ml gives an effect roughly equivalent to 5-FU while doses above 0.4 mg/ml give profound inhibition of wound healing and a relatively high incidence of prolonged postoperative hypotony[26]. The intraoperative application technique is identical to that for 5-FU and again the exact time is probably not crucial, with 1–2.5 minutes seeming to be as effective as 3.5–5.0 minutes[27]; 3 minutes again appears to be becoming the standard. It should be noted that MMC must not get into the anterior chamber, and if there is an aqueous leak on raising the scleral flap it must not be given at this site.

Indications for antimetabolite use

Intraoperative use of 5-FU or MMC should be considered for all cases where there is an increase in risk of failure (Table 23.1). The Moorfields Eye Hospital/University of Florida (More Flow) regimen is an intraoperative single-dose regimen which grades the strength of the antimetabolite to the risk of failure (Table 23.2).

POSTOPERATIVE CARE

Excessive drainage

This can be considered normal with some trabeculectomy techniques and usually lasts 7–10 days; the pressure then rises with the development of episcleral/subconjunctival scar tissue. As long as antimetabo-

Table 23.1   Stratification of risk of failure for trabeculectomy (by permission of Shah and Papadopoulos)**

Condition	Relative risk of failure
Large increase in risk of failure	
Neovascular glaucoma	+++++
Aphakic glaucoma	+++++
Previous failed surgery	+++++
Uveitic glaucoma	+++(++)
Age (< 40 years)	+++(++)
Afro-Caribbean race	+++(+)
Iridocorneal endothelial (ICE syndrome) and posterior polymorphous dystrophy (PPMD)	+++(+)
Cicatricial conjunctival disease	+++
Previous cataract surgery (conjuctival incision)	+++
Phakolytic glaucoma	+++
Sturge–Weber syndrome	++(+)
Post-keratoplasty	++(+)
Moderate increase in risk	
Acute or chronic angle closure glaucoma	++
Angle recession	++
Carotico-cavernous fistula	++
Inferior location of trabeculectomy	++
Aniridia	++
Anterior segment dysgenesis	++
Previous topical medication	+(++)
Atopy	+(++)
Pseudo-exfoliation	+(++)
Diabetes mellitus	+(+)
Asian (Indian race)	+(+)
Small increase in risk	
Previous diode laser	+(+)
Marked blepharitis (rosacea)	+(+)
Previous argon laser trabeculoplasty	+
Thyroid eye disease	+
Hispanic	+
Oriental race	+
High preoperative pressure	+

Table 23.2   Moorfields Eye Hospital/University of Florida (More Flow) Regimen[28].

Risk of failure	Use of antimetabolite
Low risk	25–50 mg/ml of 5-fluorouracil[ab]
Intermediate risk	25–50 mg/ml of 5-fluorouracil[ab] or mitomycin C 0.2 mg/ml[b]
High risk	Mitomycin C 0.4 mg/ml[b]

[a]Intraoperative β-radiation of 750 cGy is an alternative
[b]Postoperative 5-fluorouracil injections may be given in addition to the intraoperative applications of antimetabolite.

lites have not been used and there is no lenticular-corneal touch, this is usually self limiting.

Persistent hypotony (lasting more than 4 weeks) is a serious complication and requires intervention. The idea of injecting autologous blood into the bleb was first proposed for this indication[29]. It gives good short-term results and probably acts to buy time while the episcleral resistance forms. Otherwise, it is sensible to reoperate with a view to resuturing the scleral flap.

Poor drainage

The causes of poor drainage can be subdivided into early, within the first week postoperatively, and late. Early poor drainage implies either that the resistance at the level of the scleral flap is too high or that the internal ostium is blocked, while late poor drainage is usually due to episcleral/subconjunctival scar tissue formation.

The key feature of poor drainage is failure to achieve the target pressure. The immediate postoperative pressure will be zero if the trabeculectomy is draining freely. The tension in the scleral flap sutures can be reduced by gentle ocular massage just behind the posterior border of the scleral flap; the tension cannot however be increased, so this should be done gently. When standard sutures have been used, argon laser suturolysis can be considered.

Late poor drainage is usually due to scar tissue formation at the level of Tenon's and conjunctiva. There are two manoeuvres available: the first is to give a wound-modifying agent (usually subconjunctival 5-FU), and this is most effective during the cellular phase of wound healing; the second is needling, which can be tried at any time after surgery.

Adjunctive 5-fluorouracil

Further 5-FU injections can be given postoperatively if there is evidence of excessive healing, and the judgement of this is made on the basis of bleb morphology. The best single measure of wound healing activity is probably bleb vascularity, and a second feature is rising intraocular pressure. These injections can be given as often as required. The early Fluorouracil Filtering Surgery Study's regime for 5-FU was twice-daily subconjunctival injections of 5 mg for 1 week and then once daily for 1 week, but it is rare for that amount of 5-FU to be given nowadays[25].

The injection should ideally be sited posterior to the bleb. A typical dose is 2.5 mg in 0.1 ml, and the injection is given with an insulin syringe.

Needling

There are two distinct types of needling; the first is to break down the 'ring of steel' causing bleb encystment, and the second is to try and raise the scleral flap.

Needling for bleb encystment
Here, the resistance to aqueous outflow is not at the level of the tra-becular meshwork or scleral flap but is due to a dome of episcleral scar tissue (the 'ring of steel' concept), and the purpose is to make a hole in it. This is in effect a fistulizing procedure, and accordingly can cause hypotony and introduce infection. Needling can be considered an option for any encysted bleb, no matter how long after the initial surgery. The details of the procedure are:

1. Consider where to do it. It can be done on the slit lamp, but for difficult cases it should be performed in theatre.
2. Potential complications are the same as for a trabeculectomy (i.e. endophthalmitis and hypotony), and so proper informed consent should be obtained.
3. Topical anaesthesia with amethocaine is sufficient on a co-opera-tive patient, otherwise a peribulbar block or, exceptionally, a gen-eral anaesthetic may be used.
4. Prepare the eye. If it is being done on the slit lamp, a drop of a broad-spectrum antibiotic such as ofloxacin, chloramphenicol or aqueous povidone-iodine should be given. If it is in theatre, then prepare the eye as for any other intraocular procedure.
5. Use a fine needle such as an orange needle (25 G) for the needling. Introduce it under the conjunctiva and Tenon's some distance from the bleb, and advance it under Tenon's to puncture the episcleral tissue around the encysted bleb. The tip of the needle must be visualized at all times. The needle can be attached to a syringe containing local anaesthetic such as lignocaine 2% with adrenaline to balloon up Tenon's and conjunctiva and thereby give anaesthesia and prevent accidental puncturing of the conjunc-tiva around the bleb. However, as the conjunctiva/Tenon's is stuck down, this refinement rarely helps.
6. Following a successful needling, give a subconjunctival injection of 5-FU (2.5 mg in 0.1 ml) to try and prevent reformation of the scar tissue.

Follow-up after a successful needling should be almost as intensive as for a primary trabeculectomy.

Raising the scleral flap
The initial procedure is the same as for an encysted bleb, but the aim is to try and manoeuvre the tip of the needle under the scleral flap to try and raise it. Doing this, it is not uncommon for the needle tip to enter the anterior chamber. Again, following a successful needling, give a subconjunctival injection of 5-FU. Intensive follow-up is required.

The leaking bleb
Leaking blebs have two serious consequences: first, they are a risk for late onset endophthalmitis; secondly, they are a risk factor for pro-longed hypotony. Action depends upon when they are noted.

A conjunctival leak noted at the time of surgery should be repaired, as should any leak that is causing prolonged hypotony or one that has occurred because the conjunctival sutures have cut out causing the flap to dehisce.

A leak noticed after surgery without hypotony can be simply observed in the short term. Early leaks from the edge of the conjunctival/Tenon's flap are not uncommon, and usual stop spontaneously as the flap edge heals.

A particular problem is the late micro-leak, and it can occur:

1. In association with the encysted bleb
2. Secondary to a 'blow hole'
3. With dehiscence of the conjunctival flap.

Bleb morphology is dictated by mechanical factors. If there is a leak where the aqueous can freely enter the bleb but due to its encysted nature cannot exit, it behaves like an acquired fistula. Needling such a bleb alone may allow the aqueous to drain posteriorly and the conjunctival defect to heal, although this is not proven. The needling can be combined with injection of autologous blood (obtained by venous puncture from any convenient vein of the patient such as in the antecubital fossa, making sure that sterility is maintained) into the bleb. The idea is straightforward in that the blood will clot and block off the anterior leak while the posterior flow is being established from the associated needling, and although the technique was initially described to treat chronic postoperative hypotony, its application in this setting seems very reasonable[29]. It follows the basic principle that applies to any acquired fistula; direct closure always fails unless an alternative drainage pathway is established.

A host of other manoeuvres have been suggested, including gluing, cautery, laser photocoagulation and compression shells; as always when there is a long list of alternatives, it means that none work very well. The problem with all of these is that not one of them addresses the issue of establishing an alternative drainage pathway, with the implication that they would all work a lot better if they did. When all else fails, consider surgical revision.

If a full-thickness sclerostomy has been achieved, then a direct jet of aqueous will thin the overlying conjunctiva and will in time cause a defect. Not all jets give rise to problems, but if so the only way to fix this is to close off the full-thickness sclerostomy with a scleral patch graft.

COMPLICATIONS

The major complications are:

1. Failure
2. Hypotony
3. Suprachoroidal haemorrhage
4. Cataract
5. Visual loss

6. Encysted bleb
7. Late-onset endophthalmitis.

CATARACT AND GLAUCOMA

Cataract and glaucoma often coexist, creating further problems:

1. The presence of cataract makes assessment of visual fields problematic. In general, if the visual acuity is 6/12 or worse due to cataract, then any deterioration of visual fields is more likely to be due to cataract progression than to glaucoma progression.
2. Glaucoma surgery can cause cataracts, with reports of one-third of eyes requiring cataract surgery within 6 years of trabeculectomy[17,30]. The long-term results for the 'modern trabeculectomy' have yet to be reported.
3. Cataract surgery can cause trabeculectomies to fail. All types of cataract surgery would appear to decrease bleb function to some extent, and techniques that disturb the conjunctiva result in a 30–50 per cent bleb failure rate[31,32].

There are no universally accepted solutions to the problems. Perhaps the simplest situation is the presence of a symptomatic cataract, when cataract surgery should precede trabeculectomy, ideally by 4 months. In this situation cataract surgery should be via a corneal incision and the conjunctiva left undisturbed. Cataract surgery can cause a modest drop in intraocular pressure in chronic simple glaucoma, and therefore the need for glaucoma surgery should be reviewed after the cataract surgery. If drainage surgery is still required, then it should be done with a wound-modifying agent.

A second scenario is the presence of uncontrolled pressure and a clear lens. Proceed with trabeculectomy and try to avoid a period of hypotony and accept that there is a chance of causing cataract. If subsequent cataract surgery is required, then consider protecting the bleb with a wound-modifying agent such as 5-FU at the time of surgery and as necessary postoperatively.

The third scenario is the most complex, and is uncontrolled intraocular pressure and an asymptomatic cataract. With current knowledge, it is open to personal preference whether to follow the plan outlined in scenario one or two. An alternative to staged surgery is to perform combined surgery. The success rate of the drainage surgery is undoubtedly lower when combined with cataract surgery, but the key question is whether it is also lower than with staged surgery; the unproven suspicion is that it is.

If combined surgery is planned, the cataract surgery should be by phakoemulsification as it is less inflammatory than extracapsular surgery.

There are two ways to perform combined surgery. It can be done as two separate operations – a routine cataract operation by phakoemulsification through a clear corneal temporal incision followed by a routine trabeculectomy superiorly. Alternatively, perform the phakoemulsification procedure and, at the end of the cataract procedure, turn the scleral tunnel into a flap by two relieving incisions. The tunnel should be into clear cornea and the first cut has been made. An internal opening is most easily made at this stage with a scleral/Descemet's punch. The initial entry into the anterior chamber is designed to be parallel to the iris and is self sealing; this should be ignored and a second incision, angled downwards as for a standard/modern trabeculectomy, made before continuing the operation as for a modern trabeculectomy. Either way, current opinion is that the trabeculectomy should be augmented with a wound-modifying agent[33].

REFERENCES

1. Cairns, J. E. (1968) Trabeculectomy – preliminary report of a new method. *Am. J. Ophthalmol.*, 66(4) 673–9.
2. Watson, P. (1970). Trabeculectomy – a modified *ab externo* technique. *Ann. Ophthalmol.*, 2, 175.
3. Lewis, R. A. and Phelps, C. D. (1984). Trabeculectomy versus thermosclerostomy: a five-year follow-up. *Arch Ophthalmol.*, 102, 533–6.
4. Konstas, A. G. P. and Jay, J. L. (1992). Modification of trabeculectomy to avoid postoperative hyphaema: the 'guarded anterior fistula' operation. *Br. J. Ophthalmol.*, 76, 353–7.
5. Raina, U. K. and Tuli, D. (1998). Trabeculectomy with releasable sutures: a prospective, randomized pilot study. *Arch. Ophthalmol.*, 116, 1288–93.
6. Jay, J. L. and Murray, S. B. (1999). Early trabeculectomy versus conventional management in primary open-angle glaucoma. *Br. J. Ophthalmol.*, 72, 881–9.
7. Watson, P. G. and Grierson, I. (1981). The place of trabeculectomy in the treatment of glaucoma. *Ophthalmology*, 88, 175–96.
8. Lavin, M. J., Wormald, R. P., Migdal, C. S. *et al.* (1990). The influence of prior medical therapy on the success of trabeculectomy. *Arch. Ophthalmol.*, 108, 1543–8.
9. Quigley, H. A. (1997). Reappraising the risks and benefits of aggressive glaucoma therapy (editorial). *Ophthalmology*, 104, 1985–6.
10. Gunning, F. P. and Greve, E. L. (1998). Lens extraction for uncontrolled angle-closure glaucoma: long-term follow-up. *J. Cataract Refract. Surg.*, 24, 1347–56.
11. Jampel, H. D., Pasquale, L. R. and Dibernardo, C. (1992) Hypotony maculopathy following trabeculectomy with mitomycin C. *Arch. Ophthalmol.*, 110, 1049–50.
12. Stamper, R. L., McMenemy, M. G. and Lieberman, M. F. (1992). Hypotonous maculopathy after trabeculectomy with subconjunctival 5-fluorouracil. *Am. J. Ophthalmol.*, 114, 544–53.
13. Ticho, U. and Ophir, A. (1993). Late complications after glaucoma filtering surgery with adjunctive 5-fluorouracil. *Am. J. Ophthalmol.*, 115, 506–10.
14. Watanabe, J., Iwata, K., Sawaguchi, S. and Nanba, K. (1991). Trabeculectomy with 5-fluorouracil. *Acta Ophthalmol. Copenh.*, 69, 455–61.
15. Allan, B. D., van Saarloos, P. P., Cooper, R. L. and Constable, I. J. (1994). 193-nm excimer laser sclerostomy in pseudophakic patients with advanced open-angle glaucoma. *Br. J. Ophthalmol.*, 78, 199–205.
16. Wise, J. B. (1993). Mitomycin-compatible suture technique for fornix-based conjunctival flaps in glaucoma filtration surgery. *Am. J. Ophthalmol.*, 111, 992–7.
17. Vernon, S. A., Gorman, C. and Zambarakji, J. J. (1998). Medium- to long-term intraocular pressure control following small flap trabeculectomy (microtrabeculectomy) in relatively low-risk eyes. *Br. J. Ophthalmol.*, 82, 1383–6.
18. Vernon, S. A. and Spencer, A. F. (1995). Intraocular pressure control following microtrabeculectomy. *Eye*, 9, 299–303.
19. Hoskins, H. D. Jr and Migliazzo, C. (1999). Management of failing filtering blebs with the argon laser. *Ophthalmic Surg.*, 15, 731.
20. Simmons, R. J. and Savage, J. A. (1991). The shell tamponade technique for glaucoma filtration surgery. *Aust. NZ J. Ophthalmol.*, 19, 101–3.
21. Vyas, A. V., Bacon, P. J. and Percival, S. B. (1999). The benefits of phakotrabeculectomy using 10/0 polyglactin sutures. *Eye*, 13, 215–20.
22. Lard, J. and Coles, R. S. (1953). Role of cortisone in glaucoma surgery. Experimental results. *Arch. Ophthalmol.*, 49, 168–81.

23. Starita, R. J., Fellman, R. L., Spaeth, G. L. *et al.* (1985). Short- and long-term effects of postoperative corticosteroids on trabeculectomy. *Ophthalmology*, **92**, 938–46.
24. Miller, M. H., Joseph, N. H., Wishort, P. K. and Hitchings, R. A. (1987). Lack of beneficial effect of intensive topical steroids and β-irradiation in eyes undergoing repeat trabeculectomy. *Ophthalmic Surg.*, **18**, 508–12.
25. The Fluorouracil Study Group (1993). Three-year follow-up of the Fluorouracil Filtering Surgery Study. *Am. J. Ophthalmol.*, **115**, 82–92.
26. Chen, C. W., Huang, H. T., Bair, J. S. *et al.* (1990). Trabeculectomy with simultaneous topical application of mitomycin-C in refractory glaucoma. *J. Ocul. Pharmacol.*, **6**, 175–82.
27. Kalina, P. H. and Bellows, A. R. (1995). Use of antimetabolites in the surgical correction of glaucoma. In: *Recent Advances in Ophthalmology*, 1st edn (B. Jay and C. M. Kirkness, eds), pp. 105–15. Churchill Livingstone.
28. Khaw, K. T. and Wilkins, M. (1998). Antifibrotic agents in glaucoma surgery. In: *Ophthalmology*, 1st edn (M. Yanoff and J. S. Duker, eds), p. 1231. Mosby Year Book.
29. Wise, J. B. (1993). Treatment of chronic post-filtration hypotony by intrableb injection of autologous blood. *Arch. Ophthalmol.*, **111**, 827–30.
30. Lieberman, M. F. and Rich, R. (1996). Complications of glaucoma filtration surgery. In: *The Glaucomas*, 2nd edn (R. Rich, M. B. Shields and T. Krupin, eds), pp. 1703–44. Mosby.
31. Chen, P. P., Weaver, Y. K., Budenz, D. L. *et al.* (1998). Trabeculectomy function after cataract surgery. *Ophthalmology*, **105**, 1928–35.
32. Katz, J. L., Costa, V. P. and Spaeth, G. L. (1996). In: *The Glaucomas*, 2nd edn (R. Ritch, M. B. Shields and T. Krupin, eds), pp. 1661–1702. Mosby.
33. Hitchings, R. A. (1998). *Glaucoma Management. Focus from the Royal College of Ophthalmologists*. Royal College of Ophthalmologists.

24

CATARACT SURGERY

HISTORY

The earliest operation for cataract was couching, when the lens was simply pushed into the vitreous on the basis that the lens was the organ of seeing and the cataract a coagulum of fluid that occupied the space between the lens and the iris. Needless to say, the long-term results were poor due to the subsequent inflammation and glaucoma. Not until the seventeenth century was it realized that a cataract formed in the lens of the eye, and Daviel (1692–1762) first described extra-capsular surgery.

Intracapsular surgery was seen as a significant advance as complete removal of the cortex was guaranteed and the complication of posterior capsular opacification could not occur. A problem with this, however, was the high incidence of vitreous loss. It was the development of posterior chamber lens implantation combined with an improvement in microscopes and instruments that resulted in the return to extracapsular surgery. With these improvements, the problem of residual soft lens material could largely be avoided, and an intact posterior capsule provided excellent support for an intraocular lens. The development of the YAG laser meant that posterior capsular opacification could be managed on an outpatient basis with an extremely low complication rate.

Routine intracapsular surgery is no longer considered acceptable. Extracapsular surgery is still being performed in many places, but it is rapidly becoming superseded by small incision surgery and phako-emulsification.

EXTRACAPSULAR SURGERY VERSUS PHAKOEMULSIFICATION

Few surgeons doubt that phakoemulsification is significantly better than extracapsular surgery for the following reasons:

1. There is less surgically-induced astigmatism.
2. The self-sealing wound is much stronger and there is no restriction on immediate postoperative activities; there are also fewer

problems with wound leaks and iris prolapses and virtually no late wound ruptures following blunt trauma.

3. Refraction stability is achieved much more rapidly, so glasses can be dispensed as early as 1 week following surgery (compared to 3–6 months).
4. There are no sutures requiring routine removal, and no late suture-related complications.
5. It avoids periods of hypotony and so suprachoroidal haemorrhages are both rarer, and, given the self-sealing incision, less serious.
6. It is more controlled. As the eye remains effectively a closed system, patient movement is not dangerous.

EXTRACAPSULAR CATARACT EXTRACTION

SUPERIOR RECTUS SUTURE

The superior rectus suture allows mechanical rotation of the eye so that it points downwards. The surgical approach is superiorly, and there is a tendency for the threatened eye to look up (Bell's phenomenon); this will result in the wound disappearing under the upper lid and make its closure impossible. Clearly with a good local block this should not happen, but it is a potentially dangerous scenario.

The traction suture (e.g. 4/0 silk on a cutting needle) should incorporate the superior rectus insertion. If it is placed only in the conjunctiva and Tenon's it is useless, as it will not rotate the globe. To identify the superior rectus insertion, rotate the globe downwards by grasping the inferior limbus at the 6 o'clock position using a pair of toothed forceps. The superior rectus inserts 7.5 mm from the superior limbus, and the anterior ciliary vessels running on the surface of the muscle/tendon can usually be seen through the conjunctiva and Tenon's. Grasp the tendon through the overlying conjunctiva and Tenon's using another pair of toothed forceps (e.g. Lister's forceps) and check that the tendon is held by trying to rotate the globe with the forceps. Next, pass the needle just under the point of grasping.

A superior rectus suture is not needed for uncomplicated phakoemulsification surgery.

THE SECTION

There are two classic approaches to extracapsular surgery; limbal and corneal. The corneal section is described here. The advantage of corneal surgery is that the conjunctiva is left untouched, and this is particularly important in patients with glaucoma.

The earliest sections were forward sloping, and this is the essential morphology of the section for small incision surgery. However, the forward sloping section has been superseded by the reverse sloping section for extracapsular surgery (Figure 24.1). The purpose is to try

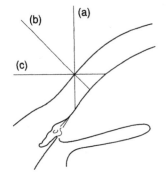

Figure 24.1 The corneal section. (a) The reverse sloping corner section had the blade orientated vertically with the eye looking straight up. The blade should not face further back or it will end up in the iris root. (b) Straight in at 45°. There is no flap valve effect, and a watertight closure will only be achieved by tension stitches causing astigmatism. There is a high risk of iris prolapse. (c) The forward sloping or 'Graefe' section. The blade is horizontal and parallel to the iris.

and create a flap valve, and the value of this is seen when it comes to wound closure. The sutures that close the wound can induce astigmatism and this is kept to a minimum if these sutures are appositional rather than tension. Good wound construction will allow a watertight closure to be achieved with appositional sutures.

Make the incision with a sharp blade. The ideal orientation is with the globe looking straight up and the blade perfectly vertical. The initial incision should be around 80 per cent depth and, as in most forms of surgery, it is ideal if the groove can be made with a single cut. There is significant risk of causing 'tramlines' if multiple cuts are required and these make wound closure difficult and predispose to postoperative leaks. In order to make a single cut, take a firm grip of the globe with a pair of microgroove forceps so that the globe can be moved in one direction while the blade is moved in the other. It is hard to get a firm grip on the conjunctiva, and one solution is to start the section with a partial thickness stab incision, and then hold onto the edge of this with a pair of microgroove forceps and complete the groove.

After making the groove, enter the eye. This time the blade changes orientation and faces forward into the anterior chamber. Its tip should be as close as possible to the base of the initial groove, and once the tip is in the eye, open the section by running it along to the left and right. The easiest way to finish the section is with corneal scissors.

Once the anterior chamber is entered, it tends to flatten due to loss of aqueous. As soon as this starts happening, inject viscoelastic into the anterior chamber to maintain it and protect the corneal endothelium from damage.

The chord length of the section is around 12 mm.

CAPSULOTOMY

A good capsulotomy is arguably the most important step in the operation. This can be done with either a preformed capsulotomy needle or one made by bending the needle on an insulin syringe (see Figure 24.2). The sharp tip will puncture the capsule and the cutting edge of the needle tip can make small linear cuts.

Beer-can capsulotomy

The beer-can capsulotomy is performed by using the capsulotomy needle to make a circle of punctures, giving a string of perforations. If each puncture is then followed by a little lateral movement, it is possible to join up the puncture marks and do a complete capsulotomy. When doing this the last bit is the hardest to complete, so start at the 6 o'clock position (which is the furthest away) and do the half circle to the 12 o'clock position and then start again at 6 o'clock for the other semicircle (Figure 24.3).

Complete the capsulotomy by making the 'sign of the cross' (Figure 24.4). Grab the centre of the capsule with a pair of angled smooth-tipped forceps (e.g. Macpherson's) and pull the tips to the left, to the

Figure 24.2 Making a
capsulotomy needle from an
insulin syringe.

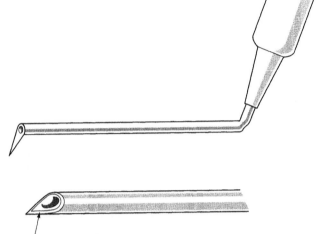

Hypodermic needles have a cutting edge. This is useful for starting the CCC.

Figure 24.3 Starting the beer-
can capsulotomy. (a) Perforate
the capsule at 12 o'clock, then
move the cutting edge of the
needle sideways to join with the
previous cut. (b) Do the
capsulotomy in two halves,
finishing nearest to the section.

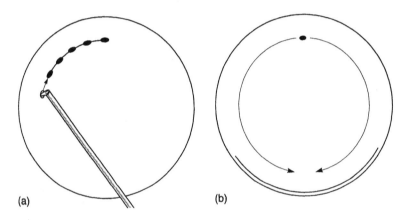

(a)   (b)

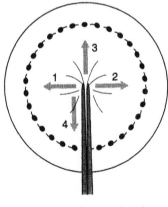

Figure 24.4 Completing the
beer-can capsulotomy. Grab the
capsule at the centre and pull to
the left (1), and then to the right
(2), then up (3) before finally
pulling it out. The purpose of
making the 'sign of the cross' is
to make sure all the perforations
are torn.

right, then up and down until all the perforations are torn and then, without relaxing the grip, pull the capsule out of the eye.

Endocapsular technique
The technique with the capsulotomy needle is very similar, but the anterior capsule is not removed at this stage. The shape of the resulting incision is a 'smile' (Figure 24.5). The idea behind the endocapsular technique is to remove the anterior capsule after the intraocular lens has been implanted and therefore ensure in-the-bag placement of the lens implant. However, the consensus position is that there is significant postoperative migration of lens implant haptics with this technique, and that the results are equivalent to the extracapsular technique. Accordingly, this is treated here as a variant on a theme.

NUCLEUS EXPRESSION

Remove the nucleus by squeezing it out. This is the most uncontrolled step of the operation, and it is at this stage that there is the greatest

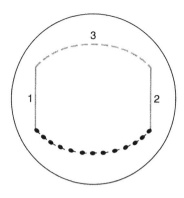

Figure 24.5 Capsulotomy for the endocapsular technique. The capsulotomy is a 'smile' incision through which the nucleus is expressed. The soft lens matter is aspirated and the intraocular lens implanted, then the capsulotomy is completed by making two cuts [(1) and (2)] with straight intraocular scissors and finally by tearing (3) as for CCC.

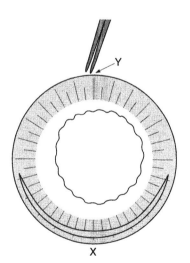

Figure 24.6 Method for nucleus expression. Grasp the limbus with the forceps and, after pressing at X to tilt the pole of the nucleus up, press at Y to express.

damage done to the corneal endothelium. First apply counter-pressure behind the section to tip the presenting pole of the nucleus up towards the section and then press at the inferior limbus to express (Figure 24.6). Although any instrument can be used, the irrigating instrument is particularly useful (e.g. a Simcoe) for applying the counter-pressure. Expression is most easily achieved by grasping (which prevents migration of the pressure point onto the cornea, thus distorting it) the conjunctiva/Tenon's at the inferior limbus with a pair of microgroove forceps and pressing gently.

The slower the expression, the less pressure is required and the greater the control. The nucleus can be helped through the section by 'dialling' if it gets stuck. The tip of the Simcoe can be placed behind the nucleus in the anterior chamber and the irrigation used both to help express it and to reform the anterior chamber; this will also prevent the anterior chamber collapsing when the expressing pressure is released.

The beer-can capsulotomy has a number of jagged edges from which a number of radial tears can propagate, and this is necessary for nucleus expression. If a continuous circular capsulorhexis is performed, then a number of relieving cuts must be made before expression.

CORTICAL CLEAN-UP

The cortex is also referred to as soft lens matter, and it is the ability to ensure its complete removal that distinguishes modern extracapsular cataract surgery from its earlier version.

Soft lens matter is removed by aspiration, and this must be done in association with an infusion line so as to maintain the anterior chamber throughout. A number of devices have been developed, but perhaps the simplest is the Simcoe cannula. This contains an infusion solution and an aspiration port, and the aspiration line is connected, via plastic tubing, to a 5-ml syringe.

The cannula is curved to allow easy angulation. Use the curve to place the tip inside the bag and engage the soft lens matter, being careful not to engage any tag of anterior capsule. When the curve is placed such that it is towards the periphery the aspiration port is facing laterally, and this is an excellent position to engage the soft lens matter. By a combination of rotation and translation, pull the engaged soft lens matter towards the central axis of the eye with the curve now facing forwards and the aspiration port facing vertically upwards. In this position there is very little chance of aspirating the posterior capsule by mistake. This technique exploits the fact that the cortical lens fibres are arranged radially, and are therefore easiest to aspirate in this direction.

Small amounts of soft lens matter can be left and will largely resorb. It is certainly better to leave a small amount than to risk rupturing the posterior capsule by prolonged attempts at complete aspiration. Incomplete cortical clean-up is a risk factor for early posterior capsular opacification, but with the development of the YAG laser this can hardly be considered a major problem.

When aspirating, look for radial folds appearing in the posterior capsule (Figure 24.7). These indicate that the posterior capsule is incorporated in the aspiration port, and any further aspiration or movement while it is impacted will lead to its rupture. If seen, perform immediate reflux to disengage it.

A collapsing bag is a feature of zonule dehiscence, and makes removing the soft lens matter very difficult. Continued aspiration of the soft lens matter tends to exacerbate the problem, and a capsular tension ring should be considered.

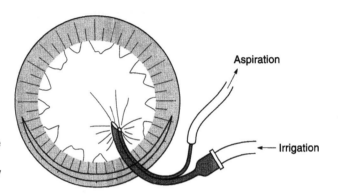

Figure 24.7 A star fold. This is indicative of the posterior capsule being aspirated and, if seen, the aspiration line should immediately be refluxed to disengage.

LENS IMPLANTATION

The standard lens for extracapsular surgery is a large diameter (8-mm optic) one-piece PMMA lens. This is because with extra/endocapsular surgery it is not possible to guarantee long-term in-the-bag implantation, and the commonest result is for one haptic to be in the bag and one in the ciliary sulcus, resulting in a mild degree of lens decentration. The standard technique is to reform the anterior chamber with viscoelastic. Post the lens into the eye through the section and place the leading haptic directly into the bag/ciliary sulcus (Figure 24.8). Place the trailing haptic behind the iris in one of two ways: either simply use

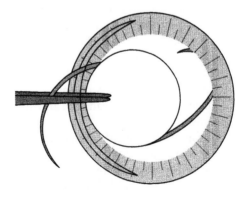

Figure 24.8 Insertion of an intraocular lens by holding the optic and placing the leading haptic into the capsular bag.

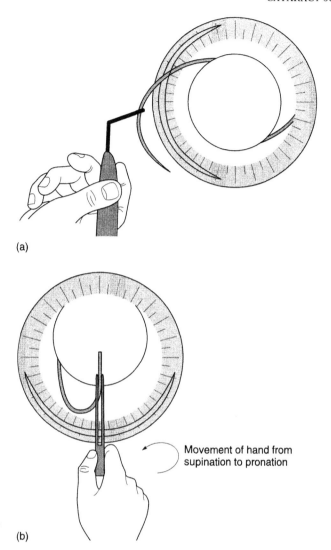

(a)

Figure 24.9 The trailing haptic can be placed by holding it approximately halfway along its length with angled forceps with the hand in supination (a). On rotating the hand into pronation (b), the bend of the haptic will rotate posteriorly and can then be released behind the iris.

Movement of hand from supination to pronation

(b)

a dialler and rotate the lens while pressing down, or grasp the haptic halfway along its length with a pair of angled forceps (e.g. MacPherson forceps) with the wrist in supination (Figure 24.9) and introduce it into the eye. Pronate the wrist to angle the haptic back, and release it so it springs back behind the iris.

SECTION CLOSURE

The usual choice of suture is 10/0 nylon or 11/0 Mersilene® on a microspatulate needle, using either a continuous 'bootlace' or an interrupted suture.

For a continuous suture, start at one end and take four or so bites along the section. Start the first bite in the wound as the suture must be

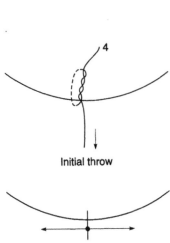

Initial throw

Figure 24.10   Tightening the second throw. By pulling at right angles to the stitch, the chance of accidental over-tightening is reduced.

buried, then on the return trip take a bite bisecting the bites of the first pass.

For interrupted sutures, take in both sides of the wound in each bite and rotate the knot after tying, trying to give minimal postoperative astigmatism. Features that make this easier are good wound architecture (so the stitches can be appositional and excessive tension is not required to make the wound watertight) and a reformed anterior chamber (usually with viscoelastic). There is no reliable technique that allows perfect control of astigmatism, and this is one of the reasons why phacoemulsification is seen as a significant step forward. However, if tension lines are visible in the cornea, this suggests that the stitch is overtightened.

To check if the section is too loosely sutured, see if it is watertight by dabbing the section with a dry cellulose swab so that the outside is bone dry and then applying a little pressure to the eye to see if any fluid seeps out.

With a bootlace suture, tie a basic surgical knot. Nylon has relatively poor knot security, so make three throws on the first loop i.e. a three–one–one. With interrupted sutures do the same, but there are methods to try and maintain control on the tension. Once the knot is laid, use three throws to hold the tension; alternatively, tie a slipknot to allow adjustment of the tension and then a square knot to make it secure. This may cause the suture to overtighten, but the risk can be minimized by pulling the knot tight at right angles to the direction of the suture (Figure 24.10).

AFTERCARE AND COMPLICATIONS

The major postoperative problem is iritis, so at the end of the operation give a subconjunctival injection of an antibiotic (e.g. cefuroxime 250 mg) and a corticosteroid (betnasol 2–4 mg). It is not clear how effective the antibiotic is at endophthalmitis prophylaxis[1].

Prescribe 6–8 weeks of topical steroids for all cases and, for the first week, consider a cycloplegic. Although it is usual to prescribe a topical steroid anti-inflammatory (such as dexamethasone 0.1%), topical non-steroidal anti-inflammatory drops (such as diclofenac 0.1%) may be just as effective[2,3]. Topical antibiotics are also routinely prescribed, but what protection they offer from endophthalmitis is far from clear. To continue with topical antibiotics for longer than 1 week, by which time the wound has epithelialized, seems illogical.

The number of postoperative visits required is not clear. The first day postoperative visit serves little useful purpose and is against the whole spirit of day-case surgery[4]. Often people like to review their cases at 1–2 weeks, but it is very unusual that any intervention is required at this stage. The next decision is at 10–12 weeks, when the question of suture removal to control astigmatism arises. Following suture removal, most cases can be safely discharged.

INTRAOPERATIVE COMPLICATIONS OF EXTRACAPSULAR SURGERY

Difficulty in expressing the nucleus

If there are problems with nucleus expression, stop! The commonest causes are:

- Too small a section. In this situation, enlarge the section. To continue to try and express through too small a section can result in the lens dislocating into the vitreous.
- A poor capsulotomy. If necessary, repeat the steps of the capsulotomy.
- The nucleus wants to tumble rather than be expressed. Very occasionally in highly myopic eyes or eyes that have been previously vitrectomized it is impossible to express, in which case use a vectis (which looks like a wire spoon and is used as such). Use an irrigating vectis attached to a syringe of viscoelastic, and insert it by pressing on the posterior lip of the wound so as to tip up the leading pole of the nucleus and slide the vectis in underneath it. Then inject viscoelastic to help express the nucleus, and withdraw the vectis and the nucleus together.

The moving patient

The moving patient presents a particularly difficult situation for extracapsular surgery. The operation requires a stage of hypotony, and movement will usually result in vitreous loss or, worse, an expulsive choroidal haemorrhage. One alternative is to convert to a general anaesthetic, but ophthalmology is a 'geriatric' speciality and many of the most mobile patients are the least fit for general anaesthesia. The best solution is not to perform extracapsular surgery, as phakoemulsification is much safer under these conditions given the self-sealing wound.

If neither of these options are available, then speed is everything and the surgery should be performed by an experienced surgeon.

Vitreous loss

Vitreous loss occurs as a result of zonule dehiscence or posterior capsule rupture. It can be difficult to recognize because vitreous is transparent and can look very like viscoelastic. Loss of a large amount of vitreous can be recognized because it deforms the pupil, but smaller losses are difficult to recognize; if in doubt, dab the edge of the wound with a dry cellulose sponge swab and watch to see if the pupil margin moves. If it does, then vitreous is present.

The key principle in dealing with vitreous is never to pull it, as this is the presumed mechanism for causing the major complications of cystoid macular oedema and retinal tears. If there is vitreous, do not pull the swab away, but cut off the vitreous with a pair of scissors (e.g. DeWecker's). Kasner first demonstrated that meticulous vitreous 'debridement' with cellulose sponges and scissors improved the final results[5]. Automated vitrectomy was introduced by Machemer in 1970[6], and the principle behind the automated vitrector is that there is an aspiration port and a guillotine cutter inside it to cut the vitreous as it enters the vitrector and so prevent traction. As with any aspiration line in the eye, there must be a separate infusion line to prevent ocular collapse. The infusion line may be on the outside of the cutter, or completely separate. With a combined cutter and infusion system, it is important to ensure that it is correctly set up; if the infusion is coming out of the cutter port, then it has been incorrectly set up and will not work.

When using dry swabs and scissors, vitrectomy results in pulling more forward and it can be a very time-consuming process. With an automated cutter, the tip of the cutter should be placed through the defect in the zonules/posterior capsule and as close to the geometric centre of the eye as possible. A typical cut rate is 400 per minute, and in this position the vitreous is removed from behind so the anterior hyaloid face will fall back into the eye rather than encouraging further prolapse. The process can be completed very quickly, usually in just a few minutes.

After the automated vitrectomy, decide whether to proceed with lens implantation. If it is possible to implant a posterior chamber lens, then it is worth checking with a dry swab that there is still no obvious vitreous going to the section. If it is not suitable for a posterior chamber lens, then constrict the pupil with acetylcholine 1% (Miochol®). Acetylcholine has a half-life of only a few minutes and must not be made up until it is required, and the miosis it produces only lasts 10 minutes. Once the pupil is constricted, check again for any residual vitreous with a dry swab to make sure that removal is complete. Then consider an anterior chamber lens implantation, but this may be better as a secondary procedure (see page 260).

PHAKOEMULSIFICATION

This is now the preferred technique for cataract surgery.

SECTION

Astigmatic surgery can be achieved by either a temporal corneal approach or a superior scleral tunnel.

Scleral tunnel
The advantage of the scleral tunnel is that the section is covered with conjunctiva at the end of surgery. Anecdotal evidence suggests that endophthalmitis is rarer with a scleral tunnel, but this has never been confirmed. The disadvantages of this approach are that the conjunctiva is disturbed and access can be poor for sunken eyes, particularly with standard lid speculums. There is a special wire speculum for this approach to help improve access.

The correct placing for the incision to be astigmatically neutral is shown in Figure 24.11. For a larger incision (e.g. 6 mm, when using a rigid lens) a frown incision is usually used so that there is the required length within the astigmatically neutral zone. The approach is very similar to that of raising a scleral flap for trabeculectomy:

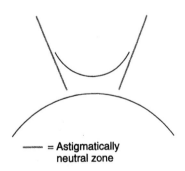

—— = Astigmatically
neutral zone

Figure 24.11 The 'frown' incision keeps the centre of the incision near the cornea while keeping the required cord length within the astigmatically neutral zone.

1. Perform a conjunctival peritomy at the limbus.
2. Diathermy the vessels over the proposed scleral incision site.
3. Make the partial-thickness incision.
4. Use a pocket blade and tunnel forward to the tip of the limbus vessels, then change direction at the limbus so as to stay within the cornea.
5. Next use a keratome to enter the anterior chamber. This is a pointed blade, the width of which determines the incision size (2.5–3.2 mm, depending upon the type of phako needle used).

Corneal section

This should be located at the temporal limbus. Not only is the access better, but it is also less astigmatic for two reasons:

1. The cornea has a larger horizontal (compared to vertical) diameter.
2. The visual axis does not pass through the geometric centre of the cornea but nasal to it (the angle kappa of strabismologists).

Therefore, a temporal incision is placed at the maximal distance from the visual axis.

The standard incision is a three-step incision:

1. Step one is the initial groove. It is good practice to measure the length of this with a pair of callipers; the exact length depends upon the requirements for lens implantation. This step should be performed with the cornea dry so as to be able to judge the depth of the groove.
2. Step two is to make the pocket with a pocket knife. The tunnelling is made in the plane of the cornea. The pocket only has to be 1 mm which, as a rule of thumb, is only about the length of the bevel on the blade of most crescent knives.
3. Step three is to enter the anterior chamber using a keratome. This determines the incision size, which is extremely important – too small and it is impossible safely to insert the phako tip; too large and the leakage of infusion solution will cause serious problems with the stability of the anterior chamber. Steady the eye by holding it at the limbus at the point opposite the entry site using a pair of microgroove or fine-toothed forceps, and make a quick stab incision in the plane of the iris.

An alternative to the three-step incision is a single stab incision with a keratome.

PARACENTESIS

The next step is to perform the paracentesis for the second instrument. Inflate the anterior chamber fully with viscoelastic before sticking a sharp blade in the cornea so as to minimize the chance of accidentally impaling any internal structure.

The paracentesis should be on the left if the surgeon is right-handed and *vice versa*. It should be orientated at 45–90° from the primary section.

CIRCULAR CONTINUOUS CAPSULORHEXIS

Phakoemulsification was first described using a beer-can capsulotomy with the nucleus prolapsed into the anterior chamber. Accordingly, it was only safe to tackle the softest nucleus because of the risk of corneal damage. The development of circular continuous capsulorhexis (CCC) was a major advance, as it permitted in-the-bag phakoemulsification. The principle is clear-cut in that capsular tears propagate from a pre-existing tear or sharp edge, and it is much stronger when there are none. CCC was described simultaneous by Gimbel and Neuhann[7].

When performing CCC, it is important to make a clear distinction between shear and rip. The generic term tearing is used here to describe CCC formation, and the tear point is the point of extension of the CCC.

Shearing occurs with the flap folded over (Figure 24.12a). All the shearing force is concentrated at the tear point, and accordingly it

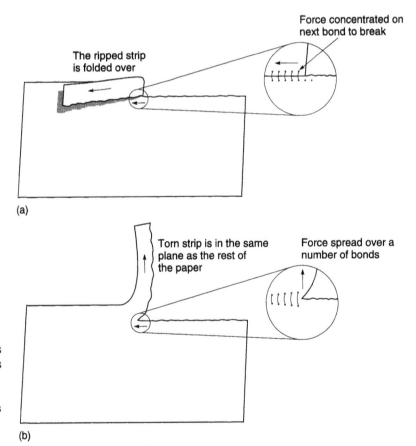

Figure 24.12 Mechanisms of tearing. (a) Piece of paper being torn by shearing. The tear point is travelling in the same direction as the applied force. (b) A piece of paper being torn by ripping. The direction of pull is at right angles to the direction of movement of the tear point.

takes relatively little force to propagate it. Pure shear occurs in a straight line, and any change of direction requires a component of 'rip'. It requires the least force to advance the tear point and accordingly is the more controlled techique.

Ripping occurs when the direction of pull is radial (Figure 24.12b) and the direction of the rip is at right angles to the direction of pull. The force is not concentrated at the point of rip, but spread out. Accordingly more force is required than for shearing, and the greater the force, the less the control. The natural path for a rip is at right angles to the force. If the direction of pull remains toward the centre of a circle, then the tear point should be circular. However, as the tear propagates there is a natural tendency for the direction of pull not to change, and so it will go in a straight line.

It is also important to be clear about the difference between initiating a tear and propagating it. It takes much less force to propagate a tear than to initiate one, and this is particularly true for ripping. Accordingly, to initiate a tear by ripping is potentially dangerous because the situation is unstable, resulting in the capsulorhexis tearing out and 'losing it'.

There are a number of variations described but most are modifications of this basic technique:

1. Start the CCC with a sharp instrument such as a bent insulin syringe (Figure 24.13). Make the initial stab in the geometric centre of the eye and then make a radial cut and end it with a dog-leg manoeuvre to generate a small flap.

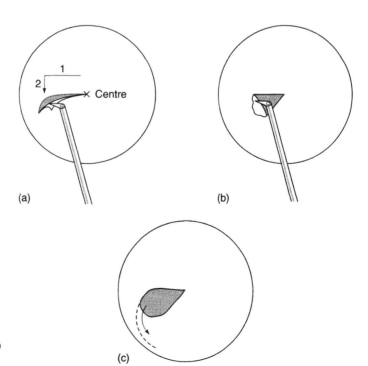

Figure 24.13 Starting the capsulorhexis. (a) Start radially using the cutting edge of a needle (1), then make a dog-leg to crease a flap (2). (b) Occasionally a V-flap will be created if the needle fails to cut. This needs to be recognized so that (c) the orientation of the flap can be changed by 90°.

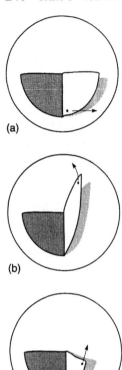

Figure 24.14 Performing the capsulorhexis. (a) When the instrument is close to the tear point this is the condition for shear, and the direction of force is the direction of tear. (b) Here the instrument is a greater distance from the tear point than the radius of curvature, and these are the conditions for rip. The direction of pull is at right angles to the direction of tear. (c) Between these extremes, the force vector takes up an intermediary position.

2. Always make sure that the anterior chamber is fully formed with viscoelastic. Keep the anterior chamber deep and prevent the nucleus from coming forward; lifting the flap up or letting the nucleus come forward results in a strong tendency for the tear to extend out radially.
3. Fold the flap over and then gently nudge the flap round. This is a slow technique, but is very controlled and essentially uses pure shear. Note that the vector changes direction and shear turns to rip with increasing distance of the instrument from the tear point (Figure 24.14). At the edge, the direction of pull is in the direction of the tear (i.e. it is tangential), and these are the conditions of shear. When the distance from the tearing edge is equal to or greater than the radius of the CCC, then the direction is at right angles to the direction of rip (i.e. radial or towards the centre of the eye), and these are the conditions for ripping. Between these two extremes the vector takes up an intermediate position, so periodically change the point of fixation (the usual advice is every three clock hours) and regrasp the capsule as close as possible to the tear point so as to maximize the component of shear.
4. As well as regrasping the capsule every three clock hours, regrasp the capsule as close as possible to the rip point if there is any tendency towards loss of control or for the capsulorhexis to tear out.
5. The diameter of the CCC should be in the region of 5–6 mm. The ideal CCC should be centred on the optical axis and just cover the edge of the optic of the lens implant. If smaller than this, the subsequent surgery is more difficult and there is a tendency for anterior capsular phimosis postoperatively. Too large a CCC and the area where the zonules start to insert into the lens capsule may be affected; in this situation there is a strong tendency for it to tear out radially and it is best to switch to forceps to bring the capsulorhexis back in.

The two commonly encountered problems when performing CCC are making it too small or for it to tear out (i.e. too big). If too small, make a cut in the CCC with a pair of intraocular scissors to create a new flap. This can then be used to initiate a second CCC.

Tearing out radially is a particular problem with the ripping technique. If the tear is not too peripheral, then the situation can be readily rescued by reverting to shearing (i.e. regrasp the flap as close as possible to the tear point). If the tear has run into zonules, then significant force is often required and this is easier with forceps rather than a needle.

A third situation occurs when the lens comes forward. This gives a second radial force vector directed out, and is resolved by anterior chamber reformation with viscoleastic.

Anterior capsular dyes

CCC is usually done under conditions of retro-illumination, when the edge of the CCC and the capsular flap can be readily visualized. It is much harder to perform on dense cataracts where there is no red reflex. There are two approaches to help visualization; the use of oblique illumination with a light pipe[8] and the use of substances to dye the anterior capsule (e.g. indocyanine green[9], subcapsular fluorescein[10,11], autologous blood[12] and trypan blue[13]).

Trypan blue is a logical choice as it is routinely used in eyebanks and therefore is known not to cause endothelial cell toxicity. Its use is straightforward. First, fill the anterior chamber with air (in order to minimize staining of the cornea) and then inject a small amount of trypan blue 0.1% (commercially available as Vision Blue™) underneath the air and spread it to ensure that the whole of the capsular surface has been exposed to it. After a short period of time (30 s) the trypan blue should be washed out. Initially the staining does not look very impressive, as it only poorly stains basement membrane. However, on starting the CCC it stains the underside of the flap, where the lens epithelial cells will take up the dye much more intensely. Its use can be combined with a dense viscoelastic such as Healon GV® to prevent leakage of lens milk into the anterior chamber, which will obscure the view. The combination allows CCC without any further modification in technique.

HYDRODISSECTION

The term 'hydrodissection' incorporates three distinct manoeuvres:

1. Hydrodelineation, which is the separation of the nucleus from the epinucleus (and gives rise to the golden ring sign).
2. 'Classic' hydrodissection, which is the separation of the epinucleus from the cortex.
3. Cortical cleavage, which is the separation of the cortex from the capsule[14].

The key aim is to allow the nucleus to rotate, and all three achieve this end.

Hydrodelineation should not be performed as a sole manoeuvre, as afterwards there will still be an epinucleus that needs to be mobile, as it is usually too hard to be dealt with by aspiration and needs to be emulsified.

The cortical cleavage technique will result in most of the cortex being removed in the phakoemulsification stage, and greatly shortens the cortical clean-up stage. Use balanced salt solution in a 5-ml syringe with a luer lock, and there are a number of specially designed hydrodissection cannulas that can be used. High flow is required, so they have quite a wide bore and a flattened section that will slip easily under the capsule.

For cortical cleavage the idea is to get a wave of fluid to travel around the lens between the capsule and the cortex, and the ideal conditions for this are high flow and low pressure – the exact opposite of viscoelastics. Accordingly, first remove any viscoelastic from the anterior chamber. Next:

1. Pass the cannula under the edge of the capsulorhexis and give a small injection to make a pocket; place the cannula in this. Inject and look for a wave of fluid going behind the lens.
2. After the injection the nucleus tends to come forward and can cause impact on the CCC, resulting in high intra-bag pressures and the risk of rupture; therefore, press the nucleus back after each small injection of fluid to decompress the lens bag.
3. Repeat this process again at another site.
4. This can be combined with hydrodelineation/hydrodissection by inserting the cannula into the lens and injecting.

It is not essential for the nucleus to be freely mobile at this stage. If it is proving difficult, return to this step after doing the initial grooving, when it is often easier to complete.

PHAKOEMULSIFICATION

The key issue for safe phakoemulsification is anterior chamber stability. A suddenly collapsing anterior chamber is the recipe for accidental aspiration or emulsification of the posterior capsule, or damage to the corneal endothelium.

Three factors are important in maintaining anterior chamber stability:

1. Infusion pressure. There is a standard height for the infusion solution, which can be increased if there is tendency for the anterior chamber to collapse.
2. The vacuum setting on the pump. When the tip is occluded the static pressure generated inside the tubing is increased, causing a small degree of collapse of tubing. When the occlusion clears, the static pressure drops and the tubing expands, causing a sudden increase in the aspiration rate and collapse of the anterior chamber. The degree of post-occlusion surge is dependent upon the vacuum setting. This factor can be partially compensated for by sophisticated software, by the surgeon taking pressure off the pedal when the port is about to become unblocked, or by a built-in resistance in the phako needle, achieved by having a small bore.
3. The leakage of fluid around the probe through the incision site. This is determined by the phako tip size; the smaller the incision size, the less the leak and the greater the anterior chamber stability.

Components of a phakoemulsification machine
The machine can irrigate, aspirate and emulsify. The surgeon switches between these modes using a foot pedal. There are two basic set-ups for the foot pedal. The commonest is to have the functions arranged linearly so they occur in order (Figure 24.15). At position 0, all three functions are off, position 1 is just irrigation, between 1 and 2 aspiration comes on in a graded fashion to be maximal at position 2,

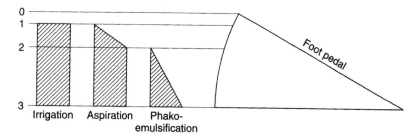

Figure 24.15 The foot pedal settings linearly arranged.

and then phakoemulsification occurs between positions 2 and 3. At position 3, all three functions are maximal. In positions 2 and 3 there is the option for fixed rather than graded functions. A limitation of this set-up is that there must be maximum aspiration before the emulsification function will start. This is not a problem when starting to emulsify a fragment, but is a potential problem when finishing emulsifying due to the post-occlusion surge (see below).

A dual linear set-up has been recently introduced (The Storz Millennium machine®). The aspiration is under linear control vertically and the emulsification is under linear control laterally (Figure 24.16). This gives exquisite control and is ideal for chopping techniques when a high vacuum is required to impact the nucleus and to perform the chopping, but lower levels of vacuum are needed for emulsification.

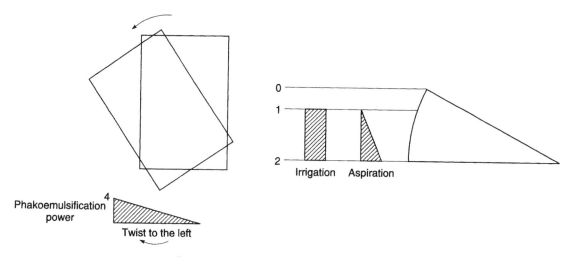

Figure 24.16 The foot pedal settings for dual linear control.

Irrigation and anterior chamber maintenance
For irrigation, the pressure is generated simply by hydrostatic pressure (Figure 24.17), and is determined by the height of the infusion bottle. An initial setting is 67 cm above the eye, but it can be increased or decreased as required. Flow is simply on/off, controlled by a pinch valve. It should be noted that the maximum hydrostatic pressure is only achieved under conditions of no flow. Under conditions of flow the pressure achieved is less because:

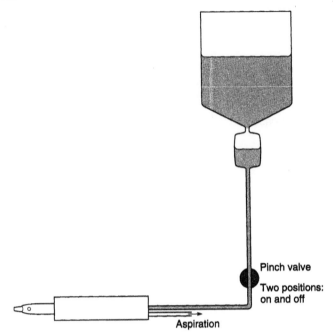

Figure 24.17 The irrigation pressure is determined by the height of the infusion bottle/bag.

- There is a pressure drop across the perfusion line, which is proportional to the resistance of the tubing.
- In a body of fluid, the total pressure is divided into static pressure (the hydrostatic pressure) and 'kinetic' pressure. The total pressure remains constant, and therefore the development of flow results in a decrease in the static pressure (Bernoulli's principle). Bernoulli's principle states that the greater the flow of fluid, the lower the static pressure. The relationship is not linear and follows a square relationship, so a small increase in flow can result in a large drop in pressure. This is why even a small leak of fluid can make it very hard to maintain the anterior chamber depth.

Aspiration and vacuum

There are two conflicting considerations with aspiration. High aspiration certainly helps with cataract removal, but can also result in the removing more than required. The associated high flow rates also reduce the pressure in the anterior chamber and accordingly compromise its stability.

A particular problem is surge, which occurs when an occluded phako needle tip becomes unblocked. How this is handled depends upon the type of pump. It is because of these conflicting requirements that different machine settings are required at different stages during the operation. The aspiration rates and/or vacuum levels can be changed from the machine's control panel.

Types of pump

There are two basic pumps, which work on fundamentally different physical principles and have different properties.

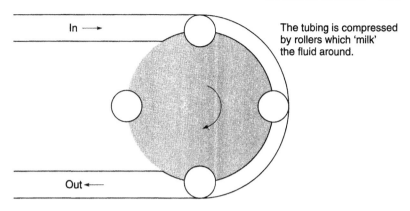

Figure 24.18 The peristaltic pump.

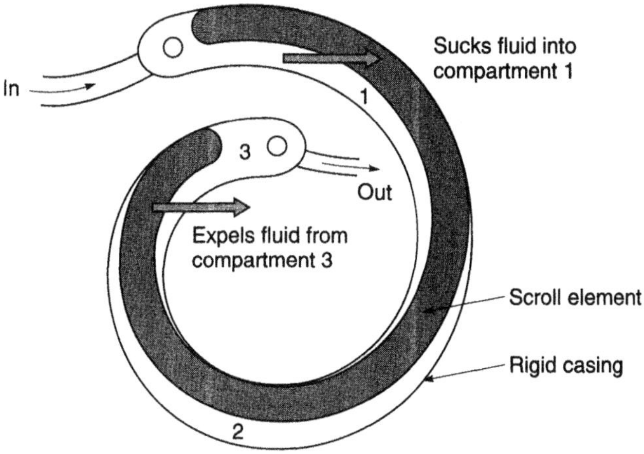

The tubing is compressed by rollers which 'milk' the fluid around.

Sucks fluid into compartment 1

Expels fluid from compartment 3

Scroll element

Rigid casing

Figure 24.19 The scroll pump. The fluid travels in boluses from compartment 1 to 2 to 3. It is like the peristaltic pump but the element that milks the fluid along is on the inside of the tubing and not the outside. This means that none of the parts are compressible so helps both back leak and post-occlusion surge.

The most commonly used flow pumps are the peristaltic pump (Figure 24.18) and its potential successor, the scroll pump (Figure 24.19). It has been said that a peristaltic pump will not generate pressure unless the tip is occluded, but this is clearly wrong because fluid will only flow from an area of high pressure to one of low pressure. The flow rate is constant, so the pressure generated will vary depending upon the resistance (i.e. whether the phako needle tip is occluded or not). It takes a little time for it to generate high pressures, and this is called the rise time. However, it does have limitations in that it works by compressing the aspiration tubing (and compressible tubing predisposes to post-occlusion surge) and it can be inefficient, with significant pump leakage. The scroll pump largely eliminates these problems.

Whereas the peristaltic and scroll pumps create constant flow, the vacuum pumps create constant pressure. There are three basic designs: the Venturi (based on Bernoulli's principle; Figure 24.20); the diaphragm pump (Figure 24.21); and the rotary vane pump (Figure 24.22).

For a vacuum pump the rise in pressure is close to instantaneous, but modern machines allow this to be varied. It is suggested that when changing from a machine with a peristaltic pump to a vacuum pump, a

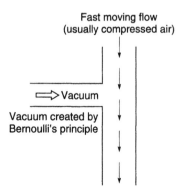

Fast moving flow (usually compressed air)

Vacuum

Vacuum created by Bernoulli's principle

Figure 24.20 The Venturi pump.

BERNOULLI'S PRINCIPLE

Bernoulli, circa 1740, derived a relation between pressure and velocity in different parts of an incompressible liquid in which resistance to flow was negligible. It is based on the conservation of energy. The energy of a fixed unit volume of fluid is comprised of three things:-

1. The hydrostatic pressure which is simply the gravitational constant (g) times the height (h) or gh.
2. The kinetic energy which is $\frac{1}{2}mv^2$ (m = mass and v = velocity) and the mass of a unit of liquid is simply one times its density (r) or $\frac{1}{2}rv^2$.
3. Work done by the liquid. Work is force times distance and force is pressure times area. Now area times distance is volume so the work done is pressure times volume, which for unit volume of fluid is simply the same as the pressure or p

Thus in a closed system, these three terms are constant:-

$$P + gh + \frac{1}{2}rv^2 = A \text{ constant}$$

In the anterior chamber of the eye, there is clearly no change in height so this expression can be simplified to :-

$$P + \frac{1}{2}rv^2 = A \text{ constant}$$

So the pressure in the anterior chamber will drop proportional to the square of the flow rate.

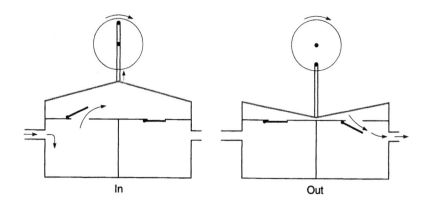

Figure 24.21 The diaphragm pump.

In

Out

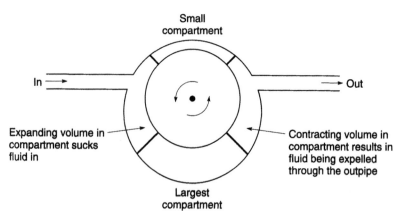

Small compartment

In

Out

Expanding volume in compartment sucks fluid in

Contracting volume in compartment results in fluid being expelled through the outpipe

Figure 24.22 The rotary vane pump.

Largest compartment

rise time of 2–3 s should be programmed to start with. Once used to it, most surgeons tend to choose a short rise time of 1 s.

The distinction between these two pump types is now of less significance as the manufactures of phakoemulsification machines are using increasingly sophisticated autoregulation and software so that the behaviour of the one type of pump can be made to mimic the behaviour of the others.

Types of phakoemulsification needle

The difference between the types of phakoemulsification needle hinges on the size of the incision they will fit through. The smaller the incision, the smaller the leak of infusion fluid and the greater the anterior chamber stability. There are three basic types (Figure 24.23):

1. The standard needle that fits through a 3.2-mm incision. The needle gets hot, and one of the functions of the infusion solution is to act as a coolant. The needle can fit through a smaller incision, but this may cause tissue burns.
2. The Microseal® (Mackool) system. This is characterized by having a reverse thread and fits through a 2.8-mm incision. It is designed with a polyimide sheath, which is both non-compressible and an insulator (which reduces the requirement for cooling). It has a significantly smaller internal bore than the standard needle, and this protects against post-occlusion surge.

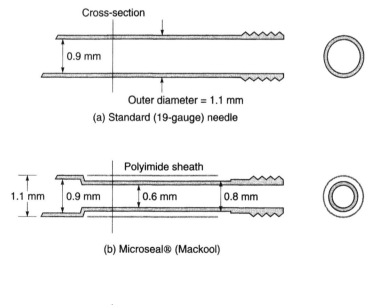

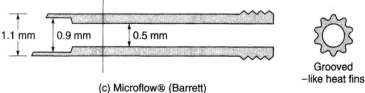

Figure 24.23 Types of phakoemulsification needle.

3. The Microflow® (Barrett) needle. This is grooved, which helps heat loss and also ensures that a tight fit does not compress the irrigation sleeve to the point that there is no flow. This will fit through a 2.5–2.8-mm incision. It also has a small internal bore to protect against post-occlusion surge.

The correct position of the irrigation sleeve is with the irrigation ports facing sideways when the needle bevel is facing up. There should be 0.5–1 mm of needle tip showing. If the end of the infusion tip is too near the tip of the needle, then grooving is difficult. The needle is entered through the section and the tip advanced with the bevel facing down. Once in the eye, the bevel is rotated to face up so the procedure can begin.

Delineating the capsulorhexis

It is sensible to delineate the margins by simply aspirating the soft lens matter and the epinucleus within the CCC, and the remaining anterior soft lens matter will act as a marker for the location of the CCC. This helps prevent accidental damage to the anterior capsule with the probe, resulting in an anterior radial tear (a common error when learning the technique). This is not particularly significant in itself, and the procedure can usually be completed successfully if the tear is recognized. The major problem is if it is not recognized, because any stress on the capsule will lead to the tear propagating to involve the posterior capsule – a major complication.

Bowel technique

This is the simplest and most intuitive technique, but it is the least reliable and is only suitable for the softest lens.

Make an initial trench and enlarge it to either side. The technique only works well if the lens is very soft, in which case at this point the walls will fall in, allowing the rest of the lens to be safely aspirated in the centre of the bag.

Divide and conquer

Gimbel developed and popularized this technique of 'trench, divide and conquer', abbreviated to 'divide and conquer'. For this and the 'stop and chop' technique, the key step is to perform the grooving correctly with a view to cracking the nucleus into sections. High phako power and low aspiration are required for this and the basic procedure is as follows:

1. Hold the probe in the dominant hand with a precision (i.e. pen) grip and then steady it with the thumb, middle and index fingers from the other hand orientated at right angles to the dominant hand (Figure 24.24). Make sure the forearms are supported (if operating superiorly use the patient's forehead, or temporally use a chair with arm rests).

2. Perform all phakoemulsification within the CCC. Depth is much more important than length. The initial aim is to split the nucleus in half. Since the halves are held together by radially orientated

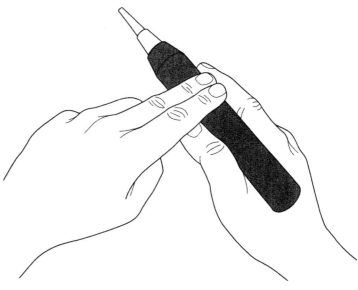

Figure 24.24 Two-handed grip for probe for initial grooving.

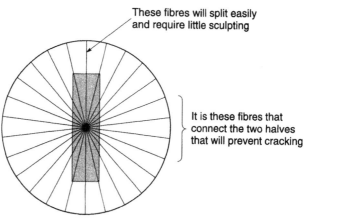

These fibres will split easily and require little sculpting

It is these fibres that connect the two halves that will prevent cracking

Figure 24.25 It is the transverse fibres that will make cracking difficult.

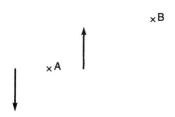

Figure 24.26 Creating a torque. Two equal forces in opposite direction will generate a couple or turning force but no translational force. This couple is identical for all the axes perpendicular to the this paper, and are the same for both point A and point B. The axis of rotation is *not* dependent on the points where the forces are applied.

lens fibres, the important ones are the transverse fibres (Figure 24.25). The suggested strategy is to groove downwards to the midline (downslope sculpturing), as this facilitates removal of the deeper layers[15], and then rotate the nucleus 180° and groove the second half of the trench in the same manner. The grip is the pen grip, and the instrument tip should face down. It is important that the width of the trench is about one and a half times the probe width so the tip can reach the bottom of the trench and is not held back by the needle sheath.

3. Rotation should be as atraumatic as possible, and best way to do this is to use two instruments. For the same force, the greater the separation of the two instruments, the greater the couple or turning force (Figure 24.26). As long as the two forces are equal in size and are in opposite directions, then the result will be to generate a pure turning force (or torque) and no translational force, with the result that very little stress will be placed on the zonules. If any degree of force is required, stop and repeat the hydrodissection step.

4. The most difficult stage is estimating the depth of the groove, and it is reassuring to note that 'phakoing out the back' is an extremely rare way to rupture the posterior capsule. There are a number of helpful pointers to estimate depth. The initial groove should be at least two and a half times the probe width. Fine white striations visible at the bottom of the trench suggest that the needle is still within the nucleus. Finally, once through the nucleus, a constant, clear red reflex appears.

5. With the divide and conquer, aim to split the nucleus into four by making a second trench at right angles to the first.

6. The cracking stage requires two instruments, one of which can be the phako probe. Place the two instruments in one of the trenches, against the nucleus and as close to the base of the trench as possible, and then slowly push them apart. If the nucleus does not crack easily, the groove is not deep enough. Do not try and crack too soon, as this may damage the walls of the trench and prevent good purchase. The crack usually starts at one end of the trench, and once it starts, move the instruments so as to run the crack along the base of the trench. The crack must be complete and a 'river of red' visible between the two halves.

7. Once the nucleus is cracked into four, each quadrant is emulsified in turn. All the emulsifying is done at the six o'clock position, to which each segment is rotated in turn. Remember that the fibres are orientated radially and accordingly the segments are most easily emulsified/aspirated from their 'noses' (Figure 24.27). Once a segment has been rotated to the six o'clock position, it is presented to the phako tip by tipping the nose up (Figure 24.28). Once it is engaged, pull the segment into the centre of the bag and emulsify it. For this manoeuvre less power is required, but much more aspiration. To facilitate rapid changing of the settings, most phako machines are pre-programmable. Typical settings for primary phako are 70 per cent phako power and 30–50 mm Hg aspiration, and for secondary phako are 40 per cent phako power and 140–280 mm Hg aspiration, but these can be altered as required.

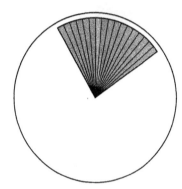

Figure 24.27 The lens fibres are orientated towards the 'nose'.

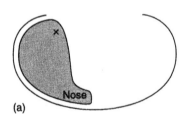

(a)

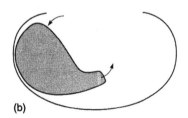

(b)

Figure 24.28 Pressure at X will lead the fragment to rotate and cause the 'nose' to move up and away from the posterior capsule.

During the grooving phase, the probe should cut the nucleus. If the probe pushes the nucleus away, then more phako power is required; if it pulls the nucleus, less aspiration is required.

During emulsification of the quadrants phase, pulsed phako is often more economical and effective. The short pulses followed by pauses result in the quadrant being continually disimpacted and re-impacted on the phako tip, thus facilitating its removal. With hard nuclei take care, as the quadrant does not aspirate and the probe may simply bore a hole through it and out the other side; it is easy to damage collateral structures in this way without realizing. If this does happen, mechanically disengage the quadrant with the second instrument and then re-engage it.

Stop and chop

Initially the process is the same as the divide and conquer technique as far as splitting the nucleus in half (see steps 1–4 above). The next step is to 'stop and chop'[16]. The idea of chopping the nucleus originated with Nagahara, but this left a number of fragments totally interlocked and immobile. Koch's idea was to start with a trench and do the initial split to create space in the bag for chopping. This technique has two major advantages over the divide and conquer technique:

1. Phakoemulsification times are consistently shorter (usually half those seen with the divide and conquer technique). The upper limit of safe phakoemulsification is around 4 minutes, and while this is readily achieved in most cases it can present a problem with hard nuclei. In principle, the shorter the phakoemulsification time the better. The trend towards shorter phakoemulsification times may account for the anecdotal observation that the occurrence rate of retinal detachments seems to be lower than the early reports of 1.17 per cent[17].
2. With the chopping action there is no stress on the zonules because the force is directed to the centre rather than outwards as in cracking.

The technique is as follows:

1. Switch to secondary phako settings (high aspiration and low phako power).
2. Orientate the groove to be at 30° to the surgical axis.
3. Tilt the heminucleus back and then impale it with the phako probe so that the tip is buried, using emulsification initially to embed the tip and then holding it there with maximum aspiration.
4. Pull the heminucleus gently towards the centre of the eye and simultaneously push slightly down (the natural tendency is to pull towards the wound, which is slightly upwards, and this will cause the heminucleus to impact on the anterior capsule) so as to create a little space between the nucleus and the anterior capsule to allow access for the chopper.
5. Pass the chopper under the lens capsule behind the nucleus and bury the end of the chopper in the soft lens matter.
6. Pull the chopper towards the phako tip (which acts as a chopping board), making a deep cut, and then at the last minute perform a dog-leg manoeuvre and pull the chopper at right angles to the initial chopping motion (Figure 24.29). The initial chopping action effectively makes a deep groove, and the second action then splits the heminucleus into two. This leaves a big portion in the bag and a small portion impaled on the tip of the phako needle.
7. Pull the impaled fragment to the geometric centre of the bag and safely emulsify it. The second instrument should be placed between the fragment and the lens capsule to act as a guard against accidental aspiration of the lens bag.
8. Once the first fragment has been emulsified, there is plenty of space to repeat the process as many times as required until all the nucleus has been removed.

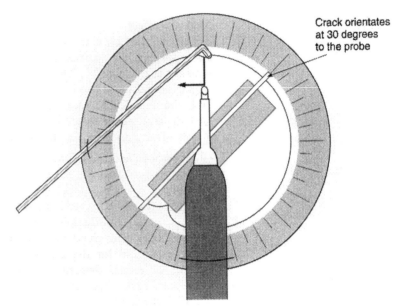

Crack orientates
at 30 degrees
to the probe

Figure 24.29 The chopping action is initially towards the phako tip and then, at the last minute, to form a dog-leg. The idea is for the chopper to make a groove and then, with the dog-leg, turn the groove into a crack.

Occasionally it is impossible to chop the nucleus neatly, in which case resort to the divide and conquer technique or a combination of the two.

The significant point regarding both the divide and conquer and the stop and chop techniques is to get a clean break into two heminuclei. If a bowel technique is attempted on a hard nucleus, the 'spinning saucer' phenomenon may result; this is a plate of nucleus that is too thin to phakoemulsify safely but too hard to implode or be aspirated. In this case, try viscoexpression by injecting viscoelastic behind it to prolapse it into the anterior chamber where it is possible to get the probe behind it safely and emulsify it.

The epinucleus, if present, can be dealt with by 'flip and chip'. Aspirate the top edge of it, which underlies the anterior capsule, and pull it whilst simultaneously using a blunt second instrument (e.g. mushroom) to push the deep part of the epinucleus overlying the posterior capsule away. This will cause the epinucleus to rotate (flip) over, and it can then be removed by what is essentially phako-assisted aspiration. If there is a problem, viscoexpress it into the anterior chamber.

Once the nucleus has been aspirated, the soft lens matter can then be dealt with as in extracapsular surgery. All machines come with automated aspiration attachments, but some still prefer manual aspiration (e.g. with a Simcoe cannula). The paracentesis site can be slightly enlarged to let the Simcoe fit through and enable easy aspiration at the twelve o'clock position.

LENS IMPLANTATION

There are basically three implantation techniques, depending upon the lens type: rigid lenses (implanted as for extracapsular surgery), injectable lenses (loaded into the injector and implanted by passing the tip of the injector through the corneal wound into the bag and injecting it) and folding lenses. The latter are inserted by the following method:

1. Inflate the capsular bag with viscoelastic.
2. Fold the lens along its long axis with a pair of folding forceps.
3. Grab the lens with a pair of lens forceps, pushing what will be the trailing haptic to the left so that when the lens is posted through the wound it will be touching the floor of the incision.
4. Post the leading haptic and the optic through the corneal wound, making sure that the leading haptic is in the bag and in the correct orientation. Some lenses are vaulted, so it is important that these lenses should not unfold incorrectly and end upside down.
5. Make sure the optic is in the bag. If not, encourage it to enter the bag (assuming the leading haptic is already in it) by pressing back on it.
6. Place the trailing haptic in the bag using the same technique as for a rigid lens, using a pair of MacPherson forceps.

An alternative method is to fold the lens at right angles to the above technique. This will result in the haptics being folded. The ends can then be tucked in to the folded lens, which is inserted through the wound and released in the bag. The idea behind this is that both haptics are simultaneously implanted in the bag at the time of lens unfolding.

CLOSURE

The wounds are usually self-sealing and do not require closure. If there is a microleak, close it by hydration of the wound. This is done by injecting balanced salt solution into the walls of the wound so that the cornea hydrates (it becomes white and can form a crystalline pattern, as in the keratopathy of that name). Clearly this is only a temporizing measure, and it almost certainly works by predicting which leaks will be self-limiting when the wounds hydrate over the first 24 hours.

Occasionally a suture is needed (e.g. 11/0 Mersilene®, which can usually be removed at one week).

AFTERCARE AND COMPLICATIONS

Postoperative care is minimal. It is standard practice to give topical antibiotics for a week (e.g. chloramphenicol q.d.s.), but this need not be continued for any longer than it takes the wounds to epithelialize. It is usual to provide topical steroids for the first 4–5 weeks but, as with extracapsular surgery, the use of a topical non-steroidal anti-inflammatory can be considered as an alternative[2,3].

An uncomplicated procedure can give very rapid visual rehabilitation and refraction and dispensing of glasses can occur as soon as week two. The only complication that occurs with any frequency is a postoperative pressure rise, which has two causes: first, failure to remove the viscoelastic at the end of the procedure (aspiration of viscoelastic from behind the lens implant can be helped by gently pressing up and down on the implant with the aspiration cannula, a process termed 'rock and roll'); and secondly, generating very high pressures when injecting fluid into the eyes to test if the wounds are watertight. It is worth making sure that the eye is soft at the end of surgery by releasing some fluid if necessary.

There is no need for routine review on the following postoperative day. If concerned about a possible pressure spike, then give 24 hours of oral acetozolamide (e.g. 250 mg t.d.s.). All pressure spikes are self-limiting, even without treatment. It is reasonable to review the patient at some point in the first 2 weeks, and most will have 6/12 unaided vision for distance at that visit and can be discharged safely back to the care of their optician. The technique therefore greatly reduces the out-patient follow-up required.

As there are no stitches used, there is no limitation on postoperative activity and the patients should simply be counselled to avoid activities that cause pain. With an aggressive discharge policy, it is important that patients are told when to seek help because there are two rare but serious complications that can present after early discharge; retinal detachment and endophthalmitis. The eye should get less red and painful, and the vision should remain stable or improve with time. All patients should be advised to seek urgent attention if the eye becomes increasingly red or painful, or if the vision deteriorates over time.

CONVERSION TECHNIQUE TO EXTRACAPSULAR SURGERY

The easiest way to convert from a scleral tunnel is to enlarge the scleral tunnel to make a giant pocket through which the nucleus can be expressed. The easiest way to convert from a temporal corneal pocket is simply to close the section with a single stitch (e.g. 11/0 Mersilene®), reinflate the eye and then start again as a routine extracapsular procedure superiorly. Try not to make the corneal section cross the paracentesis or join the original wound, as the combination of a forward sloping paracentesis/temporal corneal pocket and a reverse sloping extracapsular corneal section will make subsequent watertight closure difficult. The CCC must also be converted to a beer-can capsulotomy by making multiple relieving incisions in the anterior capsule. The nucleus will not express through an intact CCC and a single relieving tear is not sufficient – it will frequently wrap round to the posterior capsule.

MANAGEMENT OF POSTERIOR CAPSULE RUPTURE AND VITREOUS LOSS

Posterior capsular rupture without vitreous loss requires great care. If the cataract can be removed without provoking vitreous loss and enlarging the capsular tear, then in-the-bag or sulcus-fixated lens implantation can be performed. Small posterior capsular tears can be stabilized by converting them into a primary posterior capsulorhexis. The key point is where to implant the lens. If it is only a small tear, or if it can be stabilized, then it is reasonable to continue with implanting into the capsular bag; otherwise a sulcus fixated lens is more appropriate.

INTRAOPERATIVE COMPLICATIONS OF PHAKOEMULSIFICATION

The results of phakoemulsification are truly impressive in skilled hands. The major problem with the technique is not the results, but that it is difficult to learn and the operation is unforgiving. The complication rates when learning phakoemulsification are similar to when learning extracapsular surgery, but while a good phakoemulsification is much better than a good extracapsular operation, a poor phakoemulsification is much worse than a poor extracapsular operation. This leads to an unresolved ethical dilemma regarding how to teach and learn this technique.

The complications are potentially more serious in phakoemulsification than in extracapsular surgery, because in the former not all of the nucleus of the lens may have been removed. Retained nucleus (even a single quadrant) is a potent cause of phakoanaphylactic uveitis, and thus the main aim in complicated phakoemulsification surgery is to try and ensure complete nucleus removal.

Although much has been written regarding surgical technique, relatively little has been written about how the surgeon can extricate him- or herself from trouble. Therefore, this subsection is almost completely anecdotal.

Failure to complete capsulorhexis
The management decision is between continuing with phakoemulsification and converting. When phakoemulsification was first described it was a technique for lens removal in young patients; the nucleus was expressed into the anterior chamber, where the procedure was performed. It is therefore very reasonable to do this if there is a soft cataract that will largely aspirate with minimal ultrasound time.

It is not an appropriate technique for hard cataracts or for elderly patients, when the alternative is to convert to extracapsular surgery. Conversion is particularly easy at this stage.

Anterior chamber instability
A formed anterior chamber is essential for safe phakoemulsification. Loss of anterior chamber is usually due to excessive leakage of fluid from the section, and this is the rationale for developing the smaller 2.5-mm incisions with the newer phako needles. The first thing to check with a shallow anterior chamber is that the eye is soft and can be reformed with viscoelastic.

To deal with a shallow anterior chamber and a soft eye:

1. Check height of the infusion bottle and increase it as appropriate.
2. Reduce the vacuum on the aspiration.
3. Consider reducing the size of the section with the help of a stitch.

A shallow anterior chamber and a hard eye suggest either malignant glaucoma or a suprachoroidal haemorrhage, and conversion is therefore not an option because an expulsive is the likely outcome. A suprachoroidal haemorrhage usually presents as a slowly shallowing anterior chamber, and one solution is to wait for 30 minutes (the average clotting time is 6 minutes) and then restart the operation. An advantage of phakoemulsification is that it is a closed system, so the expanding haemorrhage is self-limiting due to the rise in intraocular pressure that it induces. The diagnosis can be confirmed by fundal examination in the immediate postoperative period. Malignant glaucoma is a complication that can occur during hydrodissection, and the attack can usually be broken by reforming the anterior chamber with a viscoelastic.

Small pupil

A small pupil is a recognized risk for vitreous loss[19], and is the only risk factor that is directly under the surgeon's control. Phakoemulsification is frankly dangerous if the surgeon cannot see what is happening. Pupils may be small because:

1. No dilating drops have been given – the pupil is still responsive to light.
2. Some pupils simply dilate poorly – this is a feature of ageing (senile meiosis) and some conditions such as diabetes and pseudoexfoliation.
3. The pupil is stuck down due to posterior synechiae formation.

In the first case, simply give further dilating drops. In the other two situations, the pupil can be stretched (posterior synechae can usually be easily broken by injecting viscoelastic under the iris and then sweeping with a blunt instrument such as an iris repositor) and kept in the enlarged position by the use of iris hooks, and this provides an excellent solution. The capsulorhexis should be around 5 mm in diameter, and this therefore represents the minimum desired pupil size. In cases of doubt use iris hooks, as it is easier to place them before CCC than after. There are two types of hooks available, they are similar both in cost per case and in the manner of application:-

1. Gold iris hooks. These are single use, and once inserted, are bent for retention. Once in place, they are not easy to adjust.
2. Cat gut with rubber bungs. These are more expensive, but can be reused up to a recommended maximum of three times. Their container comes with three white plastic balls attached on a piece of thread, so one ball should be cut off each time they are used.

To use iris hooks, make four holes (with a 25-gauge – orange – needle) marking out a square in the cornea close to the limbus. Make the first hole aiming for the centre of the anterior capsule, then line up the second hole with the first and the centre of the pupil. Make a note of the axis of the first pair of holes at the pupil centre; the next axis must be at right angles to this. Make the last two holes. Then insert the hooks and adjust the tension to enlarge the pupil without overstretching, which would cause the iris to tear. They are not difficult to use, just fiddly.

Hydrodissection

Hydrodissection is performed to allow the nucleus to rotate freely. If the nucleus will not rotate one way, then try the other. Failing that, hydrodissection can be repeated as often as required until the nucleus does rotate freely. Do not try to force the nucleus to rotate, as too much force will simply cause zonule dehiscence or capsular rupture.

Inability to groove and crack the nucleus

If the ultrasonic hand-piece will not groove the nucleus, turn the power up. The routine setting on most machines is in the region of 70 per cent, and occasionally 100 per cent power is required. There is the odd exceptional nucleus that will not even be dented by 100 per cent power, and this is an indication for conversion. A key point is that the phako needle should cut into the nucleus and not need to be pushed into it; if despite 100 per cent power the needle is tending to push the nucleus away, then phakoemulsification is inappropriate. This is becoming less of a problem with improving technology.

Zonule dehiscence and capsular tension rings

If zonule dehiscence occurs the capsular bag collapses and it is very hard to remove its contents. The problem may be recognized preoperatively in patients with iridodenesis or frankly dislocated lenses, or it may result from surgical complications. The solution is the use of capsular tension rings, which were first introduced by Hara in 1991[19] and have been variously termed equator rings or endocapsular rings. However, if there is severe zonular dehiscence, then consideration should be given to a vitreo-lensectomy in young patients, or an intracapsular procedure in elderly patients with either an anterior chamber lens or a sutured posterior-chamber lens implant. Endocapsular rings that can be sutured to the scleral have been developed for patients with severe zonular dehiscence.

Capsular tension rings are made of PMMA (Figure 24.30) and are currently made by Morcher GMPH and OPHTEC (Groningen, Holland); they differ very slightly in that the OPHTEC ring has a larger gap[20] and is slightly more rigid than the Morcher version. The rings come in different sizes and the most commonly used is 12–12.5/10, where the first number refers to the diameter (in millimetres) of the ring when opened and the second to the diameter that the ring can be compressed to. If too large a ring is inserted the ends will overlap, but this does not appear to be a problem[21]. For large eyes a larger ring should be used to ensure that the bag is properly supported. OPHTEC suggest using a 13/11 ring for highly myopic eyes, while Gimbel and colleagues[21] suggest 14.5/12 for eyes that measure 12.5 mm or more from 'white to white'.

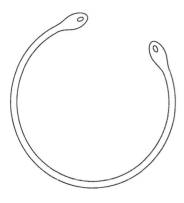

Figure 24.30   Capsular tension ring.

Insert the rings as soon as zonular dehiscence is diagnosed, or, if pre-existing, immediately after completing the capsulorhexis stage. Post the end of the ring just under the anterior capsule and dial it in, or inject the OPHTEC ring straight into the bag. When used just after capsulorhexis stage, insert the ring and then inject viscoelastic to allow the ring to slip round to the equator.

Capsular rings are an extremely effective way of converting a dangerous and difficult situation to a safe and stable one. However, they are not a universal panacea and should be used with extreme caution if there is a posterior capsular tear or more than 180° of zonular dehiscence.

Posterior capsular rupture

If posterior capsular rupture occurs during phakoemulsification, the eye is closed and there may be no vitreous loss. It has even been known for phakoemulsification to proceed smoothly on an intact anterior vitreous face and the lack of posterior capsule to be diagnosed only when implanting a posterior chamber lens.

However, the same rules apply as in extracapsular surgery, and the primary aim is to ensure that all nuclear material is removed. Step one is to recognize rupture early, and suggestive signs are:

1. Lens instability
2. Sudden deepening of the anterior chamber
3. Sudden shallowing of the anterior chamber when hydrodissecting
4. The phakoemulsification probe stops working (it will not cut vitreous)
5. Direct visualization of a vitreous or capsular tear.

Vitreous will delay or prevent nuclear material from falling, but its presence will prevent the phakoemulsification probe from working and irrigation will tend to increase the nuclear instability. If the vitreous is removed, the nuclear material will probably dislocate backwards. Little is published on how to deal with this situation, but experience suggest the following:

1. Inject viscoelastic behind the nuclear material with the dual aim of trying to prevent the vitreous coming forward and, at the same time, viscoexpress as much of the nuclear material as possible into the anterior chamber. If the problem has occurred after successfully cracking the nucleus, it is relatively straightforward to inject viscoelastic through a Rycroft cannula directly behind the nucleus. If it occurs before cracking, then try viscoexpression and the lens may come forward; if this fails, refer to a vitreoretinal surgeon.
2. Once the lens material is in the anterior chamber, pass a lens slide through a 5-mm wound and behind the lens fragments to cover the defect in the posterior capsule. Open up the wound to viscoexpress (if the cataract is hard) or emulsify (if soft) the lens fragments.
3. Once the nucleus has been removed, make sure that any vitreous in the anterior chamber is also removed.

4. Try to remove as much soft lens matter as possible while doing no further damage to any remaining capsule (if there is no chance of having enough capsule to support a posterior chamber lens then it is probably best to remove it with the vitreous cutter during the vitrectomy stage).

5. Decide on the merits of lens implantation.

Lens implantation in complicated cases

If there is only a very small break in the posterior capsule without vitreous loss, in-the-bag implantation can be performed. If there is a large posterior capsule tear with much of the anterior capsule intact (which is often the case with complicated phakoemulsification surgery), safe implantation of a sulcus fixated lens is possible. The minimum overall diameter for the lens should be 13 mm; if it is smaller than this the lens can rotate (causing pigment dispersion and iris chafing/iritis) and decentre. The fixation can be further enhanced, if the anterior capsulorhexis is intact and smaller than the optic, by pushing the optic through the CCC opening so that the optic is in the bag, leaving the haptics in the sulcus.

If there is insufficient capsule for a posterior chamber lens, then the choice is between a sutured posterior chamber lens and an anterior chamber lens. It is much easier to implant an anterior chamber lens than to suture a posterior chamber lens, and this is the preferred option in an elderly patient. However, there is a problem of long-term complications with an anterior chamber lens (particularly Fuch's corneal dystrophy), and for this reason they are usually considered inappropriate in patients under the age of 60 years. A sutured posterior chamber lens is extremely difficult on a soft eye and should not be done at the same time as a complicated cataract operation, but as a secondary procedure.

The merits of primary anterior chamber lens implantation are uncertain. Accurate positioning of an anterior chamber lens is not straightforward and can be particularly difficult to do on a soft vitrectomized eye. There is evidence that postoperative inflammation is more severe with a primary lens implant in this position, and that it is less likely to be accurately sized and positioned; it also seems that cystoid macular oedema may be more common[22]. This would argue for a secondary lens implantation in this situation, although visual rehabilitation is significantly delayed in those having a secondary lens implantation procedure[22].

If there is no posterior capsule but still a small incision of 5 mm or less, then the eye can be readily reformed and accurate sizing and placing is no more difficult than in a secondary procedure. If there is little or no retained lens matter and the vitreous has been adequately dealt with, then it is reasonable to proceed with anterior chamber lens implantation.

If a posterior chamber lens is implanted when there is insufficient capsular support and it prolapses into the vitreous, then the key point is never to try to retrieve a dislocated lens implant. The lens material is inert and, being heavier than vitreous, usually sinks to the dependent position. Patients may have odd symptoms on rising from the horizontal position, but they rapidly resolve as the lens sinks and the dislocated lens is then asymptomatic. Implant a second lens (an anterior chamber lens in an elderly patient or a sutured posterior chamber in a younger patient) as a secondary procedure.

Anterior chamber lens implantation

Anterior chamber lenses are vaulted anteriorly and have four footplates that should sit in the angle. Many of the complications of anterior chamber lens use are thought to result from the lens rubbing on the iris or the corneal endothelium, or from movement of the lens in the angle. For this reason, one anterior chamber lens size will not fit all eyes and the correct size lens must be used. The key measurement is the horizontal corneal measurement (from 'white to white') plus one in millimetres. The lens must also be inserted the correct way up (vaulting away from the iris and towards the cornea). The procedure is much easier with a small pupil, so constrict the pupil with Miochol, insert a lens slide through the wound across the pupil, inflate the anterior chamber with viscoelastic and then slide the lens in. If the footplates catch and ruck the iris, use a lens hook and gently pull the haptic towards the pupil; this usually releases the iris, which then springs back into position. Releasing the haptic will then allow it to sit in the angle. It is important to release any 'iris tucks', as this is a reported risk factor for accelerated corneal endothelial cell loss[23,24].

There is a risk of the optic occluding the pupil despite the anterior vaulting of the lens, and a peripheral iridectomy must be performed. The neatest way to do this is to use the cutter used for performing the vitrectomy, with the cutting rate turned down to the lowest rate. Use suction to aspirate the iris into the cutting port and then make a single cut to give a round iridectomy. Alternatively, grasp the iris with a pair of fine forceps and tent it through the wound and then, using a pair of scissors (either Vanna's or DeWecker's), make the iridectomy.

POSTOPERATIVE COMPLICATIONS OF CATARACT SURGERY

REFRACTIVE ERROR

Refractive error may be spherical or cylindrical (astigmatism).

Spherical error

Spherical error implies either aphakia or an error in the power of the implanted lens. The management of postoperative spherical error is currently under evolution. With small incision techniques and in-the-bag lens implantation, the refraction stabilizes much more quickly than after extracapsular surgery and large spherical errors are usually detected much more quickly. In this situation, implantation of a second lens (piggybacking) or lens exchange are the first-line treatments.

In planning a lens exchange, it is important to check that the power of the implanted lens corresponds to that planned. If it was simply human error, then the exchange is straightforward. If the intended implant was indeed implanted, then the problem is more complex. There are two approaches:

1. The required power of the new implant can be calculated from the refraction. There are formulae to calculate the required lens implant power from the refraction (such as the Holladay Consultant program), but the general rule is that it is 1.5 times the spectacle error if the patient is hypermetropic, and the spectacle error if the patient is myopic. The advantage of using a piggy-back lens is that, although unlikely, the biometric error may have been caused by mislabelling of the implanted lens. A distinct disadvantage is the potential of interface problems where the two optics touch.
2. The second approach is to assume that the biometric error was due to an error in the axial length measurement. Accordingly, back calculate to see what value of the axial length was required to obtain the observed refractive outcome, and then use this axial length to re-perform the lens calculations and assess which lens should have been used.

The alternative to lens exchange is to use the appropriate refractive correction and consider corneal refractive techniques.

Astigmatic error
Postoperative astigmatism is a well recognized feature of extracapsular surgery, where an average of 2 D of surgically-induced astigmatism is not uncommon. The usual tendency is for the stitches to be on the tight side and cause with-the-rule astigmatism (that is, the steep meridian is vertical). If using positive cylinders, then the axis marks the steep meridian. Routine suture removal cannot be considered until 8 weeks, and many surgeons prefer to wait longer; following suture removal, it is at least 2 weeks before refractive stability is achieved. This is one of the drawbacks of extracapsular surgery – it takes at least 3 months to achieve refractive stability, and longer if selective suture removal is performed.

Against-the-rule astigmatism following extracapsular surgery is associated with wound dehiscence and, if detected early, is best managed by resuturing the wound.

The management of pre-existing astigmatism is discussed in Chapter 27.

POSTERIOR CAPSULAR OPACIFICATION

Posterior capsular thickening is the commonest complication of extracapsular surgery. Risk factors for it include poor cortical clean-up at surgery and young age of the patient. It presents as progressive, painless blurring of vision, and the symptoms are very similar to those of the original cataract (it is often referred to as 'after-cataract'). Management has been greatly simplified by the development of the YAG laser, and posterior capsulotomy can easily be performed as an outpatient procedure.

This is a much greater problem in the developing world, where there is lack of access to such lasers and to health care in general, and therefore many surgeons still perform intracapsular surgery.

POSTOPERATIVE CYSTOID MACULAR OEDEMA

Angiographically detectable cystoid macular oedema was almost universal in the days of intracapsular surgery, but the incidence has dropped with improved techniques. With extracapsular surgery angiographic cystoid macular oedema (CMO) occurs in 20–30 per cent of cases, but clinically significant macular oedema occurs in just 1–2 per cent. As might be expected, cystoid macular oedema is much more common if there have been operative complications – particularly vitreous loss.

It is a complication that is better prevented than treated and, while its exact aetiology is unknown, inflammation and vitreous traction are recognized predisposing factors. If there is vitreous loss, then a thorough anterior vitrectomy must be performed to prevent the formation of traction bands (which increase the risk of retinal detachment as well as CMO). Suppression of inflammation is also important, and systemic non-steroidal anti-inflammatory drugs (NSAID) have been shown to provide effective prophylaxis[25] and should be routinely prescribed if there has been a significant surgical complication.

There is no proven effective treatment of established postoperative cystoid macular oedema and, while oral NSAIDs, carbonic anhydrase inhibitors[26,27] and hyperbaric oxygen[28] have all been tried, the benefits are small at best. Fortunately most cases are self-limiting and will resolve over a variable period of time.

CORNEAL DECOMPENSATION

Postoperative corneal oedema is a potentially serious complication. There seems to be a different mechanism for the corneal oedema associated with phakoemulsification as opposed to extracapsular surgery, as the former is more common and tends to be more severe, yet clears more rapidly. However, the management is clear-cut; always check the ocular pressure and treat appropriately. Many would prescribe increased topical steroids for severe corneal oedema, but there seems little rationale for this and there is no evidence that it improves the final outcome.

The only treatment for persisting oedema is a corneal graft but, as recovery can be delayed, at least 3 months should elapse before even considering this.

VISUAL PROGNOSIS WITH VITREOUS LOSS

There is the idea that properly handled vitreous loss is not associated with a poor outcome, but this is erroneous. The best results showed that nearly 90 per cent of patients achieved 6/12 or better following posterior capsular rupture, and this series was associated with a very low rate of vitreous loss of only 38 per cent[29]. However, overt vitreous loss is associated with only 60–65 per cent of patients achieving 6/12[22,30,31]. It is also common knowledge that this group require multiple outpatient appointments and are often required to be on topical medication for a prolonged period for postoperative uveitis and ocular pressure, and have delayed visual rehabilitation due particularly to cystoid macular oedema.

There are also potential long-term problems with the use of anterior chamber lenses, particularly pseudophakic bullous keratopathy.

RETINAL DETACHMENT

Javitt et al.[17] reported retinal detachment rates 4 years after cataract surgery of 1.55 per cent following intracapsular surgery, 0.9 per cent following extracapsular surgery and 1.17 per cent after phakoemulsification. The rate after cataract surgery complicated by vitreous loss was 5 per cent. The rates for detachment following phakoemulsification may now be lower than this, as techniques improve and operation and phakoemulsification times get shorter.

ENDOPHTHALMITIS

This is discussed fully on pages 306–10.

SUPRACHOROIDAL HAEMORRHAGE

This complication occurs in 0.2 per cent of cataract operations[32], and is also seen in other intraocular procedures such as penetrating keratoplasty and glaucoma drainage surgery. The common factor is thought to be the period of hypotony. During the hypotonous period, fluid collects in the suprachoroidal space; this puts stress on the bridging emissary vessels, which can then rupture. In extracapsular surgery the open wound means that this can result in an expulsive haemorrhage with extrusion of the retina, and the only point of management on which all are agreed is immediate and rapid closure of the wound, if necessary using stronger than normal suture material (e.g. 7–9/0 rather than 10/0 nylon), as significant tension may be required. Rapid closure can be difficult, and the use of the suture needles across the wound (like staples) has been advocated[33]. As always, pressure stops bleeding. Once closure has been achieved, the merits of any further intervention are far from certain. A sclerostomy will help drain the blood, but some surgeons suggest waiting 10 minutes before draining because early drainage may cause further bleeding, exacerbating the situation[35]. However, by 10 minutes much of the blood will have clotted and not be drainable.

The self-sealing wound in phakoemulsification results in a better outcome following suprachoroidal haemorrhage, as the bleed will immediately result in a rapid rise of the ocular pressure; this in turn will tamponade the bleed. The operation should be cancelled and performed (or completed) after having allowed time for the blood to clot (a delay of half-an-hour may be sufficient, although most surgeons would prefer longer!).

THE LEARNING CURVE

The vitreous loss rate for surgeons when learning extracapsular surgery is in the order of 3–10 per cent[35-37], and for phakoemulsification is 6–15 per cent[38-40]. The rate is similar for an experienced extracapsular surgeon learning phakoemulsification[41,42]. For experienced surgeons, the vitreous loss rate for extracapsular surgery is under 3 per cent[43] and for phakoemulsification is in the region of 1 per cent[44]. It should be noted that there is almost certainly a degree of publication bias, with only the better surgeons submitting their results to the public gaze. This leads to the unresolved issue of getting truly informed consent from patients whilst giving trainee surgeons the opportunity to learn.

REFERENCES

1. Lehmann, O. J., Roberts, C. J., Ikram, K. *et al.* (1997). Association between non-administration of subconjunctival cefuroxime and postoperative endophthalmitis. *J. Cataract Refract. Surg.*, **23**, 889–93.
2. Italian Diclofenac Study Group (1997). Efficacy of diclofenac eyedrops in preventing postoperative inflammation and long-term cystoid macular edema. *J. Cataract Refract. Surg.*, **23**, 1183–9.
3. Demco, T. A., Sutton, H., Demco, C. J. and Raj, P. S. (1997). Topical diclofenac sodium compared with prednisolone acetate after phakoemulsification lens implant surgery. *Eur. J. Ophthalmol.*, **7**, 236–40.
4. Tufail, A., Foss, A. J. E. and Hamilton, A. M. P. (1995). Is the first day postoperative review necessary after cataract extraction? *Br. J. Ophthalmol.*, **79**, 1646–8.
5. Kasner, D. (1969). A new approach to the management of vitreous (interview). *Highlights Ophthalmol.*, **11**, 304.
6. Machemar, R., Buettner, H., Norton, H. W. D. and Parel, J. M. (1971). Vitrectomy: a pars plana approach. *Trans. Am. Acad. Ophth. Otolaryngol.*, **75**, 813–20.
7. Gimbel, H. V. and Neuhann, T. (1990). Development, advantages and methods of the continuous circular capsulorhexis technique. *J. Cataract Refract. Surg.*, **16**, 31–7.
8. Mansour, A. M. (1989). Anterior capsulorhexis in hypermature cataracts (letter). *J. Cataract Refract. Surg.*, **19**, 435–7.
9. Horiguchi, M., Miyake, K., Ohta, I. and Ito, Y. (1998). Staining of the lens capsule for circular continuous capsulorhexis in eyes with white cataract. *Arch. Ophthalmol.*, **116**, 535–7.
10. Fritz, W. L. (1998). Fluorescein blue, light assisted capsulorhexis for mature or hypermature cataract. *J. Cataract Refract. Surg.*, **24**, 19–20.
11. Hoffer, K. J. and McFarland, J. E. (1993). Intracameral subcapsular staining for improved visualization during capsulorhexis in mature cataracts (letter). *J. Cataract Refract. Surg.*, **19**, 566.

12. Cimetta, D. J., Gatti, M. and Lobianco, G. (1995). Haemocoloration of the anterior capsule in white capsule CCC. *J. Cataract Refract. Surg.*, **7**, 184–5.

13. Melles, G. R. J., de Waard, P. W. T., Pameyer, J. H. and Beekhuis, W. H. (1999). Trypan blue capsule staining to visualize the capsulorhexis in cataract surgery. *J. Cataract Refract. Surg.*, **25**, 7–9.

14. Fine, I. H. (1992). Cortical cleaving hydrodissection. *J. Cataract Refract. Surg.*, **5**, 508–12.

15. Gimbel, H. V. (1992). Downslope sculpting. *J. Cataract Refract. Surg.*, **6**, 614–18.

16. Koch, P. S. (1997). Anterior chamber irrigation with unpreserved Lidocaine® 1% for anesthesia during cataract surgery. *J. Cataract Refract. Surg.*, **23**, 551–4.

17. Javitt, J. C., Vitale, S., Canner, J. K. *et al.* (1991). National outcomes of cataract extraction I. Retinal detachment after inpatient surgery. *Ophthalmology*, **98**, 895–902.

18. Guzek, J. P., Holm, M. Cotter, J. B. *et al.* (1987). Risk factors for intraoperative complications in 1000 extracapsular cases. *Ophthalmology*, **94**, 461–6.

19. Hara, T. and Yamada Y. (1991). 'Equator ring' for maintenance of the complete circular contour of the capsular bag after cataract removal. *Ophthalmic Surg.*, **22**, 358–9.

20. Sun, R. and Gimbel, H. V. (1998). *In vitro* evaluation of the efficacy of the capsular tension ring for managing zonular dialysis in cataract surgery. *Ophthalmic Surg. Lasers*, **29**, 502–5.

21. Gimbel, H. V., Sun, R. and Heston, J. P. (1997). Management of zonular dialysis in phacoemulsification and IOL implantation using the capsular tension ring. *Ophthalmic Surg. Lasers*, **28**, 273–81.

22. Hykin, P. G., Gardner, I. D., Corbett, M. C. and Cheng, H. (1991). Primary or secondary anterior chamber lens implantation after extracapsular cataract surgery and vitreous loss. *Eye*, **5**, 694–8.

23. Ambrose, V. M., Walters, R. F., Batterbury, M. *et al.* (1991). Long-term endothelial cell loss and breakdown of the blood–aqueous barrier in cataract surgery. *J. Cataract Refract. Surg.*, **17**, 622–7.

24. Walters, R. F., McGill, J. L., Batterbury, M. and Williams, J. D. (1989). Complications of anterior chamber lens implants and their effects on the endothelium. *Eye*, **3**, 690–95.

25. Rossetti, L., Chaudhuri, J. and Dickersin, K. (1998). Medical prophylaxis and treatment of cystoid macular edema after cataract surgery. The results of meta-analysis. *Ophthalmology*, **105**, 397–405.

26. Cox, S. N., Hay, E. and Bird, A. C. (1988). Treatment of chronic macular edema with acetozolamide. *Arch. Ophthalmol.*, **106**, 1190–95.

27. Tripathi, R. C., Fekrat, S., Tripathi, B. J. and Ernest, J. T. (1991). A direct correlation of the resolution of pseudophakic macular edema with acetozolamide therapy. *Ann. Ophthalmol.*, **23**, 127–9.

28. Pfoff, D. S. and Thom, S. R. (1987). Preliminary report on the effect of hyperbaric oxygen on cystoid macular edema. *J. Cataract Refract. Surt.*, **13**, 136–40.

29. Osher, R. H. and Cionni, R. J. (1990). The torn posterior capsule: its intraoperative behavior, surgical management, and long-term consequences. *J. Cataract Refract. Surg.*, **16**, 490–94.

30. Claoue, C. and Steele, A. (1993). Visual prognosis following accidental vitreous loss during cataract surgery. *Eye*, **7**, 735–9.

31. Frost, N. A., Sparrow, J. M., Strong, N. P. and Rosenthal, A. R. (1995). Vitreous loss in planned extracapsular cataract extraction does lead to a poorer visual outcome. *Eye*, **9**, 446–51.

32. Payne, J. W., Kameen, A. J., Jensen, A. D. *et al.* (1985). Expulsive haemorrhage: its incidence in cataract surgery and a report of four bilateral cases. *Trans. Am Acad. Ophth. Otolaryngol.*, **83**, 181–204.

33. Pannu, J. S. (1992). Handling expulsive choroidal haemorrhage (brief communication. *Phaco. Foldables*, **5**, 2.

34. Lakhanpal, V., Schocket, S. S., Elman, M. J. and Nirankari, V. S. (1989). A new modified vitreoretinal surgical approach in the management of massive suprachoroidal haemorrhage. *Ophthalmology*, **96**, 793–800.

35. Browning, D. J. and Cobo, L. M. (1985). Early experience in extracapsular surgery by residents. *Ophthalmology*, **92**, 1647–53.

36. Jaffe, N. S. (1978). Results of intraocular lens implant surgery. The third Binkhorst medal lecture. *Am. J. Ophthalmol.*, **85**, 13–23.

37. Pearson, P. A., Owen, D. G., Van Meter, W. and Smith, T. J. (1989). Vitreous loss rates in extracapsular cataract surgery by residents. *Ophthalmology*, **96**, 1225–7.

38. Allinson, R. W., Metrikin, D. C. and Fante, R. G. (1992). Incidence of vitreous loss among third-year residents performing phakoemulsification. *Ophthalmology*, **99**, 726–30.
39. Cruz, O. A., Wallace, G. W., Gay, C. A. *et al.* (1992). Visual results and complications of phacoemulsification with intraocular lens implantation performed by ophthalmology residents. *Ophthalmology*, **99**, 448–52.
40. Thomas, R., Naveen, S., Jacob, A. and Braganza, A. (1997). Visual outcome and complications of residents learning phacoemulsification. *Ind. J. Ophthalmol.*, **45**, 215–19.
41. Dayton, G. O. and Hulquist, C. R. (1975). Complications of phacoemulsification. *Can. J. Ophthalmol.*, **10**, 61–8.
42. Hiles, D. A. and Hurite, F. G. (1973). Results of the first year's experience with phacoemulsification. *Am. J. Ophthalmol.*, **75**, 473–7.
43. Jaffe, N. S. (1984). *Cataract Surgery and its Complications*. Mosby Year Book.
44. Kratz, R. P. (1976). Teaching phacoemulsification in California and 200 cases of phacoemulsification. In: *Current Concepts in Cataract Surgery: Selected Proceedings of the Fourth Biennial Cataract Surgical Congress* (J. M. Emery and D. Paton, eds), pp. 196–200. Mosby Year Book.

25

INTRAOCULAR LENS DESIGN

HISTORY

Harold Ridley performed the first modern-day intraocular lens (IOL) implantation at St Thomas's Hospital on 29 November 1949. A large posterior chamber lens was inserted following extracapsular surgery. He came under severe criticism from the establishment, particularly for not performing animal experimentation first. There were marked problems with postoperative iritis and lens dislocation with the Ridley lens, but despite this it generated enough interest for others to try implantation.

The evolution of intraocular lens implantation has been divided into five generations by Apple and colleagues[1]; a sixth generation can now be added:

Generation 1	1949–54	The original Ridley posterior chamber lens implant
Generation 2	1952–62	The early anterior chamber lens implants
Generation 3	1953–73	Iris-supported lenses
Generation 4	1963–present	Modern anterior chamber lens implants (AC-IOL)
Generation 5	1975–present	Modern posterior chamber rigid lens implants
Generation 6	1984–present	Posterior chamber folding lenses

ANTERIOR CHAMBER LENS IMPLANTATION

Baron was credited with performing the first anterior lens implantation on 13 May 1952 in France. The lenses were used initially as a planned procedure, either combined with or following ICCE. They are now used most often in conjunction with vitreous loss and anterior vitrectomy, which is clearly a less favourable setting.

The early anterior chamber lenses ran into a number of problems. For example, the Stampelli lens was rigid with a radius of curvature of the non-optical portion of 13 mm. The extremities were thin at 0.3 mm. If the lenses were too thick (0.8 mm or more), it resulted in iris atrophy and distortion and corneal endothelial damage. However, an advantage with a rigid lens is that it is not physically possible to get an oversized lens in. Too large a lens with flexible haptics (e.g. a Dannheim lens) will bow forward and damage the corneal endothelium, while too small a lens can rotate (causing angle damage) and decentre.

Choyce solved the problem of lens sizing problems, with research culminating in the rigid mark VIII, which had four footplates and came in a number of sizes. Most modern AC-IOLs follow his design, but with slightly flexible haptics to facilitate fit (e.g. the one-piece Kelman lens). They too have four footplates, which should all rest in the angle. Too small a lens can be diagnosed gonioscopically by finding only two or three footplates resting in the angle, and by the change in the lens axis between clinic visits. He used a horizontal corneal diameter measurement in millimetres, to which he added one ('white to white plus one') to get the appropriate overall size for the lens.

There were two major designs of fixation elements:

1. Haptics or spatula footplates. These were present on the Strampelli and Choyce lenses and are now the accepted design.
2. Lens loops. The Dannheim lens (an AC-IOL) was the earliest prototype with small-diameter closed loops, and the Barraquer AC-IOL with open loops. They have been associated with a number of problems of persisting iritis and features of the UGH (uveitis, glaucoma and hyphaema) syndrome, although this is rare with modern manufacturing techniques. This is due to a number of factors, including the fact that the small diameter of the loops can induce pressure effects such as angle recession, descemetization of the angle and iris wrap-around, causing persisting inflammation and PAS formation. The loops often became embedded in a 360° fibro-uveal capsule or 'cocoon'. In 1987 the FDA put all closed-loop designs on a 'core investigation basis', which effectively removed them from the market.

LATE CORNEAL DECOMPENSATION

Progressive corneal endothelial damage also plagues anterior chamber lens implants, causing late corneal decompensation. While there is a reduction in endothelial cell number with age, this loss is accelerated in those with anterior chamber lenses[2] but not in those with posterior chamber lenses. Thus while the endothelial cell loss with surgery is similar in the immediate postoperative period, there is greatly increased endothelial cell loss at 10 years in those with AC-IOLs[3]. The rate of endothelial cell loss can be slowed by AC-IOL removal[4], suggesting a direct causal relationship. Poor positioning of the AC-IOL with an iris tuck is further associated with increased rates of endothelial cell loss[5,6] because of iris chafing and long-term breakdown of the blood–aqueous barrier.

Due to the problem of long-term corneal decompensation, an anterior chamber lens is only considered when there is insufficient lens capsule to support a posterior chamber lens. Even so, most would not recommend implanting an anterior chamber lens in a patient aged under 60 years.

MODERN POSTERIOR CHAMBER RIGID INTRAOCULAR LENSES

Pearce pioneered the return to posterior chamber lens (PC-IOL) in 1975. His implant was a rigid tripod design with two inferior feet implanted in the capsular bag and a superior foot implanted in front of the anterior capsule and sutured to the iris. The major breakthrough in design was by Shearing in 1977, with his J-loop PC-IOL, followed shortly by Simcoe, with a C-loop. Most modern lens designs resemble these J- and C-loop lenses.

The original J- and C-loop lenses were three-piece lenses with the haptics made of polypropylene (Prolene®). Prolene® is slowly biodegradable, and some explanted lenses do show early degradation of the haptics. However, spontaneous breakage has yet to be reported and implants have been in some patients for over 20 years. The present trend is for rigid lenses to be one-piece and made completely of PMMA.

CAPSULAR VS SULCUS FIXATION

The posterior chamber lens was developed for use with extracapsular cataract surgery and the beer-can capsulotomy. In this scenario it is relatively easy to achieve in-the-bag fixation for the inferior haptic, but the tendency was for the superior haptic to be in the sulcus.

The original Shearing lens had a total diameter of 12.5 mm. The crystalline lens is 9.6 mm (SD 0.4 mm), the evacuated lens bag is 10.5 mm and the ciliary sulcus is 11.0 mm (SD 0.5 mm). If the implanted lens is too small it will move around and the loose haptic can give a 'windshield wiper effect', causing such problems as pigment dispersion and iritis. This can also happen if the other haptic erodes into the ciliary body, and accordingly the manufacturers tended to increase the total lens size to 13.75–14.5 mm. Lenses designed for in-the-bag fixation tend to have a smaller diameter (10.0–12.5 mm). A lens that it is to be implanted into the sulcus should have a diameter of at least 13 mm.

Another problem with one haptic in the bag and one in the sulcus was the potential for late lens decentration due to capsular bag contracture.

One of the advantages of CCC and the use of folding lenses is that in-the-bag fixation can be guaranteed[7].

TYPES OF LENSES

FOLDABLE LENSES

Charles Kelman pioneered phakoemulsification as a technique for cataract extraction in the 1960s, but the small incision only offered a major advantage in those cases when no lens was to be implanted; the advantage was lost if the eye had to be opened in order to implant a lens. This was the driving force to develop a folding lens. Thomas Mazocco implanted the first folding lens in 1984, using a lens made out of a silicone elastomer[8].

The obvious advantages of small incision surgery (low induced astigmatism, fewer postoperative complications, greater wound strength, possibly less inflammation, and faster visual rehabilitation) have now made phakoemulsification and foldable lens implantation the technique of choice.

OPTICS

In discussing optics, there are four main issues; lens diameter, surface properties, edge effects and monofocal versus multifocal lenses.

Optic diameter
The basic principle is the larger the optic the better, as there are less problems with lens decentration, but clearly this means a larger incision. For this reason most foldable or injectable lenses have an optic diameter of 5–6 mm.

In younger patients, a second factor that would favour the implantation of a larger lens is that the pupil dilates more widely in dim illumination in the young, often exceeding 5 mm.

Materials
Ideally, lens materials should be:

- Translucent
- Of high refractive index
- Mechanically stable
- Foldable
- Biologically inert.

Most of these properties are self-evident, with the possible exception of a high refractive index. A high refractive index means that the lens can be thinner for the same refractive power, and this has two favourable consequences; thinner lenses fold into a smaller shape and they have less optical aberration.

When assessing the refractive index, most materials are in the range of 1.4–1.6. This may seem a small variation, but the actual refractive power depends upon the difference of the refractive index from water, which has a refractive index of 1.0. Thus a material with an index of 1.6 has 50 per cent more refractive power than a material of 1.4.

Silicone

Silicone lenses were the first foldable lenses to be used. A direct comparison of the optical properties of the commonly used materials shows little difference between them, but acrylic performed significantly better than silicone under bright light conditions and PMMA performed significantly better than silicone under low contrast conditions[9]. However, these differences were small and probably not clinically significant.

The first silicone lenses had a refractive index of 1.41, making them relatively thick and difficult to fold for the high powers. Difficulty in handling these lenses was compounded by their being very springy, and if the lenses became wet they became slippery and unfoldable. A solution to these problems was injectors, which allow controlled opening by slowly extruding the lens.

A second consequence of slippery lenses is that they are difficult to explant. The standard way to explant a lens is to cut it into two and then retrieve each half though the wound, but slippery lenses are hard to cut with scissors; however, a device has been designed for this purpose.

There are two other unfavourable surface properties of silicone; it may enhance bacterial growth[10], and silicone oil suspension can bind to silicone lenses.

Acrylates/methacrylates

Acrylics are a new category of material and they have distinctive properties. They tend to be of higher refractive index and less slippery compared to silicone. One of the acrylics, AcrySof, not only has the highest refractive index (n = 1.55) of any of the foldable materials, but it has also been reported to have a number of favourable surface properties:

1. There was less giant cell reaction on AcrySof lenses than on silicone or PMMA lenses in a randomized study[11].
2. In diabetic eyes with pre-proliferative or proliferative retinopathy, there was less anterior segment inflammation in eyes undergoing cataract surgery by phakoemulsification and with AcrySof lenses implanted than with heparin-coated PMMA[12].
3. There was less posterior capsular opacification with AcrySof than with PMMA and silicone lenses[13] and low capsulotomy rates were reported[14,15], but this may be related to their square edge design rather than the material.
4. There was greater anterior capsular stability with AcrySof than PMMA and silicone lenses[16]. Differential contraction or retraction of the capsular bag is the mechanism for late lens decentration.

It should be noted that three of the above references came from a group whose work was partially sponsored by an unrestricted grant from the manufacturers of AcrySof, and they only chose the one acrylic lens for their studies. Thus it is not clear how many of these properties are generic to acrylic and how many are specific to this particular type of acrylic. Some of the observed differences may also have been due to the lens profile (with the AcrySof lens having a square edge) rather than the material.

SURFACE MODIFICATION

There have been attempts to make the surfaces of lenses more favourable by coating them, for two reasons: to reduce the inflammatory reaction and to reduce posterior capsular opacification rates.

While work is in process to see if posterior capsular opacification can be prevented by coating lenses in such substances as 5-fluorouracil, the only surface modification that is currently being used clinically is heparin, with the rationale of reducing postoperative inflammation.

PMMA lenses, although well tolerated, are not completely inert, and do generate a foreign body reaction with the deposition of giant cells on them. This is usually only mild, but there are some patient groups with a predictably more marked inflammatory reaction to surgery, including uveitic patients, diabetic patients with proliferative retinopathy, and children. It has been suggested that in this situation while surgery may be an initiating feature, it is exacerbated by a foreign body reaction, possibly as a consequence of complement activation[1].

Heparin was discovered by McLean in 1916. He found that an extract of liver not only failed to accelerate clotting but actually inhibited it (Greek for liver is hepar). Its major clinical use is still as an anticoagulant, but it was known from work on other implants (such as tubing and stents) that a heparin coating improved biocompatibility[17]. It was therefore natural to try heparin coating intraocular lenses, and such lenses were shown, *in vitro*, to be much weaker at activating compliment[18]. In addition, such lenses were shown to have reduced cell and bacteria adhesion.

All subsequent *in vivo* studies have shown the same or lower levels for all assessed inflammatory parameters for heparin-coated lenses compared to uncoated PMMA lenses. However, the advantage of using these lenses seems to be relatively small compared to the need to control pre-existing disease processes prior to surgery. This means making sure that there is no active uveitis at the time of surgery in uveitic patients and covering the surgery with a course of systemic prednisolone or, for diabetics, making sure that any proliferative retinopathy is adequately treated by pan-retinal photocoagulation prior to surgery. The use of oral prednisolone for uveitic patients (e.g. 40 mg per day started 1 week prior to surgery and tailed off over 6–8 weeks after surgery) and the recognition that proliferative retinopathy must be controlled has dramatically improved the prognosis of cataract surgery in these patient subgroups.

There is no clear benefit of heparin-coated lenses for eyes with silicone oil[19].

HAPTICS

The major purpose of haptics is to provide stable centration of the optic. The major reason for IOL explantation is decentration and, although this is discussed here with respect to lens design, it should be noted that the major determinant is surgical technique[9].

There are two major styles of haptics; loops and plates. Loop haptics can be further subdivided into one-piece lenses (when the haptics and optics are made of the same material) and three-piece lenses (when the optics and haptics are made of different materials). They all give excellent short-term results, but plate haptics have a limitation in that they rely on accurate in-the-bag implantation. They should not be used if the capsulorhexis is not intact, and should probably also be avoided if there is even a small defect in the posterior capsule.

Haptics have been made from a number of materials. Those made from a soft material have a problem with decentration and even lens dislocation, as the haptics can deform. This has been well described for one-piece silicone lenses with plate haptics, and there have been anecdotal reports of lens decentration following contracture of the capsular bag and even frank dislocation out of the bag following YAG capsulotomy[20]. Dislocation may be a generic problem with using relatively soft material, as this was also reported for one of the early hydrogel lenses[21]. There have been attempts to compensate for this by the addition of mini-loops and large footplate-positioning holes in some designs.

There is some evidence that PMMA and polyimide haptics provide better centration than polypropylene[9]. There has also been a suggestion that polyproylene haptics may be a risk factor for endophthalmitis (with a relative risk of 4.5)[22], while a second study noted a significantly increased risk of endophthalmitis with three-piece foldable silicone lenses with polypropylene haptics compared to one-piece PMMA lenses[10].

A disadvantage of three-piece lenses is that the edge of the lens needs to be thick enough to allow insertion/attachment of the haptics. This requirement is a second determinant of lens thickness (along with refractive index of the optic).

MULTIFOCAL LENSES

These lenses have two sets of zones, arranged concentrically, of different focal power; one is for distance and the other is for near vision. Perhaps surprisingly, they do not cause double vision (Figure 25.1). Although they do give rise to a multifocal effect, they do so at the expense of loss of some contrast sensitivity.

For the multifocal effect to work it is necessary to ensure:

- Accurate centration, which means implantation in the bag
- Stable and low astigmatism
- Accurate biometery.

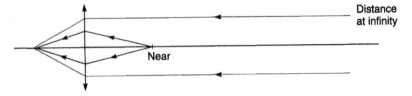

Figure 25.1 Multifocal lenses. The problem of multiple images is minimized because when looking at a distant object there is usually nothing in the way, so there is nothing at the near focal point to be seen. When looking at a new object, it will block out the distant one.

While the idea of multifocal lenses has been around for a long time, it is only with modern techniques and small inicision surgery that these criteria can be met in the majority of cases. Their exact place is still undecided, and this is an area of active development. Patients with multifocal lenses do have problems with multiple images, halos at night and reduced contrast sensitivity, but a study by Javitt et al.[23] showed that, despite these limitations, the patients scored more highly than those with monofocal lenses on a quality of life instrument – although the patients in this study were not randomized.

POSTERIOR CAPSULAR OPACIFICATION

This is the single most common 'complication' of current cataract surgery where an intact posterior capsule is required to ensure stable fixation of a posterior chamber lens. It is estimated to be around 33–50 per cent by 3–5 years. It is age-related, and posterior capsular opacification (PCO) occurs more rapidly in younger patients.

The treatment of PCO has been made much easier with the advent of the YAG laser and YAG capsulotomy, making needling an obsolete procedure, but its prevention is a major goal of modern lens research with two broad research strategies. The first is the idea that cells responsible for PCO migrate from the periphery of the bag to the centre, and that appropriate lens design can form a barrier to this happening. There is evidence of reduced PCO with the in-the-bag fixation that occurs with folding lenses, and there is a suggestion that the rate is lower with acrylic compared to silicone lenses, which has been attributed to better adhesion of acrylic to the posterior capsule[24]. The edge contour may also be helpful, with a square edge also acting as a barrier to cell migration over the posterior capsule. The use of surface modifications to prevent capsular cell proliferation is also being actively researched.

REFERENCES

1. Apple, D. J., Mamalis, N., Loftfield, K. et al. (1984). Complications of intraocular lenses. A historical and histopathological review. Surv. Ophthalmol., 29, 1–54.
2. Stur, M. (1988). Long-term changes of the corneal endothelium following intracapsular cataract extraction with implantation of open-loop anterior chamber lenses. Acta Ophthalmologica, 66, 678–86.
3. Numa, A., Nakamura, J., Takashima, M. and Kani, K. (1993). Long-term corneal endothelial changes after intraocular lens implantation. Anterior vs posterior chamber lenses. Japan. J. Ophthalmol., 37, 78–87.

4. Coli, A. F., Price, F. W. Jr and Whitson, W. E. (1993). Intraocular lens exchange for anterior chamber introcular lens-induced corneal endothelial damage. *Ophthalmology*, **100**, 384–93.
5. Ambrose, V. M., Walters, F. R., Batterbury, M. *et al.* (1991). Long-term endothelial cell loss and breakdown of the blood–aqueous barrier in cataract surgery. *J. Cataract Refract. Surg.*, **17**, 622–7.
6. Walters, R. F., McGill, J. I., Batterbury, M. and Williams, J. D. (1989). Complications of anterior chamber lens implants and their effects on the endothelium. *Eye*, **3**, 690–95.
7. Ram, J., Apple, D. J., Peng, Q. *et al.* (1999). Update on fixation of rigid and foldable posterior chamber intraocular lenses. Part 1. Elimination of fixation-induced decentration to achieve precise optical correction and visual rehabilitation. *Ophthalmology*, **106**, 883–90.
8. Mazzocco, T. R. (1985). Early clinical experience with elastic lens implants. *Trans. Ophthal. Soc. UK*, **104**, 578–9.
9. Kohnen, T. (1996). The variety of foldable intraocular lens materials. *J. Cataract Refract. Surg.*, **22**, 1255–8.
10. Bainbridge, J. W. B., Teimory, M., Tabandeh, H. *et al.* (1998). Intraocular lens implants and risk of endophthalmitis. *Br. J. Ophthalmol.*, **82**, 1312–15.
11. Hollick, E. J., Spalton, D. J., Ursell, P. G. and Pande, M. V. (1998). Biocompatibility of poly(methylmethacrylate), silicone, and Acrysof intraocular lenses: randomised comparison of the cellular reaction on the anterior lens surface. *J. Cataract Refract. Surg.*, **24**, 361–6.
12. Kamiya, I. and Kohzuka, T. (1996). Comparison of postoperative inflammation in eyes with acrylic or heparin-coated lens implantation in diabetes. *Japan. J. Cataract Refract. Surg.*, **10**, 276–89.
13. Ursell, P. G., Spalton, D. J., Pande, M. V. *et al.* (1998). Relationship between intraocular lens biomaterials and posterior capsule opacification. *J. Cataract Refract. Surg.*, **24**, 352–60.
14. Hollick, E. J., Spalton, D. J., Ursell, P. G. *et al.* (1999). The effect of polymethylmethacrylate, silicone, and polyacrylic intraocular lenses on posterior capsular opacification 3 years after cataract surgery. *Ophthalmology*, **106**, 49–55.
15. Oshika, T., Suzuki, Y., Kizaki, H. and Yaguchi, S. (1996). Two-year clinical study of a soft acrylic intraocular lens. *J. Cataract Refract. Surg.*, **22**, 104–9.
16. Ursell, P. G., Spalton, D. J. and Pande, M. V. (1997). Anterior capsule stability in eyes with intraocular lenses made of poly(methylmethacrylate), silicone and Acryosof. *J. Cataract Refract. Surg.*, **23**, 1532–8.
17. Larsson, R., Rosengren, A. and Olsson, R. (1977). Determination of platelet adhesion to polyethylene and heparinized surfaces with the aid of bioluminescence and [51]chromium-labelled platelets. *Thromb. Res.*, **11**, 517–30.
18. Pekna, M., Larsson, R., Fomgren, B. *et al.* (1993). Complement activation by polymethyl methacrylate minimized by end-point heparin attachment. *Biomaterials*, **14**, 189–92.
19. Batterbury, M., Wong, D., Williams, R. and Bates, R. (1994). The adherence of silicone oil to standard and heparin-coated PMMA intraocular lenses. *Eye*, **8**, 547–9.
20. Tuft, S. J. and Talks, S. J. (1998). Delayed dislocation of foldable plate-haptic silicone lenses after Nd:YAG laser anterior capsulotomy. *Am. J. Ophthalmol.*, **126**, 586–8.
21. Levy, J. H., Pisacano, A. M. and Anello, R. D. (1990). Displacement of bag-placed hydrogel lenses into the vitreous following neodynium:YAG laser capsulotomy. *J. Cataract Refract. Surg.*, **16**, 563–6.
22. Menikoff, J. A., Speaker, M. C., Marmor, M. and Raskin, E. M. (1991). A case—control study of risk factors for postoperative endophthalmitis. *Ophthalmology*, **98**, 1761–8.
23. Javitt, J. C., Wang, F., Trentacost, D. J. *et al.* (1997). Outcomes of cataract extraction with multifocal intraocular lens implantation. Functional status and quality of life. *Ophthalmology*, **104**, 589–99.
24. Ram, J., Apple, D. J., Peng, Q. *et al.* (1999). Update on fixation of rigid and foldable posterior chamber intraocular lenses. Part 2. Choosing the correct haptic fixation and intraocular lens design to help eradicate posterior chamber capsule opacification. *Ophthalmology*, **106**, 891–900.

26

BIOMETRY

When Harold Ridley inserted the first intraocular lens into an eye (and himself into history), he also ushered in the subject of biometric error. The postoperative refraction of his first patient was $-24\,DS + 6\,DC$ at $30°$[1]. Clearly the purpose of an intraocular lens implant is to reduce (and ideally eliminate) the requirement for 'visual prostheses' (glasses or contact lenses), so the success of intraocular lens implantation hinges upon accurate choice of lens power. The accepted standards for biometry are getting progressively more stringent – 'at least 50 per cent of patients should be ±0.5 dioptres of the planned refractive outcome after surgery, 90 per cent ±1 dioptre and 100 per cent ±2 dioptres'[2]. The key statistic is the proportion of patients within $0.50\,DS$ of target refraction, and some surgeons are claiming rates approaching 90 per cent.

Choosing the correct lens power requires accurate measurement of a number of ocular parameters – most commonly the corneal steepness (keratometry) and the axial length of the eye – and the choice of an appropriate formula.

THEORY

The effective power of any lens at a particular plane depends upon its position. The focal power of a lens is quoted from its own principle plane, but its power at any other plane can easily be calculated. In Figure 26.1, the lens is a 0.5-D lens and it will therefore bring parallel light to a point focus at 2 m. At a new plane (called A) midway between the lens and the focal point, the light will be brought to a focus at 1 m; hence the effective power of the lens at plane A is 1 D. The formula for working out the effective power of a lens of power F is:

$$F_{effective} = F/(1 - dF)$$

where $F_{effective}$ = the effective power of the lens in dioptres at a new plane; F = lens power in dioptres; d = distance of new plane from plane of lens in metres.

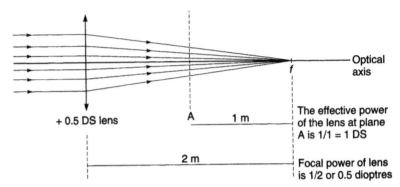

Figure 26.1 Calculating the effective power of a lens.

FORMULAE

There are two basic sets of formulae; regression and theoretical. The major advantage of regression formulae is that the required calculations are simple to perform, whereas theoretical formulae are computationally complex.

REGRESSION FORMULAE

The most commonly used regression formulae, the SRK-I[3] and its successor, SRK-II, were developed by Sanders, Retzlaff and Kraff and, although they appear in the software in most A-scanning devices, these formulae should be considered obsolete.

The SRK-I regression formula is:

$$\text{Power} = A - 2.5\,AL - 0.9\,K$$

where A = intraocular lens A constant; AL = axial length in mm; K = average of the K-readings. To calculate K in dioptres, $K = 2(K1 \times K2/K1 + K2)$; to calculate K in mm, $K = 675(K1 + K2)$.

It is a standard mathematical technique to approximate a function by a power series. The fact that this regression formulae does not include any terms other than of power one shows that it is a very simple formula, but the use of only linear terms is too great an assumption.

The SRK-II formula improved on this by adjusting the axial length in order to compensate for the observed non-linear behaviour, which they termed the corrected axial length (CAL), and using this in place of AL in the SRK-I formula. The adjustment is made on the basis of the axial length:

$$\text{CAL} = AL + 3 \text{ for axial lengths under } 20\,\text{mm}$$

where $CAL = AL + 2$ for axial lengths of 20 to < 21 mm; $CAL = AL + 1$ for axial lengths of 21 to < 22 mm; $CAL = AL$ for axial lengths of 22 to < 24.5 mm; and $CAL = AL - 0.5$ for axial lengths of 24.5 mm and over.

This formula, like the SRK-I, has the advantage of ease of calculation, which can be done without a computer. However, it does have its limitations. For example, a 0.02 mm change in axial length from 20.99 to 21.01 mm will result in a 1 D change in the power of the predicted lens implant. Notwithstanding these limitations the SRK-II works reasonably well for axial lengths of 22–24.5 mm, which is nearly 80 per cent of all eyes, but like all regression formulae it is least accurate at the ends of the range[4-6].

Although this formula is now considered obsolete, it does indicate the sort of error introduced by errors in measurement of the axial length or of the K-readings. For example a 1-mm error for an eye of axial length of 23.5 mm is 2.35 D, although it should be noted that the error does vary with the axial length. For longer eyes it is less (1.75 D for axial length of 30 mm), but for an eye of 20-mm axial length, it rises to 3.75 D.

THEORETICAL FORMULAE

There are three commonly used third-generation theoretical formulae; the SRK-T, Holladay-1 and Hoffer Q[7]. These formulae have superseded the regression formulae. The calculations are much more complex, but that is no longer an issue given the current status of computer technology. All the theoretic formulae have the following equation as the starting point for their development:

$$Power = n/(AL - ACD) - nK/(n - K.ACD)$$

where n = refractive index of media; K = average of the K-readings; AL = axial length; ACD = anterior chamber depth.

The first part of the formula, n/(AL − ACD), is the power required to focus parallel light onto the retina from the plane where the lens implant will sit (Figure 26.2). The second part, nK/(n − K.ACD), is the effective power of the cornea at this plane. Therefore the implant power is simply the total required power minus the effective power of the cornea. The key variable introduced is the anterior chamber

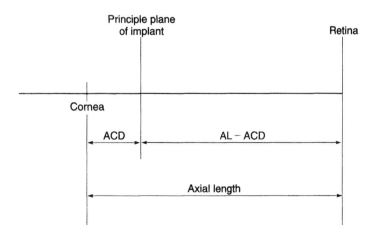

Figure 26.2 Distance from principal plane to implant is AL − ACD. Required power (to focus light) is n/AL − ACD.

depth (ACD). The ACD is defined as the distance from the apex of the anterior corneal surface to the principal plane of the lens implant along the optical axis.

Fyodorov first suggested a way of estimating the ACD by developing a 'corneal height' formula. The corneal height (H) is defined as the distance from the apex of the posterior corneal surface to the iris plane. It is shorter than the ACD, as it does not include the corneal thickness nor the distance from the iris plane to the principle plane of the lens. Fyodorov assumed that the cornea was part of a sphere and, with this assumption and given the radius of curvature of the cornea (K-readings) and the diameter of the cornea, it is easy to calculate the corneal height using the following formula (see Figure 26.3 for derivation):

$$H = K - (K^2 - \tfrac{1}{4}CD^2)^{\tfrac{1}{2}}$$

where H = corneal height (mm); K = corneal keratometry (mm); CD = corneal diameter (mm).

This height gives the distance from the posterior surface of the cornea to the iris plane. The corneal diameter can be measured directly, but it is hard to do so accurately, and the SRK-T estimates this using the axial length and the K-readings:

$$Cde = -5.41 + (0.58412 \times MAL) + (0.098 \times K)$$

where Cde = estimated corneal diameter; MAL = modified axial length; K = average keratometry.

The corneal diameter can be measured directly (e.g. with the Holladay Godwin corneal gauge or calipers) or, more commonly, it can be estimated. The relationship between axial length and corneal width is linear for small and normal eyes, but not for large eyes. This accords with clinical experience where in high myopia the posterior segment of the eye is preferentially enlarged. To allow for this, the SRK-T uses a modified axial length for the corneal width calculations:

$$\text{If } AL \leq 24.2\,\text{mm, then the } MAL = L$$

$$\text{If } AL > 24.2\,\text{mm, then the } MAL = -3.446 + 1.716\,AL - 0.0237\,AL^2$$

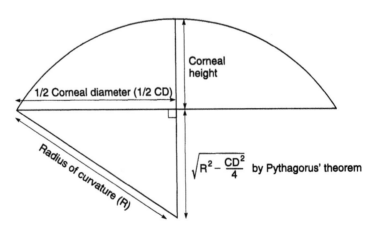

Figure 26.3 Derivation of Fyodorov's corneal height formula. The corneal height is $R - \sqrt{(R^2 - CD^2/4)}$.

With this estimate of the corneal diameter, and knowing the K-readings, the corneal height can be calculated. An offset must be added to this, which includes a term for the corneal thickness and a term to allow for the distance from the iris plane to the principle plane of the implanted lens (Figure 26.4). This offset depends upon the lens design, and in particular upon the angulation of the haptics, and there is an $ACD_{constant}$ for each lens design. An average eye has an ACD of 3.36 mm, so the calculated offset is simply:

$$Offset = ACD_{constant} - 3.336$$

A problem is that not all lenses have a reliable $ACD_{constant}$ provided. The A constant contains the same information as the $ACD_{constant}$, and accordingly one can be calculated from the other:

$$ACD_{constant} = 0.62467A - 68.747$$

where A = lens A constant.

The next refinement is to decide which AL value to take. Ultrasound reflects back most strongly from the internal limiting membrane of the retina, while the photoreceptor layer is where light is physiologically absorbed. Accordingly a term is introduced to allow for retinal thickness. Intuitively, this would be expected to have a constant value that correlated with known retinal thickness, but empirically the best predictions were given if this 'retinal thickness' correction factor (RT) was calculated as:

$$RT = 0.65696 - 0.2029\,AL$$

where RT = retinal thickness correction factor; AL = measured axial length.

The altered axial length (AAL) used for calculations is then the measured axial length plus the RT. Now the calculated ACD and the AAL can be entered into the formula that introduced this section:

$$Power = n/(AAL - ACD) - nK/(n - K.ACD)$$

All that is left to decide is what value of n (the refractive index) to use. The eye is not of uniform refractive index, and it can be divided into two major refractive elements; the aqueous and vitreous (n_a), and the cornea (n_c). The third refinement is to take this into account and optimize the value for the corneal refractive index. Empirically, a value of 1.333 was selected for the corneal refractive index. The use of more than one refractive index significantly complicates the above formula and the final published version is:

Figure 26.4 Diagram showing the difference between anterior chamber depth and corneal height. Anterior chamber depth is the combined corneal height and an offset. The offset is composed of corneal thickness and the 'surgeon factor'.

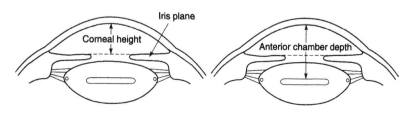

$$Power = 1000n_a(n_a r - (n_c - 1)\,AAL)/$$
$$(AAL - ACD)(n_a r - (n - 1)ACD)$$

As can be seen in the derivation, there are a number of simplifying assumptions and, despite its 'theoretical' nature, empirical factors do appear. The derivation of Holladay-1 can be found in Holladay et al. (1988)[8] and the Hoffer-Q in Hoffer (1993)[7].

The performance of the different formulae vary with the axial length of the eye, and no one formula is perfect for all situations. All the formulae work well with eyes that have healthy corneas and axial lengths within the normal range (22 – 24.5 mm). The following table gives a guide to which formula works best for which axial length.

Axial length (mm)	Method
19 >	Holladay-2
19 – 22	Hoffer-Q
22 – 24.5	Hoffer-Q, Holladay-1, SRK-T
24.5 – 26	Holladay-1
> 26	SRK-T

KERATOMETRY

Keratometry is performed by a keratometer, which works by reflecting two targets off the anterior corneal surface; the operator then aligns the reflections, from which the radius of curvature is deduced. The optical power is deduced from the radii of curvature measurements using the spherical refractive surface formula:

$$K = (n_2 - n_1)/r$$

where K = refractive power; n_2 = refractive index of 'cornea'; n_1 = refractive index of air = 1; r = measured radius of curvature.

The standard keratometric index is 1.3375, and the above equation reduces to:

$$K = 0.3375/r$$

However, the question arises as what is the appropriate value to take for n_2. The tear film has the same refractive index as aqueous and water (1.336), but the posterior surface has a radius of curvature 1.2 mm steeper than that of the anterior surface. The cornea itself has a refractive index of 1.376. If the power of the cornea is calculated exactly (allowing for its two refractive surfaces and different refractive index), and the answer is used to back calculate what would have been an appropriate value for the refractive index in the above formula, the value is almost exactly 4/3 (1.3333). This is the value that Holladay recommends using for keratometry[9]. The adjusted K-readings can be readily calculated from the values obtained by most machines by multiplying by a conversion factor:

$$K_{adjusted} = K_{measured} \times 0.98765431$$

Keratometers only sample two small areas that are actually doing the reflecting, and these points are in the region of 3 mm apart. This should be remembered for eyes with corneal diseases and is a particular problem for corneas that have had refractive surgery, when these two points may not be representative of the refracting surface.

AXIAL LENGTH MEASUREMENT

ULTRASOUND

The current standard way to measure the axial length is by A-scan ultrasonography, either by applanation (with the patient sitting upright) or by the immersion technique (Figure 26.5). Although most units use the contact method, which is quicker and easier, the latter has consistently proved to be accurate[10-13]. Place a drop of local anaesthetic in the eye and then recline the patient so that the head is horizontal. Place a small cup on the eye, and fill this with a viscous fluid such as gel tears or hypromellose. Next put the probe (a non-focused transducer of 8–10 MHz) in the fluid, and a tracing will be obtained (Figure 26.6). Orientate the probe so that the B/C and F peaks are the highest, and measure from the B-peak (the anterior corneal surface) to the F-peak (the retina). The features of a good quality A-scan are that the B/C and the F peaks are the highest and the F-peak has a vertical take-off.

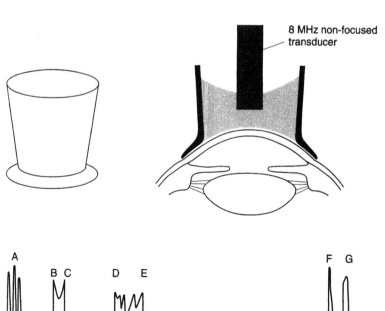

Figure 26.5 The immersion technique for A-scanning.

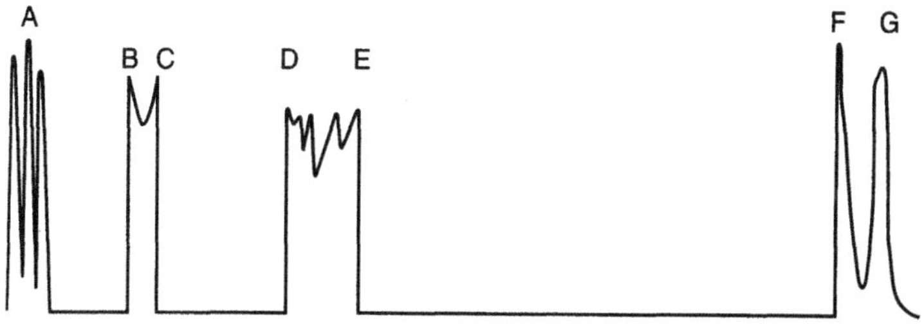

Figure 26.6 Ultrasound measurement of axial length. A, probe tip; B, anterior corneal surface; C, posterior corneal surface; D, anterior lens capsule; E, posterior lens capsule; F, retina; G, sclera.

Note that:

- The echo trace will be shifted more to the left the closer the probe is to the cornea. It is important that the trace is properly aligned with respect to the measuring gates.
- The corneal echo can be surprisingly hard to find. The corneal curvature means that there is only one correct orientation and the echoes drop off rapidly with the probe off-axis, and the anterior lens echo can then be mistaken for the corneal echo. Look for the pattern of three echoes from the anterior segment, a double-peaked echo from the cornea, and the two echoes from the anterior and posterior lens surface. In applanation biometry, there is not a clear corneal peak due to the proximity to the probe.

The quality of the A-scan is operator-dependent, with the commonest sources of error being alignment, corneal indentation (applanation only) and changes in the speed of sound through the ocular media. With the immersion technique, the probe does not touch the cornea and so eliminates indentation as a source of error.

Notwithstanding the better performance of the immersion technique, most departments use a contact method. This is performed in the upright position and the probe should be spring-loaded. Only one study has looked at hand-held versus slit-lamp supported biometry[14], and this showed no systematic difference in axial length between the machine-mounted and hand-held methods.

The problem of indentation can be compensated for by having the biometer attached to a spring mounting. Even so, great care must be taken to ensure that the probe rests lightly on the surface of the cornea with minimal pressure.

Pupillary dilatation does not alter the axial length measurement on biometry[15], but it may impair the assessment of the quality of the scan. The presence of a pre-lens blip on the A-scan shows that it is non-axial (Figure 26.7).

A-scans measure the time between the different reflections and deduce the distance on the basis of the formula:

$$\text{Distance} = \text{speed} \times \text{time}$$

The speed of sound differs for various media (Table 26.1[16,17]).

The speed of sound through water/aqueous/vitreous is 1532 m/s, while the speed through the lens and the cornea is 1641 m/s. Assuming that the time is proportional to the distance in the phakic eye, then it may appear that the thickness of the cornea and the lens is proportional to the axial length. In fact this is wrong; the velocity of sound in an eye of normal axial length is 1555 m/s, for an axial length of 30 mm is 1549 m/s and for an axial length of 20 mm is 1560 m/s. The thickness of the cornea is a constant and adds an almost insignificant error to the measurement due to its thinness (0.5 mm), but the lens thickness is significant and varies with age more than with axial length.

There are two approaches to improve upon this. The simplest is to assume a constant lens thickness and sound velocity. The axial length

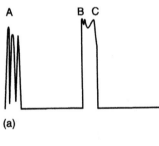

(a)

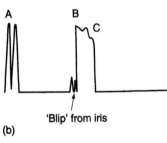

'Blip' from iris

(b)

Figure 26.7 An A-scan with undilated pupil allows assessment of whether the scan is (a) axial or (b) non-axial, depending on the absence or presence of a 'blip' from the iris in front of the B-spike.

Table 26.1 Table of speed of sound in different media

Media	Speed of sound (m/s)
Air	335
Water	1532
Cornea	1641
Aqueous	1532
Clear lens	1641
Vitreous	1532
Cataract	1590–1670
PMMA lens	2780
Acrylic lens	2180
Silicone	980

is calculated by assuming a speed of sound of 1532 m/s (i.e. for water/aqueous/vitreous) and then adding a 'correction of axial length factor' (CALF) with a value of 0.28 mm to account for the lens and cornea. The maximum error using this formula is 0.027 mm, which is well within the tolerance of the axial length measurement[9].

The second approach is to have gates that can be set to measure directly the lens thickness and apply a different velocity for that. This will work for early cataracts, but for dense cataracts there may not be a posterior lens echo and lens thickness will have to be assumed.

A further potential source of error is that the speed of sound through the lens not only varies with age but also with the type and degree of cataract, but this seems to have only a very small effect on the results of lens power prediction[18]. Given the importance of accurate axial length measurement, the following are suggested guidelines for remeasurement:

1. Axial length less than 22 mm or greater than 25 mm in either eye
2. Difference in axial length of 0.3 mm between the two eyes
3. Axial length that does not correlate with patient's refraction (short eyes should be hypermetropic and long eyes myopic).

PARTIAL INTERFERENCE TOMOGRAPHY

The longitudinal resolution of a 10-MHz probe is in the region of 200 μm, but interferometry can reduce this error to 10 μm[19]. Axial lengths obtained with this technique are consistently longer than with applanation ultrasound because interferometry is a non-contact technique and because the major signal appears to come from the retinal pigment epithelium and not from the internal limiting membrane. This is partly compensated for by the fact that the optical method measures from the secondary principle plane – a difference of 0.05 mm[9,20,21]. The recommended conversion equation is[9]:

$$\text{Axial length}_{\text{optical}} = \text{Axial length}_{\text{ultrasound}} + 0.20\,\text{mm}$$

It is well known that cataracts can cause shifts in the refractive index of the human lens (e.g. index myopia), and thus its role in patients with cataracts is not clear. Accordingly, this technique seems most applicable for aphakic eyes or for eyes requiring implant exchange. It is a new and exciting technique whose exact role is still uncertain.

SOURCES OF ERROR

There are three major sources of error and they are, in descending order of importance:

1. Axial length measurement (54 per cent)[22]
2. Postoperative anterior chamber depth estimation (38 per cent)[22]
3. Keratometric error (11 per cent).

PERSONALIZATION OF A CONSTANTS

Personalization of the A constants is rarely done, but it is important and should not be neglected. The purpose of personalization of A constants is to eliminate any source of systematic error, whether introduced by the surgeon, the biometry equipment or the formulae used.

PROBLEMS

ABNORMAL AXIAL LENGTH

All the formulae work well with eyes that have healthy corneas and axial lengths within the normal range, but long and short eyes pose particular problems and the appropriate formula should be chosen according to the axial length.

Hypermetropes did pose a second problem as many lens designs only went up to 30 DS and higher powers required piggybacking (using more than one lens implant; the program Holladay Consultant can perform the necessary calculations), but powers up to 45 DS in some lens designs are now available. There are very few eyes that require a more powerful lens, and the more common indication for piggybacking is correction of a biometric error.

ABNORMAL MEDIA – THE SILICONE-FILLED EYE

The speed of sound varies in different media (Table 26.1), and in silicone oil is approximately two-thirds of that in vitreous. A particular problem is that the fill of an eye with silicone is rarely complete, and biometry is best performed using a B-scan directed A-scan. A sharp shadow from the front surface of the silicone oil appears on a B-scan, and the distance from the front of the cornea to the front of this bright shadow plus the distance from this shadow to the back of the eye multiplied by 0.64 (the ratio of 980/1532; Table 26.1) gives the appropriate axial length. This can be cross-checked by performing biometry on the fellow eye as, in the same person, both eyes usually have axial lengths within 0.3 mm of each other. A second management problem is whether the silicone oil is going to be removed. This will clearly have a marked effect on the biometry, with a shift of 3–4 DS. Although biometry is less accurate in this situation, the visual potential is also often reduced as there is often a significant co-existing maculopathy. Thus biometric errors are of less significance.

Asteroides hyalosis may give rise to extra shadows but does not seem to affect the speed of sound significantly.

STAPHYLOMA

This is a particular problem in myopic eyes, and should be considered in any eye with an axial length greater than 26 mm. The key point is to try and establish where the fovea is, and this is done by using the cross-hair target of the direct ophthalmoscope and asking the patient to look at it, then making a note of how many disc diameters the fovea is away from the optic nerve. With this in mind, use a B-scan directed A-scan. Hold the probe horizontally so that the fovea and the optic nerve appear in the same plane, and then estimate the location of the fovea on the basis of the number of disc diameters estimated clinically. This clearly presupposes that the cataract is not advanced and that the fovea can be seen.

If the cataract is advanced, then there is little option but to warn the patient of a potential 'biometric surprise'.

THE EYE WITH PREVIOUS REFRACTIVE SURGERY

The above formulae are all valid on patients who have had refractive surgery, but the keratometry often is not. There are three methods that have been proposed to overcome this[23], and they are, in order of preference:

1. The history method
2. The contact lens method
3. The topographic method.

The history method
The best solution is for patients who are undergoing refractive surgery to have biometry done first. The really important measurements are the pre-refractive surgery K-readings and the pre- and post-surgical refractive errors.

If the pre-procedure refraction and keratometry and post-procedure refraction are known, the appropriate K-readings can be calculated as follows:

1. First correct the pre- and post-procedure refractions to the plane of the cornea. The usual back vertex distance is around 12 mm, so the formula is $F_{effective} = F/(1 - dF)$ with d = back vertex distance in metres, with a default value of 0.012 m.
2. The change in refraction is simply the best sphere equivalent before the procedure minus the best sphere equivalent after the procedure.
3. This indicates how much the vergence of a parallel beam of light has changed at the cornea. Subtract this change from the pre-operative average of the K-readings to get the adjusted K-readings for biometry.

Worked example

The required information is:

- Pre-procedure refraction = −7.00 DS (using best sphere equivalent)
- Back vertex distance = 12 mm
- Pre-procedure average of the K-readings = 44 D
- Post-procedure refraction = 0 (using best sphere equivalent).

The calculation is as follows:

1. First convert the refractions to the refraction at the corneal plane, which is still 0 for the post-procedure refraction but is −7/(1 + 0.012 × 7) = −6.5 (two significant figures) for the pre-procedure refraction.
2. The change in refraction is therefore −6.5 DS.
3. Add the change in refraction, which is −6.5 DS, to the average of the pre-procedure K-readings to get 44 + (−6.5) = 37.5 (pay attention to the signs!). This is the value to be entered into the biometry formulae.

The contact lens method

This method relies on being able to get a reliable refraction, and clearly this is not always possible in patients with a cataract. The rationale is that if the K-readings are equal to the base curve of a plano contact lens, it should have no effect on the refraction. The change in the refraction with such a lens gives a good estimate of the keratometric error. This method will work on patients who have had radial keratotomy as well as photorefractive keratectomy.

Therefore fit a plano hard contact lens (HCL) that most closely approximates to the patient's K-readings, and obtain a refraction before and after fitting the contact lens. The calculations are then as for the history method, with the following substitutions: the K-readings are substituted for the pre-procedure K-readings; the pre-contact lens refraction is substituted for the pre-procedure refraction; and the over-refraction is substituted for the post-procedure refraction.

Worked example

The post-procedure refraction, the refraction with a fitted plano rigid contact lens (RCL) and the base curve of the RCL must be known.

Consider a patient who has a refraction of -0.5 DS (best sphere equivalent) and -5.00 DS with a plano RCL with a back vertex distance of 12 mm and a base curve of 42 DS. The calculation is as follows:

1. Convert the refractions to the effective refractions at the cornea. They are $-0.5/(1 + 0.012 \times 0.5) = -0.5$ DS and $-5.0/(1 + 0.012 \times 5.0) = -4.7$ DS for pre- and post-procedure respectively.
2. The change in refraction is $-4.7 + 0.5 = -4.2$ DS.
3. The average K-reading is simply the base curve plus the change in refraction, which is $42 + (-4.2) = 37.8$ DS.

Topographic method

Use computer-assisted corneal topography and use the central Ks in a theoretical formula, and warn the patient of the potential for a 'biometric surprise'. The estimate is based on the average on the central two to four rings.

SUMMARY

1. Use theoretical formulae and use special techniques for eyes with previous refractive surgery
2. Consider Holladay's suggestion of using 4/3 for the keratometric index of refraction
3. Immersion is more accurate than applanation for axial length measurement
4. Consider adjusting the ultrasound velocity (some A-scanners do this automatically)
5. Personalize the A constant
6. Beware of staphyloma in long eyes
7. Be aware of incongruent results and be prepared to repeat the measurements.

REFERENCES

1. Ridley, H. (1952). Introcular acrylic lenses: a recent development in the surgery of cataract. *Br. J. Ophthalmol.*, **36**, 113.
2. Claoue, C. (1996). Cataract surgery. In: *Refractive Surgery*, 1st edn (C. Claoue, ed.). BMJ Publishers.
3. Sanders, D. R. and Kraff, M. C. (1980). Improvement of intraocular lens power calculation using empirical data. *J. Am. Intraocular Implant Soc.*, **6**, 263–7.
4. Norozler, A., Unlu, N., Yalvac, K. S. *et al.* (1998). The SRK-II formula in the calculation of intraocular lens power. *Ophthalmologica*, **212**, 153–6.
5. Olsen, T., Thim, K. and Corydon, L. (1991). Accuracy of the newer generation intraocular lens power calculation formulas in long and short eyes. *J. Cataract Refract. Surg.*, **17**, 187–93.
6. Yalvac, I. S., Nurozler, A., Unlu, N. *et al.* (1996). Calculation of intraocular lens power with the SRK-II formula for axial high myopia. *Eur. J. Ophthalmol.*, **6**, 375–8.

7. Hoffer, K. J. (1998). The history of IOL power calculation in North America. In: *The History of Modern Cataract Surgery*, 1st edn (M. L. Kwitko and C. D. Kelman, eds), pp. 193–208. Kugler Publications.

8. Holladay, J., Prager, T. C., Chandler, T. Y *et al.* (1988). A three-part system for refining intraocular lens power calculations. *J. Cataract Refract. Surg.*, **14**, 17–24.

9. Holladay, J. T. (1997). Standardizing constants for ultrasonic biometry, keratometry, and intraocular lens power calculations. *J. Cataract Refract. Surg.*, **23**, 1356–70.

10. Giers, U. and Epple, C. (1990). Comparison of A-scan device accuracy. *J. Cataract Refract. Surg.*, **16**, 235–42.

11. Hoffmann, P. C., Hutz, W. W., Eckhardt, H.B. and Heuring, A. H. (1998). Intraocular lens calculation and ultrasound biometry: immersion and contact procedures (in German). *Klin. Monatsbl. Augenheilkd.*, **213**, 161–5.

12. Olsen, T. and Nielsen, P. J. (1989). Immersion versus contact technique in the measurement of axial length by ultrasound. *Acta Ophthalmol.*, **67**, 101–2.

13. Schelenz, J. and Kammann, J. (1989). Comparison of contact and immersion techniques for axial length measurement and implant power calculation. *J. Cataract Refract. Surg.*, **15**, 425–8.

14. Whelehan, I. M., Heyworth, P., Tabandah, H. *et al.* (1996). A comparison of slit-lamp supported versus hand-held biometry. *Eye*, **10**, 514–16.

15. Sadiq, S. A. and McElvanney, A. M. (1996). Pupillary dilation and axial length measurement for preoperative assessment of intraocular lens power. *Eur. J. Ophthalmol.*, **6**, 147–9.

16. Retzlaff, J. A., Sanders, D. R. and Kraff, M. C. (1990). *Lens Power Implantation. A Manual for Ophthalmologists and Biometrists*, 3rd edn. Slack Inc.

17. Retzlaff, J. A., Sanders, D. R. and Kraff, M. C. (1995). Intraocular lens power. New challenges, old principles. *Ophthalmol. Clin. North Am.*, **8**, 509–15.

18. Psilas, K., Kalogeropoulos, C., Aspiotis, M. and Nikalaou, V. (1992). The effect of cataract type on the intraocular lens power calculation using the SRK formula. *Eur. J. Implant. Ref. Surg.*, **4**, 255–9.

19. Drexler, W., Findl, O., Menapace, R. *et al.* (1998). Partial coherence interferometry: a novel approach to biometry in cataract surgery. *Am. J. Ophthalmol.*, **126**, 524–34.

20. Binkhorst, C. D. (1972). Power of the pre-pupillary pseudophakos. *Br. J. Ophthalmol.*, **56**, 372–7.

21. Colenbrander, M. C. (1973). Calculation of the power of an iris clip lens for distant vision. *Br. J. Ophthalmol.*, **57**, 735–40.

22. Olsen, T. (1992). Sources of error in intraocular lens power calculation. *J. Cataract Refract. Surg.*, **18**, 125–9.

23. Hoffer, K. J. (1995). Intraocular lens power calculation for eyes after refractive keratotomy. *J. Refract. Surg.*, **11**, 490–93.

27

CORRECTION OF ASTIGMATISM

The modern goal of cataract surgery is to achieve good distance vision, and increasingly also near vision, without optical aids. The major problem with extracapsular cataract (and corneal graft) surgery is surgically-induced astigmatism. Modern cataract surgery by phako-emulsification has solved this problem, and accurate in-the-bag placement of the intraocular lens and improved accuracy of biometry has resulted in accurate correction of the spherical component of the refractive error. Accordingly, attention has turned to the problem of eliminating pre-existing astigmatism. This is a rapidly moving area.

Given the problems with developing a truly accommodating lens, it is likely that current research will continue to centre on the multifocal lens implant and that elimination of pre-existing corneal astigmatism will be a critical part of this approach. The current problems that reduce the acceptability of multifocal lenses are inaccurate biometry and astigmatism[1], and both of these problems are soluble.

VIDEOKERATOSCOPY

Keratometry has its limitations because the curvature is assessed on the basis of reflections of light that are being reflected at spots 2–4 mm from the optical centre, and in some situations these spots may not be representative of the central cornea. The problem is solved by using videokeratoscopy to measure the corneal topography. Essentially this technique uses a luminated Placido's disc, and a computer program can detect the edges of the reflections and so work out the local dioptric power. The information is presented as contour lines of equal refractive power, and high powers are given the hot colours (yellow to red) while low powers are given the cold colours (blue to green). The steeper the change, the closer together the contour lines, but there is no standardized step between the lines and the scale can change from 1-D to 1/8-D steps (Figure 27.1). Accordingly, the topogram of a cornea with a small amount of astigmatism can appear completely spherical or grossly astigmatic depending on the scale.

Videokeratoscopy provides extra information because it is able to detect if the hemi-meridians are of differing powers and whether they are directly aligned with each other (Figure 27.2), which affects man-

Figure 27.1 Corneal topography: (a) A perfectly regular cornea has circular contours. (b) The pattern of regular cornea astigmatism is the bow-tie.

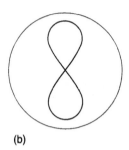

(a)

(b)

Figure 27.2 Corneal topography can detect when the hemi-meridians are of unequal power; (a) shows inferior steepening of a keratoconus suspect. (b) It will also detect when the hemi-meridians are not aligned with each other.

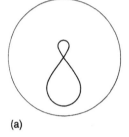
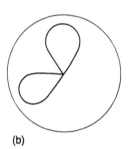

(a)

(b)

agement, or whether there is a frankly irregular component present, which predicts a poor prognostic outcome to surgical intervention.

Keratoconus has always been considered a contra-indication for refractive surgical techniques because of the unpredictability of the outcome. The features that best correlate with clinical keratoconus are[2]:

1. Central corneal curvature of greater than 46.6 D
2. A difference between eyes of central keratometry of greater than 0.8 D
3. An inferior–superior keratometry ratio of greater than 1.6 D (indicative of inferior steepening).

It has become clear that there is a large subgroup of patients presenting for refractive surgery with inferior steepening who have been termed keratoconic suspects[3], and it is not clear whether this is due to referral bias, contact lens warpage or overly sensitive diagnostic criteria. It should be noted that keratoconus is a progressive condition, and that the prognosis is dependent in part on the age at presentation[4]. Most patients presenting for cataract surgery are of an age where significant undiagnosed and progressive keratoconus is extremely rare.

It is not certain that routine videokeratoscopy is necessary in correcting astigmatism in cataract patients.

BASIC TECHNIQUES

The correction of astigmatism using laser techniques is still in its infancy, and the surgical techniques are all variants on wound resuturing, relieving incisions, compression sutures and combinations thereof.

Most surgical techniques in refractive surgery are much more effective at correcting myopia than hypermetropia, and this applies to astigmatism as much as it does to spherical error.

SUTURE REMOVAL AND RESUTURING OF WOUNDS

The first-line approach to surgically-induced astigmatism is to modify the wound, if possible. If the wound lies on the steep meridian, then suture removal will often result in its flattening. Sutures should be removed as soon as it is considered safe, and a basic principle is that the closer the wound is to the limbus, the quicker it heals. By contrast, if the wound is on the flat meridian, it suggests wound dehiscence and should be resutured as soon as the problem has been identified.

The earliest that suture removal from corneal sections for cataract surgery can be considered is 8 weeks, and many suggest 10–12 weeks for routine removal.

RELAXING INCISIONS

All incisions have the same basic effect of increasing the chord length. The effect this has on the optical zone, and therefore the final refractive effect, depends upon the orientation of the incision.

A key concept with relaxing incisions is that of 'coupling'. There is a tendency for the overall curvature of the cornea to remain constant, so a flattening of one part of the cornea is compensated for by increased curvature elsewhere.

Radial relaxing incisions

The radial cut is the relaxing incision used for radial keratometry (Figure 27.3) for the correction of high myopia, and the mechanism by which it works is well understood. The incision causes an increase in the peripheral cord length by gaping[5], and this results in a steepening (or bulging) of the peripheral cornea with an accompanying flattening of the central cornea[6-9](Figure 27.4). Regression of the effect is

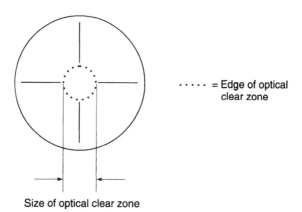

Figure 27.3 Radial incisions used to correct myopia.

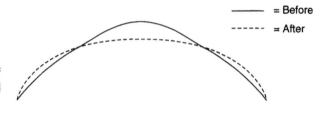

Figure 27.4 Exaggerated diagram to show the change in shape of the anterior corner surface before and after radial keratonomy. There is flattening of the central cornea with peripheral bulging.

associated with reduction of wound gaping due to contracture during the healing process[10], and accordingly is amenable to wound-modifying agents – particularly topical steroids.

With radial keratotomy there is the potential for a smooth variation in the refractive power of the cornea going out from the centre of the optical axis to the periphery, which is reminiscent of the principle underlying multifocal intraocular lenses. Thus it is not surprising that patients have been described who do demonstrate a multifocal effect[7,8,11–13].

Radial incisions have been largely superseded by laser techniques (PRK and LASIX) for the correction of myopia.

Arcuate relaxing incisions

The earliest descriptions of arcuate relaxing incisions (Figure 27.5) concerned treating gross levels of astigmatism following cataract surgery[14]. Until recently these incisions were mainly refined to deal with post-keratoplasty astigmatism, but they are now seeing a role in treating pre-existing astigmatism, particularly in association with cataract.

The incisions cause gaping and thus have a flattening effect, and the coupling effect results in a concomitant steepening of the meridian at right angles.

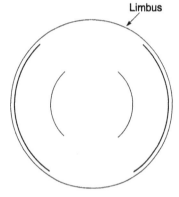

Figure 27.5 Pairs of arcuate relaxing incisions (corneal and limbal).

Corneal

Factors affecting the degree of astigmatic shift with corneal relaxing incisions (CRI) are:

1. The depth of the cut
2. The length of the cut
3. The position of the cut
4. The number of cuts
5. The age of the patient (the older the patient, the greater the effect)
6. Wound-modifying agents, which can prevent regression with healing.

It is currently accepted that the cut should be about 85 per cent of corneal thickness in depth, and this is achieved by using a pachymeter. Either determine the central corneal depth (where the cornea is thinnest) and then set the blade to that depth, which equates to around 85 per cent depth in the paracentral cornea, or measure the paracentral corneal thickness directly and set the blade at 85 per cent of this. The effect of a pair of arcuate incisions is directly proportional to their length (measured in degrees) in the range of 45–120°[15]. Cuts of

120° have the maximum effect (although most surgeons make their cuts up to 90°); longer cuts reduce their effectiveness[16]. The cuts seem to have the most effect when placed with a clear zone of 5–6 mm, but even limbal-placed cuts have some effect.

The astigmatic shift can be increased by increasing the number of cuts. The biggest effect is seen with the first pair of cuts, a second pair of cuts increases the effect by 20–30 per cent, and a third or more pairs gives less additional effect[17]. Practically speaking, close to a maximal effect is seen with two pairs of cuts of 120°. The cuts do cause a steepening in the meridian at 90° due to coupling. Coupling is not perfect, and a coupling constant can be defined as the ratio of flattening of the steep meridian to steepening at the perpendicular meridian. The ratio is around 1.5–2.0, and as a consequence a small hypermetropic shift might be expected; however, this is usually small and is often not clinically apparent[15,18].

Limbal

Limbal relaxing corneal incisions (LRI) seem particularly suitable for the correction of pre-existing astigmatism at the time of cataract surgery. The incisions are placed just anterior to the palisades of Vogt at a depth of 0.6 mm for a length of 6–12 mm (Figure 27.6). These incisions have several advantages over corneal relaxing incisions:

1. There is no risk of perforation, so there is no need for corneal pachymetry
2. The incisions are much longer than corneal relaxing incisions, so accurate placement with respect to the steep meridian is less critical

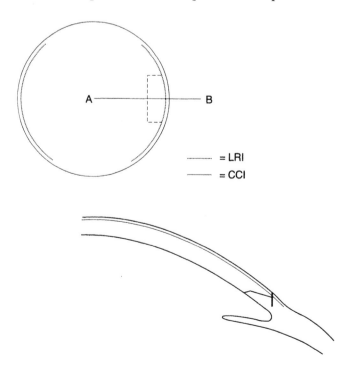

Figure 27.6 The temporal LRI can take in the clear corneal incision (CCI) for phakoemulsification.

and routine corneal topography is not required for non-complex cases

3. This is a relatively weak procedure, so over-correction is rare; if it does occur and is identified early, it can be reversed by suturing the incision closed
4. They can be readily 'augmented' (re-operated).

Several monograms have appeared, and Gills' monogram is quoted here (see website: www.stlukeseye.com/physicians.htm).

For under 4 D of astigmatism: The location is at the limbus with a depth setting of 0.6 mm and the incisions located on the steepest meridian (or hemi-meridian if just one incision is used). The variables are the number and length of incisions. For with-the-rule astigmatism, the incisions are located superiorly and inferiorly; for against-the-rule astigmatism, the incisions are located temporally and nasally. The temporal relieving incision can run through the clear corneal incision site (Figure 27.6).

Error to be corrected	Number of incisions	Length of incision(s) (mm)
1 DC	1	6
2 DC	2	6
3 DC	2	8
4 DC	2	10

For over 4 D of astigmatism:

Incisions	Blade settings	Length	Optical zone	Number of incisions
LRI CRI (for residual astigmatism)	600 μm 99 per cent depth (central corneal pacyhmetry)	10–12 mm 2 mm for every dioptre over 4 DC	At limbus 8 mm	2 Based on correction desired over 4 DC

This nomogram is for people over the age of 73 years; for younger people, longer incisions are required to achieve the same effect. There is no need to do both the LRI and the CRI at the same time. It would be reasonable to do the LRI at the time of the cataract surgery and, if the residual astigmatism was unacceptable, the CRI 3 months later.

One study on only 12 eyes using just the LRIs (and a modified nomogram) essentially substantiated Gills' claims[19].

Initially these incisions were cut freehand, but now a number of 'arcuatomes' are being produced. The idea behind them is to make incision depth and contour more reproducible and length more accurate. These improvements should all result in increased predictability of this approach.

Other incisions

The transverse incision (or T-cut) is similar to the arcuate excision, differing only by being a straight line. It has a couple of theoretical disadvantages compared to the arcuate incision, but these disadvantages can be overcome by good technique. The disadvantages are that all parts of the incision are not equidistant from the corneal centre, and accordingly the corneal thickness will vary, as will the contribution to the result from different parts of the incision. These factors suggest that the arcuate incision would give a more regular topographic effect[16]. Equally, a transverse incision must be accurately placed, otherwise it will have an oblique component with potentially unpredictable results.

Trapezoidal keratotomy and oblique incisions are now rarely used due to poor predictability of the outcome.

SURGICAL TECHNIQUE FOR ARCUATE INCISIONS

The technique for all the incisions is very straightforward in principle, though numerous refinements are described. There is little change in the best sphere correction, due to the effect of coupling, and no adjustments need to be made to the calculated lens implant power.

The basic problem is that, for CRI, the cuts must be nearly full corneal thickness to have an appreciable refractive effect, yet perforation has to be avoided because any repair will require suturing, which will undo any refractive effect. The second point is that the cuts must be carefully orientated to prevent an oblique component with unpredictable results. With these two points in mind, the procedure is:

1. For corneal relaxing incisions, mark the optical axis and the optical clear zone accurately. There are special optical zone markers for this purpose. This step is not necessary for limbal relaxing incisions.
2. Measure the central corneal thickness with a pachymeter and then set the blade to the required depth. This is usually 100 per cent of the central corneal depth which, in the paracentral location, equates to 85 per cent. For accuracy, use a guarded blade with a micrometer; it is also good practice to check the micrometer against a calibration device. Again this step is not required for limbal relaxing incisions, when the depth is pre-set at 0.6–0.7 mm.
3. Identify the steep axis, which should be known preoperatively on the basis of keratometry and/or corneal topography. In the context of cataract surgery, any lenticular astigmatism will be eliminated and accordingly surgery is based purely on the corneal findings. The direction of the steep axis should be checked in theatre with a handheld surgical keratometer (the Maloney keratometer is illustrated in Figure 27.7). There are two ways of identifying the steep axis (Figure 27.8): it is where the reflections from concentric rings are closest, and the reflection of a ring from an astigmatic cornea is oval and the steep axis is the short one.

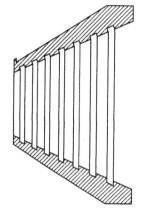
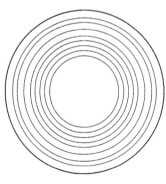

Figure 27.7 Maloney keratometer, which is used with an operating microscope. It gives rise to series of concentric reflections not unlike the Placido's disc.

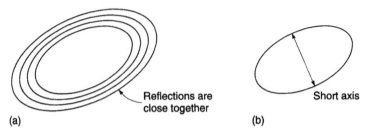

Figure 27.8   (a) The steep meridian can be identified by where the reflections are closest together. (b) It is also aligned along the short axis of the reflected oval.

4. Make the cuts using a nomogram, being sure to press firmly to ensure that the required depth of incision is achieved.
5. At the end of the procedure, irrigate the wounds in order to prevent epithelial cell implantation.

The postoperative follow-up is topical steroids, which can be used to titrate the wound-healing response to some extent, and topical antibiotics until the wounds have epithelialized over.

COMPRESSION SUTURES

Compression sutures will act to steepen the meridian on which they are placed, but isolated compression sutures rarely give rise to any significant remodelling of the cornea (the reverse of the observation that severe suture-induced astigmatism can be readily reversed by suture removal[20]).

Compression sutures should be completely non-absorbable (e.g. Mersilene®), and are rarely used in isolation. They are most commonly used in conjunction with relaxing incisions, where the effect of coupling means that the compression sutures cause the relaxing incisions to gape more and an increased gape results in corneal remodelling. It also allows for deliberate over-correction and the response can then be titrated during the postoperative period by selective suture removal.

A more extreme adjunct is to combine the compression sutures with a wedge resection. This was described by Troutman for large degrees of post-keratoplasty astigmatism, who suggested that a 0.5-mm wedge extending to 60–90° centred on the steep meridian will correct 10 D astigmatism (giving a rough estimate of 0.05 mm per dioptre to be corrected)[21].

MANAGEMENT OF SURGICALLY-INDUCED ASTIGMATISM

EXTRACAPSULAR CATARACT SURGERY

There is a natural tendency for surgeons to tie sutures too tightly, and as a consequence most extracapsular cataract extractions with a superior section result in with-the-rule astigmatism. This is managed by selective (or total) suture removal, starting 8–12 weeks after surgery.

Premature suture removal can result in wound dehiscence and require resuturing.

Marked against-the-rule astigmatism is usually due to wound dehiscence or gaping, and this should be managed by wound resuturing as soon as the problem is identified.

It is not uncommon for 1–3 D of astigmatism to persist even after all the sutures have been removed. This is usually managed by spectacle correction.

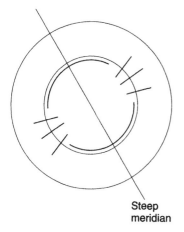

Steep
meridian

Figure 27.9 An example of treating post-keratoplasty astigmatism. A pair of 120° arcuate CRI are located 0.5 mm inside the graft–host junction in association with compression sutures on the perpendicular (flat) meridian.

POST-KERATOPLASTY

Most of the techniques for correction of surgically-induced astigmatism were developed for post-keratoplasty patients.

Short-term adjustment of astigmatism can be performed by suture manipulation[22]. For interrupted sutures, this is simply selective suture removal of stitches on the steep axis. With a continuous suture, this can be manipulated to transfer the tension from the steep axis to the flat axis. This can be done on the slit lamp using blocked microforceps under topical anaesthesia, and can be undertaken as soon as the astigmatism is detected.

If this fails the next step is to consider arcuate relaxing incisions, usually in association with compression sutures (Figure 27.9). The relaxing incisions were first described as being placed at the graft–host interface, but this is a site of great variation both in the degree of scar tissue formation and the thickness, with resulting unpredictability of the result. It is more sensible to place these incisions just within (e.g. 0.5 mm) the graft. The optimum timing for arcuate incisions and/or compression sutures is 1–3 months after all the sutures have been removed.

PHAKOEMULSIFICATION AND PRE-EXISTING ASTIGMATISM

Now that small incision surgery has solved the problem of surgically-induced astigmatism, the next goal is to eliminate pre-existing astigmatism. At the moment the need to do this routinely is questionable, but this may change if multifocal lenses become more acceptable.

The simplest approach is to place the incision on the steep axis, which is not necessarily the temporal meridian. The three-step incision causes about 0.50 D against-the-wound refractive shift. The degree of against-the-wound shift does depend upon wound size, and by the time the incision is below 3.25 mm it is close to being astigmatically neutral. Accordingly the trend is increasingly to ignore the effect of the surgical wound and concentrate on the appropriate placement of relaxing incisions. Gills' LRIs seem particularly suitable for this purpose.

REFERENCES

1. Williamson, W., Poirier, L., Coulon, P. and Verin, P. (1994). Compared optical performances of multifocal and monofocal intraocular lenses (contrast sensitivity and dynamic visual acuity). *Br. J. Ophthalmol.*, 78, 249–51.
2. Rabinowitz, Y. S. and McDonnell, P. J. (1989). Computer-assisted corneal topography in keratoconus. *Refract. Corneal Surg.*, 5, 400–408.
3. Waring, G. O. (1993). Nomenclature for keratoconus suspects. *Refract. Corneal Surg.*, 9, 219–22.
4. Tuft, S. J., Moodaley, L. C., Gregory, W. M. *et al.* (1994). Prognostic factors for the progression of keratoconus. *Ophthalmology*, 101, 439–47.
5. Petroll, W. M., New, K., Sachdev, M. *et al.* (1992). Radial keratotomy. III. Relationship between wound gape and corneal curvature in primate eyes. *Invest. Ophthalmol. Vis. Sci.*, 33, 3283–91.
6. Henslee, S. L. and Rowsey, J. J. (1983). New corneal shapes in keratorefractive surgery. *Ophthalmology*, 90, 245–50.
7. McDonnell, P. J. and Garbus, J. (1989). Corneal topographic changes after radial keratotomy. *Ophthalmology*, 96, 45–9.
8. McDonnell, P. J., Garbus, J. and Lopez, P. F. (1988). Topographic analysis and visual acuity after radial keratotomy. *Am. J. Ophthalmol.*, 106, 692–5.
9. Rowsey, J. J., Balyeat, H. D., Monlux, R. *et al.* (1988). Prospective evaluation of radial keratotomy: photokeratoscope corneal topography. *Ophthalmology*, 95, 322–34.
10. Jester, J. V., Steel, D., Salz, J. *et al.* (1981). Radial keratotomy in non-human primate eyes. *Am. J. Ophthalmol.*, 92, 153–71.
11. Hemenger, R. P., Tomlinson, A. and McDonnell, P. J. (1990). Explanation for good visual acuity in uncorrected residual hyperopia and presbyopia after radial keratotomy. *Invest. Ophthalmol. Vis. Sci.*, 31, 1644–6.
12. Maguire, L. J. and Bourne, W. M. (1989). A multifocal lens effect as a complication of radial keratotomy. *Refract. Corneal Surg.*, 5, 394–9.
13. Santos, V. R., Waring, G. O. 3rd, Lynn, M. J. *et al.* (PERK Study Group) (1987). Relationship between refractive error and visual acuity in the Prospective Evaluation of Radial Keratotomy (PERK) Study. *Arch. Ophthalmol.*, 105, 86–92.
14. Schiotz, H. A. (1885). *Archiv für Augenheilkunde*, 15, 178–81.
15. Duffey, R. J., Jain, V. N., Tchah, H. *et al.* (1988). Paired arcuate keratotomy. A surgical approach to mixed and myopic astigmatism. *Arch. Ophthalmol.*, 106, 1130–35.
16. Merlin, U. (1987). Curved keratotomy procedures for congenital astigmatism. *J. Refract. Surg.*, 3, 92–7.
17. Lindstrom, R. L. (1990). The surgical correction of astigmatism: a clinician's perspective. *Refract. Corneal Surg.*, 6, 441–54.
18. Lundergan, M. K. and Rowsey, J. J. (1985). Relaxing incisions. Corneal topography. *Ophthalmology*, 92, 1226–36.
19. Budak, K., Friedman, M. D. and Koch, D. D. (1999). Limbal relaxing incisions with cataract surgery. *J. Cataract. Refract. Surg.*, 24, 503–8.
20. Van Rig, G. and Waring, G. O. (1986). Suture-induced astigmatism after a circular wound in the rhesus monkey. *Cornea*, 5, 25–8.
21. Troutman, R. C. (1983). Corneal wedge resections and relaxing incisions for post-keratoplasty astigmatism. *Int. Ophthalmol. Clin.*, 23, 161–8.
22. McNeill, J. I. and Wessels, I. F. (1989). Adjustment of a single continuous suture to control astigmatism after penetrating keratoplasty. *Refract. Corneal Surg.*, 5, 216–23.

28

TRAUMA SURGERY

All structures of the eye and orbit can be subjected to trauma, which can be subdivided into blunt and penetrating injury. Blunt trauma to the globe and orbit does not usually require surgical intervention except in cases such as orbital blow-out fractures and retinal detachments. By contrast, penetrating injuries usually require urgent surgical repair.

Fortunately cases of penetrating ocular trauma requiring surgery have become relatively rare with the introduction of seatbelt regulations. The important issue is whether the patient's best interests are served by transferring to a specialist for surgery, or whether the delay would nullify this advantage. This has to be answered on an individual patient (and surgeon) basis, and depends upon the nature and severity of the injury. For example, a lid margin laceration can be closed simply along the lines described for a lid shortening procedure, while trauma to the orbital floor or to the lacrimal system will not be adversely affected by a 24–48-hour delay. The one situation where the surgery may be complex and technically demanding but any delay is potentially deleterious is in penetrating injury to the globe. Here an immediate primary repair to make the eye safe from further damage is indicated, to be followed by a definitive repair by the appropriate team.

PRIMARY REPAIR

The basic principles of primary repair are:

1. Explore the injury
2. Remove foreign material
3. Conserve as much tissue as possible
4. Debride only that tissue which is frankly necrotic and non-viable
5. Approximate the normal sclero-corneal anatomy
6. Give adequate endophthalmitis prophylaxis.

A normal eye is a structure that is pumped up to a positive pressure due to aqueous production. The major resistance to fluid outflow is the sclera and any sclera rupture will result in hypotony, which if uncorrected will lead to phthisis. The aim of primary repair is to re-establish the integrity of the sclera so as to allow the eye to reinflate.

A major cause of irreversible damage is prolapse of the intraocular contents outwards. In order to minimize this, efforts must be made to reduce any pressure being applied to the injured eye. Apply an eye shield to prevent accidental rubbing of the eye or other contact, from as soon as possible from the time of injury until the patient goes to theatre. In theatre, when preparing the eye for surgery, consider how to keep the lids apart without raising the intraocular pressure; this is a situation where lid clips may be preferable to a lid speculum.

Preoperative imaging can be helpful. The imaging of choice is computerized tomography; MRI is contraindicated if there is any chance of metal contaminating the traumatized tissue. A CT scan is very helpful in locating bony damage (such as blow-out fractures) and the presence and location of foreign bodies. It is important to be able to localize foreign bodies as in or outside of the eye, because the consequences of leaving them and the approaches to retrieving them are fundamentally different. Both CT and MRI images can suggest that scleral rupture is present, but neither technique can reliably exclude it or determine the extent. For these reasons, the first step in repairing a traumatized eye is to explore the injury.

EXPLORATION

The purpose of exploration is to see the extent of damage. The major aim of primary repair is to find and close all scleral breaks. If a scleral laceration or rupture extends to involve the insertion of an extraocular muscle, for example, then disinsert that muscle to see that the rupture of laceration does not extend underneath it.

REMOVAL OF FOREIGN MATTER

Not all foreign matter needs to be removed, or needs to be removed immediately. All organic foreign matter should be removed to reduce the risk of infection, but the decision whether to remove other foreign matter depends upon its presumed content and its location. Many pieces of metal can be left in the orbit but not in the eye, where most metals are toxic[1].

DEBRIDEMENT

This should be kept to a minimum, as the tissues are either extremely difficult (e.g. lids) or impossible (e.g. retina) to reconstruct or replace. It is easy to underestimate tissue viability. The aim of debridement is to aid wound closure.

REPAIR

Wound closure follows debridement and approximation of the tissues. The tissue that is repaired is the corneo-scleral envelope, and accordingly a non-absorbable suture (e.g. 9/0 or 10/0 nylon) on a spatulate or microspatulate needle is the suture of choice. Interrupted sutures are better than continuous as selective suture removal can be performed and, more importantly, the whole repair is not threatened if one stitch cuts out or loosens prematurely.

If a muscle has had to be disinserted, then reinsert it with 5/0 or 6/0 Vicryl® as for strabismus surgery. The conjunctiva can be sutured with 8/0 Vicryl®.

Following wound closure, give adequate endophthalmitis prophylaxis and consider intra-cameral antibiotics for high-risk cases.

SECONDARY REPAIR

The ideal time to undertake a secondary repair is around day 10–14. It usually requires an internal approach, and is often best undertaken by a vitreo-retinal surgeon. Earlier intervention is sometimes required, for instance if there is endophthalmitis.

FORENSIC MEDICINE

Trauma is often the result of assault, which is a criminal offence. The treating surgeon may therefore find that his or her involvement will extend beyond medical treatment to providing a statement to the police and even testifying in court. Therefore accurate documentation is important and a photographic record can be very helpful. Interested readers are referred to Anon (1996) and Knight (1997) for further information.

REFERENCES

1. Morris, D. A. (1994). Ocular trauma. In: *Pathobiology of Ocular Disease. A Dynamic Approach*, 2nd edn (A. Garner and G. K. Klintworth, eds), pp. 387–432. Marcel Dekker Inc.
2. Anonymous (1996). *Limitations of Expert Evidence*, 1st edn. Cathedral Print Services Ltd.
3. Knight, B. (1997). *Simpson's Forensic Medicine*, 11th edn. Dah Hua Printing Press Co. Ltd.

29

INFECTIONS

The mainstay of treatment of bacterial infections is antibiotics. Surgery is indicated if there is any collection of pus, particularly if it is not responding to antibiotics.

ABSCESSES

The principles of treating abscesses have been long established. Antibiotics do not penetrate well into the centre of abscess, so the abscess should be drained through a stab incision and a sample sent for microbiology. If there is overlying necrotic skin, this should be removed (a process called saucerization). If the cavity is of any size, it should be lightly packed with ribbon gauze to help ensure that it heals from the deep surface outwards. Tight packing of an abscess is counterproductive as it hinders drainage, delays collapse of the cavity and is extremely painful to remove.

DACROCYSTITIS

The mainstay of treatment of dacrocystitis is a broad-spectrum oral antibiotic (e.g. Augmentin^{TM}). It this fails, the pus should be drained through a stab incision at the most raised point. The subsequent management is as for any other abscess. Occasionally a lacrimal fistula will form from a spontaneously ruptured lacrimal abscess or from the stab incision, but this will usually close spontaneously following re-establishment of the normal tear drainage following a standard DCR.

Recurrent dacrocystitis is an indication for DCR.

CHRONIC CANALICULITIS – ACTINOMYCES

MICROBIOLOGY

Actinomyces are gram-positive filamentous bacteria that are facultative anaerobes. The most commonly isolated species is *Actinomyces israeli*. In culture it tends to fragment.

CLINICAL FEATURES

The canaliculitis is characterized by a sticky and watery eye with an associated conjunctivitis. The discharge from the punctum is green and stringy and may contain 'sulphur granules'. It causes dilatation of the canaliculus, which contains hard stone-like material, and this enlargement can be both seen and felt. It nearly always affects only one canaliculus, and there is just the odd case report where it has spread from an upper to a lower canaliculus. Strangely, the infection does not block the canaliculus and it is patent to syringing and to probing.

It is a chronic condition that will persist for years without the correct treatment.

INVESTIGATIONS

Microscopy rather than culture is the investigation of choice. A deep specimen must be obtained from the canaliculus; material may be very hard to express, so inserting a lacrimal cannula into the suspect canaliculus and aspirating is as good a technique as any. Following this, the contents of the lacrimal cannula can be injected directly onto a glass slide, air dried and then transported to the laboratory for gram staining. Formal expression can also work.

TREATMENT

The surgical principle is the same as for any abscess. The granules are too big to drain through either the common canaliculus or the lacrimal punctum, so make an opening via a two-snip procedure along the roof of the canaliculus (or floor of the upper canaliculus). The canaliculus is usually grossly dilated and the contents need to be expressed and curretted.

Syringe the tear duct system with benzyl-penicillin 600 mg (one vial) followed by benzyl-penicillin 0.3% drops q.d.s. for 10–14 days. Although benzyl-penicillin is the antibiotic that ophthalmologists classically give, it should be noted that some strains of A. israeli are relatively resistant to penicillin but are sensitive to amoxicillin, ampicillen or a cephalosporin. The mainstay of treatment is surgical removal of all the concretions, and antibiotics may actually not be necessary[1].

ENDOPHTHALMITIS

Endophthalmitis is one of the most serious complications following intraocular surgery. The clinical features are those of inflammation, and the diagnosis should be expected whenever there is an unexpectedly severe inflammatory reaction to surgery and always if there is a hypopyon, no matter how small (polymorphonucleocytes are denser than lymphocytes and will sediment, and their presence is an important feature of acute suppuration). Endophthalmitis due to the more virulent organisms typically presents at 48–72 hours, with only 10 per cent of cases presenting on the first postoperative day. Over half (55 per cent) present after 1 week and 20 per cent present after 2 months[2].

It is likely that inoculation occurs at the time of surgery[3]. Gram-positive organisms make up the majority (76–90 per cent) of cases of culture-positive pseudophakic endophthalmitis, and of these *S. epidermidis* (or coagulase-negative Staphylococci) make up 38–59 per cent[4–6]. An interesting point is the slow presentation, which contrasts sharply with the experience in the laboratory where most cultures show growth by 2 days. Organisms under ideal growth conditions grow exponentially in 'planktonic' form. The alternative growth form is as a 'biofilm', and this is the preferred mode of growth in many natural situations (e.g. slime in sewage pipes)[7].

Propionibacterium acnes, another gram-positive organism, is considered to be the major cause of late-onset endophthalmitis. Fox *et al.*[8] defined late-onset endophthalmitis as presenting 4 weeks after surgery; in this group of 60 cases positive cultures were present in only 21, of which 13 were due to *P. acnes*, while another series of six cases of *P. acnes* had presentation at between 2 and 6 months after surgery[9]. *P. acnes*, like *S. epidermidis*, is a normal commensal of the conjunctival mucosa[10], and it has a distinct clinical presentation. Its onset is particularly late, and it causes a granulomatous uveitis and a characteristic plaque on the posterior capsule[11]; again its growth has all the features of being a biofilm infection. It should be noted that while it may be a common cause of delayed onset endophthalmitis, it is a rare cause overall – the 13 cases reported by Fox *et al.* were from a series of 187[8].

Organisms in biofilms behave very differently from their planktonic form. They grow on surfaces and particularly implants (including hip implants, prosthetic heart valves and IOLs). Growth is contiguous and is 5–15 times slower than under planktonic conditions. Bacteria in this form require 20–1000 times higher levels of antibiotics to achieve killing, but in fact the organisms in the biofilm may be asymptomatic and it is those organisms that are shed from the surface that give rise to symptoms. This is a major explanation of recurrence of the infection after apparently successful treatment in the present of implants. This is an important and generally neglected topic, and the interested reader is referred to Elder *et al.*[12] for further information.

SAMPLE COLLECTION

If all goes well, the infection will have been successfully cured by the intravitreal injection of broad-spectrum antibiotics before any microbiological results are available. However, culture results are invaluable for non-responsive or recurrent infections, particularly where rare organisms such as fungi are involved.

The standard protocol is to perform a vitreous and anterior chamber tap first, immediately followed by the injection of intravitreal antibiotics. There are two ways of taking the sample. The easiest is with a 23-G (blue) needle through the pars plana, and this depends upon the presence of a posterior vitreous detachment, which is present in most cases of endophthalmitis. In the absence of a posterior vitreous detachment, then the sample should be taken with a vitrecter in theatre.

The protocol is as follows:

1. Perform a B-scan ultrasound to check that there is a posterior vitreous detachment. The presence of intravitreal opacities is a feature of vitreal involvement, and should be noted.
2. Anaesthetize the eye: Topical amethocaine followed by a subconjunctival injection of lignocaine over the proposed injection site is sufficient. It is sensible to choose an inferior site, as any Bell's phenomenon will act to improve exposure.
3. Prepare the eye: Clean around the eye and consider using a plastic incision drape as for any other intraocular procedure. Insert a lid speculum. Clean the ocular surface with aqueous povidone-iodine or a broad-spectrum antibiotic such as chloramphenicol.
4. Perform vitreous aspiration using a 23-G (blue) needle (vitreous can not be aspirated through anything finer) and insert it 3 mm (4 mm if the patient is phakic) from the limbus and aspirate. Not much is needed – 0.1 ml is plenty – and plate this out immediately and include a slide for a gram stain. The yield and complication rates from a needle biopsy are similar to those using a vitrecter biopsy[13].
5. Perform the anterior chamber tap with a finer needle (e.g. a 27-G insulin needle).
6. Give the intravitreal antibiotic injections after the taps and aspiration, through the pars plana, again 3 mm from the limbus.

The same procedure can be done with a vitrectomy cutter substituted for the blue needle. This time raise a small conjunctival flap and make a hole 3 mm from the limbus with an MVR blade. Enlarge the hole with a 19-G (white) needle, then insert the cutter but have the aspiration tubing disconnected from the vitrectomy machine and connected to a syringe. Switch the cutter on and gently aspirate the required sample. Perform the anterior chamber taps as above and inject the antibiotics through the pars plana incision, before closing it, the sclerostomy and the conjunctiva with 5/0 Vicryl®.

INTRACAMERAL ANTIBIOTICS

This section concentrates on post-surgical endophthalmitis, where the most common organisms are *S. epidermidis* and *aureus*, Streptocci, Propionobacterium, gram negatives and occasionally fungi. In bleb-associated infections, Streptococci and Haemophilus are the most common. The pattern of infecting organisms differs after trauma or with metastatic endophthalmitis.

Given the poor ocular penetration of most systematically administered antibiotics, direct injection into the vitreous cavity is the mainstay of treatment. As with any serious infection that has to be treated before any microbiological results are available, broad-spectrum agents must be used. A broad-spectrum penicillin and an aminoglycoside are the usual chosen combination for 'blind' treatment, and most eye units have their standard regime (e.g. vancomycin[14] and amikacin[15]). Intravitreal amphotericin should be considered if fungal infection is suspected. The therapy may have to be modified in the light of microbiological results. The most commonly used antimicrobials are, in alphabetical order:

- Amikacin – 0.4 mg in 0.1 ml
- Amphotericin – 5.0 μg in 0.1 ml
- Cefuroxime – 1.0 mg in 0.1 ml
- Clindamycin – 1.0 mg in 0.1 ml
- Gentamicin – 0.1–0.2 mg in 0.1 ml
- Vancomycin – 1.0–2.0 mg in 0.05–0.1 ml.

All these antibiotics should be drawn up in preservative-free normal saline, with the exception of amphotericin, which should be drawn up in 5% dextrose.

There is no role for topical antibiotics unless there is an associated ocular surface disorder (e.g. infected trabeculectomy bleb, corneal ulcer, leaking wound etc.).

There are no clear guidelines about the indications for repeated doses. The estimated half-life of most intravitreal antibiotics is in the region of 24 hours, and accordingly a half dose can be injected at 24 hours and a full dose after 3 days, if appropriate. The half-lives in vitrectomized and aphakic eyes are shorter, and the higher doses of gentamicin and vancomycin should be given for these.

SYSTEMIC ANTIBIOTICS

Systemic antibiotics are essential for bleb-associated endophthalmitis, as most blebs are vascular and antibiotics will penetrate them. Otherwise, systemic antibiotics penetrate poorly into the eye. Ciprofloxacin does show reasonable ocular penetration and is often prescribed routinely for endophthalmitis, as does chloramphenicol and cephazolin. It is an adjunct, and not a substitute, for intracameral antibiotics.

ANTI-BIOFILM AGENTS

Biofilm is a major cause of relapses after apparently successful treatment. The biofilm resides on the implant, and one strategy is to remove any lens implant and then treat, but clearly it would be much more desirable to treat the infection successfully without having to remove the implant.

There are agents that will reduce the amount of biofilm present, and the one that has received most attention for ocular use is clarithromycin. Clarithromycin enhances the bactericidal effect of other antibiotics by eradicating biofilm *in vitro*[16,17], and this occurs at a much lower dose than its MIC 90 for most bacteria. While the penetration of oral clarithromycin into the inflamed eye is unknown, it is encouraging that there is at least one documented case of it achieving cure as a single agent[18].

Recurrence of post-surgical endophthalmitis despite the use of an anti-biofilm agent necessitates removal of the lens implant and the posterior capsule along with repeat intravitreal and systemic antibiotics.

ANTI-INFLAMMATORY MEDICATION

Most of the ocular damage is due to the inflammatory response. There is a general principle with ocular infections that 'if it is not worse, then it is better'. If 24 hours after the commencement of antibiotics the clinical situation shows no deterioration, then it is reasonable to consider a short course of oral prednisolone starting at 60 mg and tapering over 2 weeks with the idea of 'turning off' the inflammatory response and preventing 'bystander' damage.

Steroids should be avoided for fungal infections.

ROLE OF VITRECTOMY

The management outlined above can all be done as an outpatient. The rationale for doing a vitrectomy is clear cut (if there is pus, drain it), and its role was scrutinized by the Endophthalmitis Vitrectomy Study Group[19]. Vitrectomy was found to be an advantage in only the severest cases, where the presenting vision was perception of light only.

ORBITAL CELLULITIS

This is usually secondary spread from an adjacent infective focus such as an infected meibomian cyst or sinus disease. As for any abscess or infection that either does not settle quickly with systemic antibiotics or shows evidence of ocular or optic nerve involvement, it should be scanned to look for a collection of pus. If located, this should be drained. Most collections of pus occur in association with sinus disease, and an ENT surgeon is often the appropriate person to be doing the drainage.

REFERENCES

1. Hussain, I., Bonshek, R. E., Loudon, K. *et al.* (1993). Canalicular infection caused by Actinomyces. *Eye*, 7, 542–4.
2. Fisch, A., Salvanet, A., Prazuck, T. *et al.* (1991). Epidemiology of infective endophthalmitis in France. The French Collaborative Study Group on Endophthalmitis. *Lancet*, 338(8779), 1373–6.

3. Speaker, M. G., Milch, F. A., Shah, M. K. (1991). Role of external flora in the pathogenesis of acute postoperative endophthalmitis. *Ophthalmology*, **98**, 639–50.
4. Driebe, W. T. Jr, Mandelbaum, S., Forster, R. K. *et al.* (1986). Pseudophakic endophthalmitis. Diagnosis and management. *Ophthalmology*, **93**, 442–8.
5. Olsen, J. C., Flynn, H. W. Jr, Forster, R. K. and Culbertson, W. W. (1983). Results in the treatment of postoperative endophthalmitis. *Ophthalmology*, **90**, 692–9.
6. Puliafito, C. A., Baker, S. A., Haaf, J. and Foster, C. S. (1982). Infectious endophthalmitis: a review of 36 cases. *Ophthalmology*, **89**, 921–9.
7. Costerton, J. W., Lewandowski, Z., Caldwell, D. E. *et al.* (1995). Microbial biofilms. *Ann. Rev. Microbiology*, **49**, 711–45.
8. Fox, G. M., Joondeph, B. C., Flynn, H. W. Jr *et al.* (1991). Delayed onset pseudophakic endophthalmitis. *Am. J. Ophthalmol.*, **111**, 163–73.
9. Meisler, D. M., Palestine, A. G., Vastine, D. W. *et al.* (1986). Chronic Propionibacterium endophthalmitis after extracapsular cataract extraction and intraocular lens implantation. *Am. J. Ophthalmol.*, **102**, 733–9.
10. Perkins, R. E., Knudsin, R. B., Pratt, M.V. *et al.* (1975). Bacteriology of normal and infected conjunctiva. *J. Clin. Microbiol.*, **1**, 147–9.
11. Vafidis, G. (1991). *Propionibacterium acnes* endophthalmitis (editorial). *Br. J. Ophthalmol.*, **75**, 706.
12. Elder, M. J., Stapleton, F., Evans, E. and Dart, J. K. G. (1995). Biofilm-related infections in ophthalmology. *Eye*, **9**, 102–9.
13. Han, D. P., Wisniewski, S. R., Kelsey, S. F. *et al.* (1999). Microbiologic yields and complication rates of vitreous needle aspiration versus mechanized vitreous biopsy in the Endophthalmitis Vitrectomy Study. *Retina*, **19**, 98–102.
14. Pflugfelder, S. C., Hernandez, E., Fliesler, S. J. *et al.* (1987). Intravitreal vancomycin. Retinal toxicity, clearance, and interaction with gentamicin. *Arch. Ophthalmol.*, **105**, 831–7.
15. Talamo, J. H., D'Amico, D. J. and Kenyon, K. R. (1986). Intravitreal amikacin in the treatment of bacterial endophthalmitis. *Arch. Ophthalmol.*, **104**, 1483–5.
16. Braga, P. C. and Piatti, G. (1993). Sub-lethal concentrations of clarithromycin interfere with the expression of *Staphylococcus aureus* adhesiveness to human cells. *J. Chemotherapy*, **5**, 159–63.
17. Yasuda, H., Ajiki, Y., Koga, T. *et al.* (1993). Interaction between biofilms formed by *Pseudomonas aeruginosa* and clarithromycin. *Antimicrob. Agents Chemotherapy*, **37**, 1749–55.
18. Warheker, P. T., Gupta, S. R., Mansfield, D. C. and Seal, D. V. (1998). Successful treatment of saccular endophthalmitis with clarithromycin (letter). *Eye*, **12**(6), 1017–19.
19. The Endophthalmitis Vitrectomy Study Group (1995). Results of the Endophthalmitis Vitrectomy Study Group. *Arch. Ophthalmol.*, **113**, 1479–96.

INDEX

Printed and bound by CPI Group (UK) Ltd, Croydon, CR0 4YY

08/06/2025

01896874-0007